Principles and Practice of Laparoscopic Surgery

Emeka Ray-Offor • Raul J. Rosenthal
Editors

Principles and Practice of Laparoscopic Surgery

Second Edition

Springer

Editors
Emeka Ray-Offor
College of Health Sciences
University of Port Harcourt
Choba, Nigeria

Raul J. Rosenthal
Division of General Surgery
Ronald Reagan UCLA Medical Center,
David Geffen School of Medicine
Los Angeles, CA, USA

ISBN 978-3-031-96320-9 ISBN 978-3-031-96321-6 (eBook)
https://doi.org/10.1007/978-3-031-96321-6

T&D Press Ltd, Principles & Practice of Laparoscopic Surgery, 2015

This Springer imprint is published by the registered company Springer Nature Switzerland AG
The registered company address is: Gewerbestrasse 11, 6330 Cham, Switzerland

Foreword

MD, PhD(Hon), FACS, FRCS(Eng), FRCS(Ed), FRCSI(Hon), Hon FRCS(Glasg), FRCS(Eng), MAMSE, I am gratified to my alumnus, Dr. Ray-Offor, and to my dear friend, colleague, and coworker, Dr. Rosenthal, for asking me to write this foreword to the second edition of their textbook on principles and practices of laparoscopic surgery. Not many months ago, I had the honor and privilege of authoring the Foreword to their first edition. In that Foreword I noted that the prerequisites for success for any textbook are the depth and breadth of content, the expertise of the authors, and the relevance to the reader. I stated that their first edition not only fulfilled but exceeded expectations in each of those areas through their selection of exceptionally timely topics authoritatively addressed by internationally acclaimed experts. Moreover, they successfully ensured that each topic was of tremendous current relevance and immediately translatable to each reader's clinical practice. In seemingly record time, undoubtedly due to the success of their first edition Drs. Ray-Offor and Rosenthal have amassed a collection of 22 new chapters addressing the entire gamut of principles and practice of laparoscopic surgery. In this second edition, they begin with basic principles in which the topics of the evolution of laparoscopic surgery, laparoscopic equipment and instruments, energy sources, ergonometrics, care and maintenance of laparoscopic instruments, and physiology of pneumoperitoneum are discussed. They proceed to technical aspects, including access, creation of pneumoperitoneum, port placement, suturing, tissue approximation, organ retrieval, port closure, as well as complications, and simulation and training. The next section of their second edition, application of laparoscopic techniques, delves into diagnostic laparoscopy, appendicectomy, cholecystectomy, pediatric, urologic, and gynecologic surgery as well as video-assisted thoracoscopic surgery. The third and final portion of their second edition delves into the very currently popular topics of fluorescence-guided laparoscopic surgery, robotic-assisted surgery, and artificial intelligence in surgery. I am absolutely enthused at this second edition. I am thrilled to be able to recommend this second edition to every practicing surgeon and surgeon in training. The book is comprehensive, current, authoritative, practical, and of course highly clinically relevant. Once again, I thank Drs. Ray-Offor and Rosenthal for having invited me to again author the Foreword to their textbook. Given the popularity of their work, I suspect that it will not be long until we see a third edition by these esteemed academicians, Drs. Emeka Ray-Offor and Raul J. Rosenthal.

Steven D. Wexner

Ellen Leifer Shulman, and Steven Shulman
Digestive Disease Center, Department
of Colorectal Surgery
Cleveland Clinic Florida
Weston, FL, USA

Cleveland Clinic Lerner College
of Medicine at Case Western
Reserve University
Cleveland, OH, USA

Charles E. Schmidt College of Medicine
Florida Atlantic University
Boca Raton, FL, USA

Herbert Wertheim College of Medicine
Florida International University
Miami, FL, USA

Department of Surgery
University of South Florida Morsani
College of Medicine
Tampa, FL, USA

Division of Surgery, and Interventional
Science, Department of Targeted Intervention
University College
London, UK

Department of Surgery and Cancer
Imperial College
London, UK

Preface

Laparoscopy is a paradigm shift in abdominal surgery with the surgeon sacrificing wrist movement and tactile feedback for the benefits of precision and reduced trauma. This closed-cavity surgery technique of laparoscopy with complex gadgetry has been a notable advancement in surgical practice. The benefits include reduced post-operative pain, hospital stay, early return to work, and improved cosmesis. Surgeons are challenged to operate with a magnified visual field of the abdominal cavity on a video monitor using long slender instruments inserted through miniature skin incision with a peritoneal distension medium established for the workspace.

The overwhelming evidence in medical literature favoring laparoscopic surgery has shifted from "Which procedure can?" to "Which cannot?". A wide application of laparoscopic surgery can be seen from specialty surgeons that operate within the abdominal cavity. This practice is well established in high-index countries but still budding in low-middle-income countries (LMICs). Beyond open surgery skills, laparoscopic surgeons must be familiar with complex gadgetry, specialized instruments, pneumoperitoneum, and other unique aspects of laparoscopic surgery. This requires adequate training for optimal outcomes.

Competence in laparoscopic surgery is gained from simulation training and guided practice for beginners. This book is an adjunct to proctored training for laparoscopic surgery skills. It is crafted with in-depth discussion on the basic principles of laparoscopic surgery, numerous figure illustrations, easy-to-read text, and operative details of basic laparoscopic procedures. The applications of laparoscopic techniques in pediatric surgery, urology, gynecology, and the related topic of video-assisted thoracoscopic surgery are highlighted. Additionally, newer concepts of fluorescence image-guided, robot-assisted laparoscopic surgery and applications of artificial intelligence are discussed. This book is designed for medical students, nurses, post-graduate surgical trainees, and beginner laparoscopic surgeons in the various subspecialties of surgery involved with the abdomen with extension to the thorax—General, Colorectal, Pediatric, and Thoracic Surgery, Urology, and Gynecology.

It is our sincere hope that the book meets the desired objectives.

Port Harcourt, Nigeria Emeka Ray-Offor
Los Angeles, CA, USA Raul J. Rosenthal

Acknowledgments

Profound thanks to God Almighty, the ultimate source of knowledge and wisdom.

A sincere appreciation to all medical teachers on whom a good surgical foundation has been built for the practice of laparoscopic surgery. All the authors deserve special commendation for their wealth of experience and noble efforts in compiling this textbook.

Special thank you for the expert opinion from all chapter reviewers: *Dr. Adejumo, Adeyinka* MBBS (Nig), FMCS (Nig), Dip Lap (Tai), FICS, FACS; *Prof. Boni, Luigi* MD, FRCS, FACS; *Dr. Eguare, Emmanuel* MBBS, FRCSI, MSc, MD, FRCS; *Dr. Eke, Grace Ngozi* MBBS, FWACS, FACS; *Prof. Ekeke, Ngozi O.* MBBS, FWACS, FICS; *Prof. Falase, Bode* FRCS (CTh), FWACS; *Prof. Fiebai, Preye O.* MBBCh, FWACS, FICS; *Prof. Hafez Ahmed Shoukry* MSc, FRCS (ed); *Dr. Iroatulam, Augustine* JN, MD; *Prof. Ka, Ousmane*; *Prof. Marano, Luigi* MD, PhD; *Dr. Nweze, Onochie U.* MBBS, FWACS; *Prof. Oyetunji, Tolu.* MD, MPH, MBA; *Dr. Salu, Iliya Karniliyus* MBBS (ABU), FWACS, FRCS (Eng); *Dr. Sanni, Saheed B.* MBBS (Lagos), FMCS (CTh); and *Prof. Eke, Ndu* MBBCh, FRCS (ed), FICS. Thank you to *Elektra McDermott*, *Melissa Morton*, and the entire Springer editorial team.

This acknowledgment will not be complete without the warm appreciation of the Editors' family members for their caring support.

Emeka Ray-Offor
Raul J. Rosenthal

Contents

About the Editors and Contributors

About the Editors

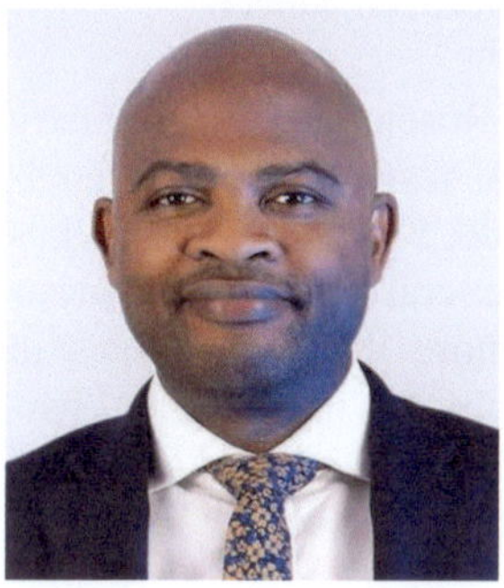

Emeka Ray-Offor Emeka Ray-Offor is an astute surgeon skilled in Endoscopy, Minimally Invasive Surgery, and Colorectal and Hernia surgeries, with a Bachelor of Medicine, Bachelor of Surgery degree -MBBS, from the University of Nigeria, Nsukka, and postgraduate surgery training acquired in India, Europe, and the United States. He recently completed a 1-year Research Fellowship in the Colorectal Surgery department of Ellen Leifer and Steven Shulman Digestive Disease Center, Cleveland Clinic, Florida, USA. He has held a faculty position in the College of Health Science, University of Port Harcourt, Nigeria, since 2011, and is currently a Professor of General & Minimal Access Surgery. In addition, he is the Director of the Minimal Access Surgery Program at the University of Port Harcourt Teaching Hospital, Port Harcourt, Rivers State, Nigeria, and a Consultant General and Minimally Invasive Surgeon in the Colorectal/ Minimal Access Surgery Unit of thc hospital.

He is a surgeon educator and has organized multiple workshops for training in Endoscopy/Minimal Access Surgery. He is a seasoned author with over 80 abstracts and peer-reviewed journal publications, in addition to being the editor of two other books on Endoscopy and Laparoscopic surgery, respectively. He is a reviewer of multiple scientific journals and Editor in Chief of the *Nigerian Journal of Gastroenterology and Hepatology* with membership in several professional societies in

Africa, Europe, Asia, and North America. These include the West African College of Surgeons (WACS), the Society of Gastroenterology and Hepatology (SOGHIN), the Nigerian Society for Colorectal Disorders (NSCD), European Association of Endoscopic Surgeons (EAES), World Association of Laparoscopic Surgeons (WALS), American College of Surgeons (ACS), Society of American Gastrointestinal Endoscopic Surgeons (SAGES), and American Society of Colon and Rectal Surgeons (ASCRS).

He is the founder of Oak Endoscopy Centre & Radiodiagnostics Port Harcourt Nigeria—a nonprofit organization for the advancement of Endoscopy and MIS.

His main professional and scientific interests focus on gastrointestinal endoscopy, minimally invasive general/colorectal surgery, and colorectal cancer.

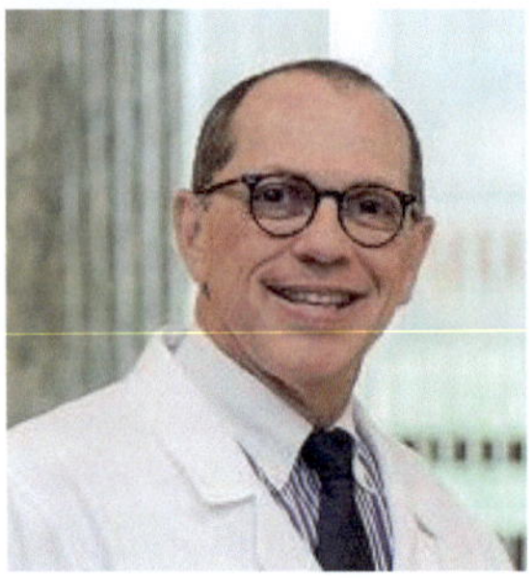

Raul J. Rosenthal Dr. Raul Rosenthal is an industry leader, prolific author, medical researcher, and attending surgeon at Cleveland Clinic, Florida, where he has conducted well over 10,000 general surgery and bariatric procedures and trained more than 50 fellows in advanced gastrointestinal, minimally invasive, and bariatric surgery. In 2018, he received the LEAD Award from the American Society of Metabolic & Bariatric Surgery (ASMBS) Foundation in recognition of lifetime contributions to the field of bariatric surgery. Also in 2018, his breakthrough research into the use of indocyanine green fluorescence imaging in laparoscopic cholecystectomy was featured during the American College of Surgeons annual Clinical Congress. Based on the results of his multinational, multi-year trial, the use of fluorescence imaging is becoming established as the gold standard of care for minimally invasive gall bladder removal and other abdominal procedures worldwide.

He completed his medical school and surgical residency in Rosario, Argentina. In 1982, after emigrating to Frankfurt, Germany, and repeating a general surgery residency, he became an attending surgeon at the Northwest Hospital. In 1993, he emigrated to the United States, where three years of minimally invasive surgery fellowship at Cedars Sinai Medical Center in LA was followed by a third general surgery residency at Mount Sinai Medical Center in New York City. After arriving at Cleveland Clinic Florida, he became Chief of Minimally Invasive and Bariatric Surgery and director of the Fellowship program. He has subsequently served as Chief of the Medical Staff, Chairman of the Department of General Surgery, Director of the General Surgery Residency Program, and Chairman of the Medical Executive Committee. Among his professional leadership roles, he served as president of the Society of American Gastrointestinal and Endoscopic Surgeons (SAGES) and the SAGES Foundation, and as a past president of the executive committee of the American Society of Metabolic & Bariatric Surgery (ASMBS) and the ASMBS Foundation. He is founding Clinical Editor of *Bariatric Times* and Associate Editor of *SOARD* and *Obesity Surgery*. He serves as the Editorial Board member of *Annals of Surgery*, *Selected Readings in General Surgery*, *Langenbeck's Archives of Surgery*, and *Surgical Endoscopy*. He is a founding member and a past President of the Fellowship Council and also served as President of the South Florida Chapter of the American College of Surgeons and Governor of the American College of Surgeons.

A polyglot, he is fluent in English, Spanish, and German. He has been granted honorary membership by professional organizations around the world, including the Federation of Latin American Surgeons, and the Argentinian, Indian, Peruvian, German, and Israeli Societies of Surgery. He is the author or co-author of over 300 abstracts and peer-reviewed publications, more than 30 book chapters, and over 100 educational videos. He has contributed over 80 book chapters and is the Co-Editor of several books including the *ASMBS Textbook of Bariatric Surgery*, *Globesity*, *Netter's Gastroenterology*, *The Pathophysiology of Pneumoperitoneum*, *Fluorescence Imaging for Surgeons*, *Operative Strategies in Laparoscopic Surgery*, *Weight Loss Surgery*, and *Mental Conditioning to Perform Common Operations in General Surgery Training: A Systematic Approach to Expediting Skill Acquisition and Maintaining Dexterity in Performance*.

Contributors

Lukman O. Abdur-Rahman, MBBS, MPH, FWACS, FMCS, FACS Division of Paediatric Surgery, Department of Surgery, University of Ilorin Teaching Hospital (UITH), Ilorin, Kwara State, Nigeria
Clinical Skills and Simulation Laboratory, College of Health Sciences, University of Ilorin, Ilorin, Kwara State, Nigeria

Ademola Adeyeye, MBBS MSc FRCS FACS FEBS FWACS Department of Colorectal Surgery, King's College Hospital, London, UK
Faculty of Life Sciences and Medicine, King's College, London, UK
Afe Babalola University, Ado-Ekiti, Ekiti State, Nigeria

Adewale O. Adisa, MBChB, FWACS, FMCS, DMAS, FACS Department of Surgery, Obafemi Awolowo University, Ile Ife, Nigeria

Mukhtar Ahmad, MBBS, MMedSci, FRCS (Gen Surg) University Hospitals Dorset NHS Foundation Trust, Poole, UK

Christian E. Amadi, MBBCh, FWACS, CTh Faculty of Clinical Sciences, University of Port Harcourt, Choba, Nigeria
Cardiothoracic/Vascular Unit, Surgery Department, University of Port Harcourt Teaching Hospital, Port Harcourt, Rivers State, Nigeria

Olanrewaju Samuel Balogun, MBBS, FWACS, FMAS, FHPBS Lagos University Teaching Hospital (LUTH), Lagos, Nigeria

Usman M. Bello, MBBS, FWACS Bayero University Kano, Kano, Nigeria
Aminu Kano Teaching Hospital, Kano, Kano State, Nigeria

Elad Boaz, MD Department of General Surgery, The Bariatric and Metabolic Institute, Ellen Leifer Shulman and Steven Shulman Digestive Disease Center, Cleveland Clinic Florida, Weston, FL, USA
Department of General Surgery, Shaare Zedek Medical Center, Faculty of Medicine, Hebrew University of Jerusalem, Jerusalem, Israel

Olujimi A. Coker, MBBS, FRCS (Gen Surgery), FWACS Sapphire Surgical Centre, Lagos, Nigeria
Laparoscopic Surgery Society of Nigeria LASSON, Lagos, Nigeria

Christopher N. Ekwunife, MBBS, DMAS, FWACS, FIAGES Department of Surgery, Federal Medical Centre, Owerri, Imo State, Nigeria

Sameh H. Emile, MBBCh, MSc, MD, FACS Cleveland Clinic Florida, Weston, FL, USA
Schmidt College of Medicine, Florida Atlantic University, Boca Raton, FL, USA
Faculty of Medicine, Mansoura University, Mansoura, Egypt

Emmanuel R. Ezeome, MA, MBBS, FWACS, FACS, FNAMed College of Medicine, University of Nigeria Nsukka, Nsukka, Nigeria
Institute of Public Health, University of Nigeria, Nsukka, Nigeria
West African College Surgeons WACS, Lagos, Nigeria

Sotonye Fyneface-Ogan, B.Med Sc MBBS PgDA FWACS, Dip Department of Anesthesia, University of Port Harcourt Teaching Hospital (UPTH), Port Harcourt, Rivers State, Nigeria
Department of Anesthesia, Faculty of Clinical Sciences, University of Port Harcourt, Choba, Rivers State, Nigeria

Zoe Garoufalia, MD Ellen Leifer Shulman and Steven Shulman Digestive Disease Center, Cleveland Clinic Florida, Weston, FL, USA

Kristine Griffin, MD Nationwide Children's Hospital, Columbus, OH, USA

Nir Horesh, MD Ellen Leifer Shulman and Steven Shulman Digestive Disease Center, Cleveland Clinic Florida,, Weston, FL, USA
Faculty of Medicine, Tel Aviv University, Tel Aviv, Israel

Patrick O. Igwe, MBBS FMCS DMAS FWACS FICS FACS Faculty of Clinical Sciences, University of Port Harcourt, Port Harcourt, Rivers State, Nigeria
Colorectal/Minimal Access Surgery Unit, Department of Surgery, University of Port Harcourt Teaching Hospital (UPTH), Port Harcourt, Rivers State, Nigeria

Rex F. O. A. Ijah, MBBS, MPH, FWACS, MS, MAS, FMAS Department of Surgery, Rivers State University (RSU)/Rivers State University Teaching Hospital (RSUTH), Port Harcourt, Rivers State, Nigeria

Noam Kahana, MD Department of General Surgery, The Bariatric and Metabolic Institute, Ellen Leifer Shulman and Steven Shulman Digestive Disease Center, Cleveland Clinic Florida, Weston, FL, USA
Department of General Surgery, Shaare Zedek Medical Center, Faculty of Medicine, Hebrew University of Jerusalem, Jerusalem, Israel

Olusegun Komolafe, FRCS NHS Lanarkshire, University Hospital Wishaw, Wishaw, Scotland, UK

Emanuele Lo Menzo, MD, PhD, FACS, FASMBS Minimally Invasive and Bariatric Surgery, The Bariatric and Metabolic Institute, Ellen Leifer Shulman and Steven Shulman Digestive Disease Center, Weston, FL, USA
Department of General Surgery, The Bariatric and Metabolic Institute, Ellen Leifer Shulman and Steven Shulman Digestive Disease Center, Cleveland Clinic Florida, Weston, FL, USA
Florida Atlantic University College of Medicine, Boca Raton, FL, USA
Florida International University College of Medicine, Miami, FL, USA

Ogbu E. Ngim, MBBS, FMCS Department of Surgery, University of Calabar, Calabar, Cross River State, Nigeria
Department of Surgery, University of Calabar Teaching Hospital (UCTH), Calabar, Cross River State, Nigeria

Benedict Nwomeh, MD, MPH, FRCS(Edin), FACS Department of Surgery, The Ohio State University, Columbus, OH, USA
Department of Pediatric Surgery, Nationwide Children's Hospital, Columbus, OH, USA

Tamunomie K. Nyengidiki, MBBS, FWACS, DMAS, FICS Department of Obstetrics and Gynaecology, Faculty of Clinical Sciences, University of Port Harcourt, Choba, Rivers State, Nigeria
Gynaecological Oncology Unit, University of Port Harcourt Teaching Hospital (UPTH), Port Harcourt, Rivers State, Nigeria

Emmanuel O. Ocheli, MBBS, FWACS, CTh Faculty of Clinical Sciences, University of Port Harcourt, Choba, Nigeria
Cardiothoracic/Vascular Unit, Surgery Department, University of Port Harcourt Teaching Hospital, Port Harcourt, Rivers State, Nigeria

Johnson Ogundare, DNP, MPH, PGDE, CNOR, RPON, RN Society for Nurses in Endoscopy and Minimally Invasive Surgery-Nigeria (SNEMIS-NG), Ibadan, Oyo State, Nigeria

Jude E. Okohue, MBBS, FWACS, FMCOG, DMAS, FICS Madonna University, Elele, Rivers State, Nigeria
Gynescope Specialist Hospital, Port Harcourt, Rivers State, Nigeria

Kelechi E. Okonta, MBBS MSc FWACS (CTh) FACS Faculty of Clinical Sciences, University of Port Harcourt, Choba, Nigeria
Cardiothoracic/Vascular Unit, Surgery Department, University of Port Harcourt Teaching Hospital, Port Harcourt, Rivers State, Nigeria

Charles P. Okpani, MBBS, M.Sc. FWACS Faculty of Clinical Sciences, University of Port Harcourt, Choba, Nigeria
Urology Division, Department of Surgery, University of Port Harcourt Teaching Hospital, Port Harcourt, Rivers State, Nigeria

Adedapo Osinowo, MBBS, FMCS, FMAS, DMAS Lagos University Teaching Hospital, Idi Araba, Lagos State, Nigeria

Chukwuemeka C. Osuagwu, MBBS(Nig), FWACS Department of Surgery, Al Quwayiyiah General Hospital, Riyadh Region, Saudi Arabia

Job G. Otokwala, MBBS, FWACS Faculty of Clinical Sciences, University of Port Harcourt, Choba, Rivers State, Nigeria
Department of Anesthesia, University of Port Harcourt Teaching Hospital (UPTH), Port Harcourt, Rivers State, Nigeria

Ana Pena, MD Department of General Surgery, The Bariatric and Metabolic Institute, Ellen Leifer Shulman and Steven Shulman Digestive Disease Center, Cleveland Clinic Florida, Weston, FL, USA

John E. Raphael, MBBS, FWACS, FICS, FACS Faculty of Clinical Sciences, University of Port Harcourt, Choba, Rivers State, Nigeria
Division of Urology, Department of Surgery, University of Port Harcourt Teaching Hospital (UPTH), Port Harcourt, Rivers State, Nigeria

Emeka Ray-Offor, MBBS(Nig) FWACS FMAS DMAS FACS College of Health Sciences, University of Port Harcourt, Choba, Rivers State, Nigeria
Minimal Access Surgery Program, University of Port Harcourt Teaching Hospital (UPTH), Port Harcourt, Rivers State, Nigeria
Department of Surgery, UPTH, Port Harcourt, Rivers State, Nigeria
Oak Endoscopy Centre and Radiodiagnostics, Port Harcourt, Rivers State, Nigeria

Raul J. Rosenthal, MD, FACS, FASMBS, MAMSE Division of General Surgery, Ronald Reagan UCLA Medical Center, David Geffen School of Medicine, Los Angeles, CA, USA

Samuel Szomstein, MD, FACS, FASMBS Department of General Surgery, The Bariatric and Metabolic Institute, Ellen Leifer Shulman and Steven Shulman Digestive Disease Center, Cleveland Clinic Florida, Weston, FL, USA
Herbert Wertheim College of Medicine, Florida International University, Miami, FL, USA

Brett P. Weiss, MD, MBA Candidate Miller School of Medicine, University of Miami, Miami, FL, USA

Steven D. Wexner, MD,PhD-Hon,FACS,FRCS,FRCSI,MAMSE Director, Ellen Leifer Shulman, and Steven Shulman Digestive Disease Center Emeritus Chair, Department of Colorectal Surgery, Cleveland Clinic Florida, USA
Clinical Professor, Cleveland Clinic Lerner College of Medicine at Case Western Reserve University
Clinical Affiliate Professor, Charles E. Schmidt College of Medicine, Florida Atlantic University
Clinical Professor, Herbert Wertheim College of Medicine, Florida International University
Affiliate Professor, Department of Surgery, University of South Florida, Morsani College of Medicine
Honorary Professor, Division of Surgery and Interventional Science, Department of Targeted Intervention, University College London, UK
Visiting Professor, Department of Surgery and Cancer, Imperial College London, UK
Past-President American Society of Colon and Rectal Surgeons
Past-President American Board of Colon and Rectal Surgery
Past-President, Society of American Gastrointestinal and Endoscopic Surgeons

Chair, National Accreditation Program for Rectal Cancer
Past Vice-Chair, Board of Regents, and Communications Consultant, American College of Surgeons
Editor-in-Chief, Surgery.

Part I
Basic Principles

Chapter 1
Evolution of Laparoscopic Surgery

Emeka Ray-Offor, Olujimi A. Coker, Emmanuel R. Ezeome, and Raul J. Rosenthal

Introduction

Minimally invasive surgery (MIS), often synonymously referred to as minimal access surgery or minimal access therapies, involves a surgical approach for diagnosis or treatment with the reduction of trauma without compromising the operating field. The term MIS was originally coined by John Wickham in 1983 [1]. This multi-specialty surgical practice uses the least disruptive route and causes the least

E. Ray-Offor (✉)
College of Health Sciences, University of Port Harcourt, Choba, Rivers State, Nigeria

Minimal Access Surgery Program, University of Port Harcourt Teaching Hospital (UPTH), Port Harcourt, Rivers State, Nigeria

Department of Surgery, UPTH, Port Harcourt, Rivers State, Nigeria

Oak Endoscopy Centre and Radiodiagnostics, Port Harcourt, Rivers State, Nigeria
e-mail: emeka.ray-offor@uniport.edu.ng

O. A. Coker
Sapphire Surgical Centre, Lagos, Nigeria

Laparoscopic Surgery Society of Nigeria LASSON, Lagos, Nigeria

E. R. Ezeome
College of Medicine, University of Nigeria Nsukka, Nsukka, Nigeria

Institute of Public Health, University of Nigeria, Nsukka, Nigeria

West African College Surgeons WACS, Lagos, Nigeria

R. J. Rosenthal
Division of General Surgery, Ronald Reagan UCLA Medical Center, David Geffen School of Medicine, Los Angeles, CA, USA
e-mail: rosentr@ccf.org

E. Ray-Offor, R. J. Rosenthal (eds.), *Principles and Practice of Laparoscopic Surgery*, https://doi.org/10.1007/978-3-031-96321-6_1

disturbance of structure and function. The scope of minimal access therapies comprises laparoscopy, thoracoscopy, arthroscopy, perivisceral and luminal endoscopies, and interventionals [2]. Laparoscopy, a fascinating interaction between technology and medicine, is derived from the Greek words 'lapara' –soft part of the belly (between the hips flanks, and rib cage and 'skopien' which means to view. The landmark advances in this field are from pioneering works in optics, lighting, peritoneal access, instrumentation, video technology, and techniques [3].

Advances in Optics and Lighting

From ancient times (circa 460–375 BC) the use of minimal access instruments in surgery is noted in literature and artifacts from Egypt, the Mesopotamian Empire, Greece, and Rome [4]. Traditionally called the 'Father of Medicine', Hippocrates reported direct vision of the inner cavity using an open tube system (rectal speculum). A historical treatise from Asia by the Indian surgeon, Sushruta (circa 600–800 BC) describes different surgical instruments including specula for inspecting the nose, mouth, ear, vagina, and anus [5]. One of the earliest reports of an examination of the internal system (vagina and cervix) using natural light reflected by a glass mirror was performed by the Arabian doctor Al-Zahrawi (AD 936–1013) [5]. Then a leap in visualization of human anatomy was made using relected light by Philip Bozzini in 1805. He projected artificial light from a wax candle into the body cavity with the aid of a concave mirror using his invention—"Lechleiter" (light conductor) [6]. This device directs light rays into the body's internal cavities and redirects them to the eye of the observer. For his effort, he was censored for "undue curiosity" by the Medical Faculty of Vienna. Further on, Antonin J Desormeaux reported the use of a lens to condense the beam of light from a kerosene lamp burning alcohol and turpentine to perform cystoscopy in 1865. Electrical illumination at endoscopy became possible with the invention of the light bulb by Thomas Alva Edison in 1879. Maximilian Nitze and his collaborators developed a cystoscopy instrument that integrated an electrical internal lighting source and an irrigation system to cool this portable device [7]. An adaptation of this device by Johann Mikulicz-Radecki (1850–1905) and Joseph Leiter, was applied to examine the upper gastrointestinal tract [8]. At this point, all these optical systems were fraught with inadequate illumination and shallow depth of penetration (Fig. 1.1). Harold Hopkins through the invention of the rod lens transformed the optical system which traditionally comprised relay and field lenses made from glass with long intervening air spaces to air lenses and long glass spaces [7]. The doubled light transmitting capacity was achieved by this telescope design as the refractive index predominantly became that of glass. An introduction of fiber optics (1954) involving a bundle of flexible, narrow glass fibers for light transmission was also pivotal [9]. In present settings, illumination in laparoscopy is achieved using an artificial

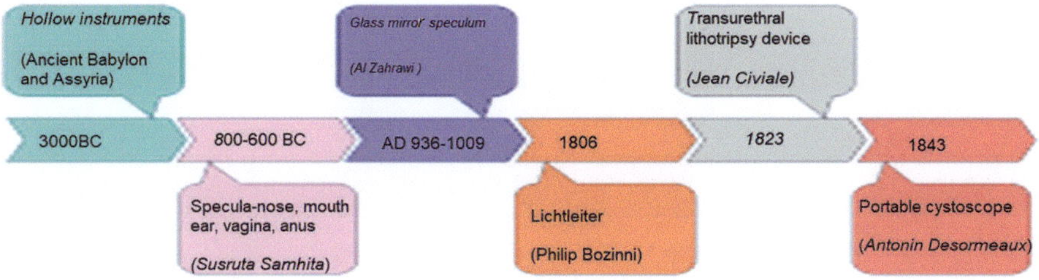

Fig. 1.1 Timeline and pioneers of internal organ visualization (Stone Copper age- nineteenth century)

external light source connected to a fiber optic cable. Based on the principle of total internal light reflection in glass fiber, the fiber optic cable conducts light into a rod-lens telescope. This is then transmitted into the peritoneal cavity.

Advances in Peritoneal Access and Instrumentation

Closed cavity operation in laparoscopic surgery requires insufflation of the abdominal cavity (pneumoperitoneum) and peculiar instrumentation. The pneumoperitoneum creates a workspace between the visceral peritoneum and parietal peritoneum. George Kelling in 1901, insufflated the abdominal cavity of a dog for visualization using a cystoscope [10]. Hans Jacobaeus, a Swedish surgeon (1910), performed the first laparoscopy on a man using an injector for air insufflations; in the United States, laparoscopy was first performed in 1911 by Bertram M Bernheim [11]. Air insufflation was observed to cause audible explosions and flashes of light in the abdominal cavity with electrocautery; Zollikoffer used carbon dioxide in 1924 [12]. At present, carbon dioxide is mostly used due to its colorless, cheap, clean, non-combustible, and blood diffusion for absorption properties. For peritoneal access, a sharp pointed pyramidal point of trocar was developed by Benzamin Orndoff (1920) for ease of passage through the abdominal wall. Janos Veress, a Hungarian surgeon, developed a spring-loaded needle for insufflation in 1938. Then following the monitoring of intra-abdominal arterial pressure (IAP) in 1944 by Raol Palmer the automatic insufflator was introduced by Kurt Semm in 1963 [13]. Automatic insufflators aid in monitoring and controlling IAP at an adequate pressure of 10–15 mmHg for most laparoscopic surgeries. Harith Hasson (1978) proposed a direct peritoneal access technique to reduce the complication rate with blind needle puncture into the peritoneum. Also, Professor Heinz Kalk made an innovative stride in instrumentation using oblique viewing optics from the longitudinal axis [14]. This permitted better inspection of organs as the image can be changed by altering the viewing direction of the optics such that the lens is moved around the object. All these developments and more from many other innovative surgeons advanced the practice of laparoscopy as an effective diagnostic tool leading to its therapeutic applications (Fig. 1.2).

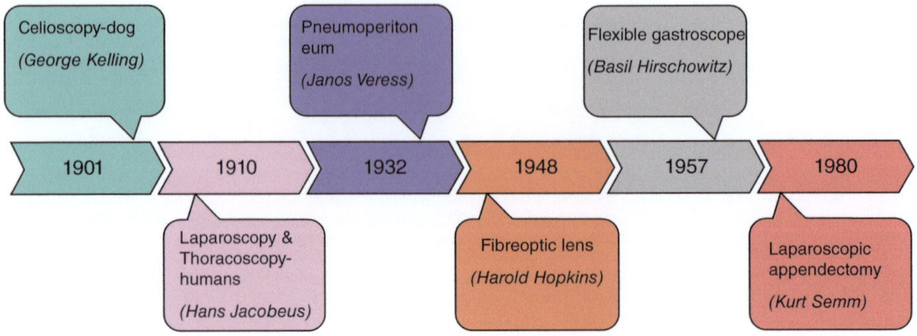

Fig. 1.2 Twentieth-century historical landmarks in Laparo- Endoscopic surgery

Video Technology and Laparoscopic Revolution

In the first part of the twentieth century, minimally invasive surgery was generally confined to urology, gynecology, gastroscopy, diagnostic laparoscopy, and some otorhinolaryngology. The ability to broadcast and publicize these technological advances with photography and video recording was pertinent to their expansion and rapid application. Notably, in the development of laparoscopic surgery, video technology was introduced in the 1970s. Computer chip technology invented by Welch Allyn (USA)-1984 was incorporated into the tip of an endoscope. A video monitor connected to the laparoscope enables a simultaneous view of the operative field between the operating surgeon and assistant. For complex surgeries, this virtual real-time image displayed on a video monitor enables effective interaction between the operating team while serving as a useful aid for students. However, there is the need to appreciate the right direction, depth, and momentum as the abdominal compartment is dynamic with peristaltic bowels, pulsatile blood vessels, elusive bleeders, and moving organs resulting from breathing and heart movement. To date, the wide application and acceptance of laparoscopic cholecystectomy has been tagged it as the 'flagship' of this closed-cavity abdominal surgical practice. The first laparoscopic cholecystectomy was performed in 1985 by Eric Muhe in Germany. However, it was the video-laparoscopic procedure of the same surgery two years later by Philip Mouret (Lyon France) that sparked the surgical renaissance all over the world [15]. In a short time, a plethora of therapeutic abdominal surgeries were reported to be successfully performed by this closed cavity technique (Table 1.1). The rapid developments in video imaging have resulted in higher-resolution video monitors with clearer images improving the operative field and making fine dissection of the tissue plane easier. Three-dimensional television monitors have been developed to counter the challenge of depth perception. The debate is no longer about which surgery can be done by laparoscopy but when the preferable choice is by open method for certain reasons.

Table 1.1 Historical landmarks in therapeutic laparo-endoscopic surgery

Year	Name	Surgery
1929	Heinz Kalk	Dual Puncture Technique
1933	Carl Fervers	Laparoscopic Adhesiolysis
1944	Raol Palmer	Laparoscopic Tubal Sterilzation
1982	Kurt Semm	Laparoscopic Appendectomy
1985	Eric Muhe	Laparoscopic Cholecystectomy
1987	Philip Mouret	Video Laparoscopic Cholecystectomy
1989	Reich H. et al	Laparoscopic Hysterectomy
1991	Moises Jacobs et al	Laparoscopic-Assisted Colectomy
1992	William Schuessler et al	Laparoscopic Prostatectomy
1992	Peter Goh et al	Laparoscopic Billroth II Gastrectomy
1995	Ming Han Chen et al	Laparoscopy-Assisted Abdominal Aortic Aneurysm repair
1997	Jacques Himpens & Guy Bernard Cardierre	Robot-Assisted Laparoscopic Cholecystectomy
2004	Anthony Kalloo et al	Natural Orifice Transluminal Endoscopic Surgery (NOTES)
2007	Jean-Claude Marescaux et al	First Human Transgastric Cholecystectomy
2007	Curcillio PG & King SA	Single Port Access Surgery

Advancing Frontiers of MIS

An advancement of the concept of MIS is introducing 3–4 trocars through one umbilical incision to perform laparoscopic procedures and this was developed by Drs. Paul Curcillo and Stephanie King in 2007—Single-port access (SPA) [16]. The synonyms for SPA surgery are Single Incision laparoscopic Surgery (SILS), Single Site Laparoscopy (SSL), Single-Port Laparoscopic Surgery (SPLS), Single-Port Laparoscopy (SPL), and Laparo Endoscopic Single-Site (LESS) surgery [17]. Further advancement of the MIS concept involving the use of multi-tasking platforms is the Natural Orifice Transluminal Endoscopic Surgery (NOTES). This hybrid procedure uses flexible endoscopic technology to perform laparoscopic surgical procedures beyond the confines of the gastrointestinal tract. Both NOTES and SILS necessitated the development of dexterous instrumentation for adequate maneuverability, independent camera articulation, triangulation, and intuitive control. These are crucial to the surgeon for performing complex bimanual surgical tasks like suturing and knot-tying.

Robotic Surgical Systems (RSS) were introduced into the theatre initially for neurosurgical, urology, and orthopedic procedures in the late 80s and early 90s of the twentieth century for programmed tasks [18]. However, the first robotic system for laparoscopic surgery, AESOP, became available in 1994 developed by Computer Motion (Santa Barbara, CA, USA). This enabled the surgeon's voice control of the laparoscope positioning. Driven by the investigational military need for urgent surgical intervention close to the battlefield, an area with the most limited resources and personnel (telepresence), the Zeus became available in the United States in 1996 [18]. The most popular RSS, da Vinci (Intuitive Surgical Sunnyvale, CA, USA), was first introduced in Europe and received US Food and Drug Approval in 2000. This stable RSS enabled with 3D vision and 7 degrees of freedom hand movement has largely dominated the RSS market. The cost of acquisition and maintenance is a major limitation in widening availability. Machine vision with artificial intelligence (AI), enables robotic systems to interpret intraoperative imagery in real time, ensuring accurate navigation, tissue identification, and execution of surgical tasks [19]. This not only aids in minimizing surgical trauma but also expedites the recovery process, underscoring the transformative impact of AI in modern surgical practices. AI is finding more applications in surgery to improve diagnosis, guide decision-making during preoperative planning/practice, provide intraoperative aides, and improve postoperative care [20]. Virtual reality applications are currently available in simulation training for essential laparoscopic skills. (See Chap. 11). Also augmented reality and fluorescence technology are becoming available in laparoscopy to aid in improved diagnosis and precision in surgery (See Chap. 19).

In summary, advancement in the closed cavity approach of laparoscopic surgery has resulted from slowly progressing research, breakthroughs, discoveries, and a rapid paradigm shift. The frontiers of minimally invasive surgery continue to unfold and so the laparoscopic surgeon is faced with more complex gadgetry and new technologies beyond traditional surgery skills. Mastery, rather than apathy or rejection, is required to harness the ultimate results of improved patient-related outcome measures and surgical health care delivery.

References

1. Wickham JEA. Phone interview by G.S. Litynski, tape recording, April 23, 1996. In: Litynski GS, editor. Highlights in the history of laparoscopy. Frankfurt/Main: B. Bernert Verlag; 1996. p. 199–202.
2. Cuschieri A. Technology for minimal access surgery. Interview by Judy Jones BMJ. 1999;319(7220):1304.
3. Gaskin TA, Ische JH, Matthews JL, Winchester SB, Smith RJ. Laparoscopy and the general surgeon. Surg Clin North Am. 1991;71(5):1085–97.
4. Hargest R. Five thousand years of minimal access surgery: 3000BC to 1850: early instruments for viewing body cavities. J R Soc Med. 2020;113(12):491–6.
5. Spaner SJ, Warnock GL. A brief history of endoscopy, laparoscopy, and laparoscopic surgery. J Laparoendosc Adv Surg Tech A. 1997;7(6):369–73.
6. Dave T, Habte A, Vora V, Sheikh MQ, Sanker V, Gopal SV. Sushruta: the father of Indian surgical history. Plast Reconstr Surg Glob Open. 2024;12(4):e5715.

7. Hargest R. Five thousand years of minimal access surgery: 1850 to 1990: technological developments. J R Soc Med. 2021;114(1):19–29. Arregui ME, Fitzgibbons RJ, Katkhouda N, Mckernan JB, Reich H (eds) New York. Springer; 1995: pp. 3–20.
8. Mikulicz J. Gastroskopie und oesophagoskopie. Verh dt Ges Chir Berlin. 1882;11:31–8.
9. Hopkins HH, Kapany NS. A flexible fiberscope, using static scanning. Nature. 1954;17:39–41.
10. Hatzinger M, Badawi JK, Häcker A, Langbein S, Honeck P, Alken P. Georg Kelling (1866–1945): the man who introduced modern laparoscopy into medicine. Urologe A. 2006;45:868–71. https://doi.org/10.1007/s00120-006-1068-9.
11. Morgenstern L. The first laparoscopist in the United States: Bertram M. Bernheim, MD. Surg Innov. 2007;14:241–2. https://doi.org/10.1177/1553350607309433.
12. Alkatout I, Mechler U, Mettler L, Pape J, Maass N, Biebl M, Gitas G, Laganà AS, Freytag D. The development of laparoscopy-a historical overview. Front Surg. 2021;8:799442. https://doi.org/10.3389/fsurg.2021.799442.
13. Litynsk GS. Endoscopic surgery: the history, the pioneers. World J Surg. 1999;23:745–53. Kelley WE. The evolution of laparoscopy and the revolution in surgery in the decade of the 1990s. JSLS. 2008;12:351–7.
14. Kalk H. Erfahrungen mit der Laparoskopie (zugleich mit Beschreibung eines neuen Instrumentes). Z Klin Med. 1929;111:304–48.
15. Kaiser AM, Corman ML. History of laparoscopy. Surg Oncol Clin N Am. 2001;10:483–92.
16. Curcillo PG 2nd, King SA, Podolsky ER, Rottman SJ. Single port access (SPA™) minimal access surgery through a single incision. Surg Technol Int. 2009;18:19–25.
17. Arkenbout EA, Henselmans PW, Jelínek F, Breedveld P. A state of the art review and categorization of multi-branched instruments for NOTES and SILS. Surg Endosc. 2015;29(6):1281–96. https://doi.org/10.1007/s00464-014-3816-z.
18. Lane T. A short history of robotic surgery. Ann R Coll Surg Engl. 2018;100(suppl 6):5–7. https://doi.org/10.1308/rcsann.supp1.5.
19. Satava RM. Surgical robotics: the early chronicles: a personal historical perspective. Surg Laparosc Endosc Percutan Tech. 2002;12(1):6–16. https://doi.org/10.1097/00129689200202000-00002.
20. Reza T, Bokhari SFH. Partnering with technology: advancing laparoscopy with artificial intelligence and machine learning. Cureus. 2024;16(3):e56076.

Chapter 2
Laparoscopic Equipment and Instruments

Rex F. O. A. Ijah

Introduction

Laparoscopy is highly technology dependent; thus, it is expected that every laparoscopic surgeon should have a reasonably good knowledge of the equipment/instruments. The availability of the right quality of equipment and instruments, a good knowledge of their use, proper ergonomics, safety precautions, and the surgeon's motivation and experiences have largely contributed to the successes recorded in modern surgical practice. The importance of this subject can be seen in the occurrence of equipment failures capable of not only affecting the outcome of surgery but also contributing to prolongation of operation time [1]. About 38.6% of laparoscopic surgeries are complicated by equipment failures [2, 3]. These equipment and instruments have few similarities to those of open surgery as seen in the tissue ends of some hand instruments. However, huge differences exist especially in the long and slender insulated shaft, specially designed handles, and tissue ends adapted for different functions. They are available in different makes and generations ranging from branded ones from highly reputable companies to low-budget qualities. Also, as the single-use disposable and the reusable ones [2].

Laparoscopic Trolley [4]

This is the platform on which some of the 'magnificent seven' (light source, fiber optic cable, laparoscope, camera head, video signal processor, video cable, and monitor) are mounted (Fig. 2.1). Other equipment on the trolley are photo printers,

R. F. O. A. Ijah (✉)
Department of Surgery, Rivers State University (RSU)/Rivers State University Teaching Hospital (RSUTH), Port Harcourt, Rivers State, Nigeria

E. Ray-Offor, R. J. Rosenthal (eds.), *Principles and Practice of Laparoscopic Surgery*, https://doi.org/10.1007/978-3-031-96321-6_2

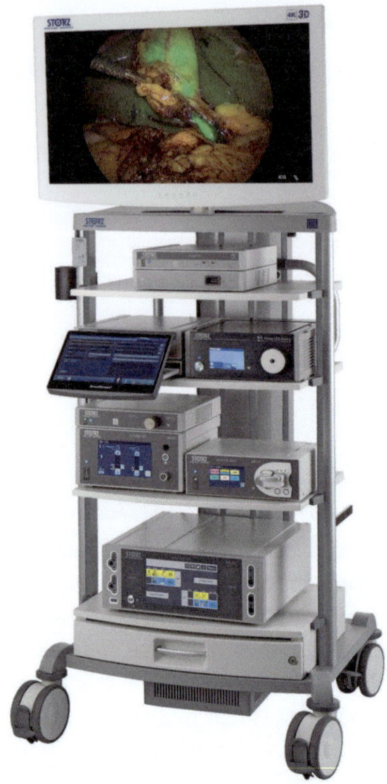

Fig. 2.1 Laparoscopy cart with equipment (©Karl Storz SE & Co. KG)

VCRs, and digital capture devices. This platform is also called a laparoscopic cart and has different designs fitted with mobile antistatic rollers. The laparoscopy cart is designed to be stationary and provides stability to the fragile equipment in use and moves en-masse when adjustment in space is needed. Irrespective of the design of the trolley, the function is the same.

Classification of Laparoscopic Equipment and Instruments

Many classifications abound based on function, arrangement in theatre, material composition, single or multiple usages, disassemblage, and manufacturer. Laparoscopic equipment and instruments can be grouped into the following categories [2]: Laparoscopic trolley; imaging systems—laparoscopic camera, telescope/laparoscope, light cable, light source, and laparoscopic video camera; insufflation system—insufflator/laparoflattor, gas tube, and gas (carbon dioxide) cylinder; suction/irrigation system—suction machine and suction/instillation tube; energy source—diathermy machine, coagulating and dissecting electrodes; instruments—laparoscopic working instruments, port access instruments (trocar and cannula), hand instruments (graspers and others), sharp dissection instruments (scissors, electrosurgical hook, HF electrosurgery spatula, HF surgery knife, knife—endoknife, scalpel, biopsy forceps, and others (aspiration needle, retractors, needle holder, laparoscopic clip applicators, knot pushers, laparoscopic auto-suturing device, fallop ring applicator, uterine manipulator, myoma fixation screw, tissue morcellator, hernia stapler, endoanchor and tacker). However, for ease of description, Oak et al. classified laparoscopic equipment and instruments into three [2]:

(a) ***Imaging System:*** This comprises a telescope and endo-vision camera; light source and fiber optic cable; and video monitor.
(b) ***Exposure and manipulation equipment/instruments:*** These include electronic carbon dioxide insufflators; suction irrigation systems; and energy sources (mono-polar cautery, bipolar cautery, ultrasound devices, lasers, argon beam coagulators, etc.).
(c) ***Hand Instruments:*** They are Veress needles; trocars and cannulas; and working instruments (dissecting instruments, scissors, hooks and spatulas, clamping instruments, stapling, suturing instruments, and miscellaneous instruments—endoscopic retractors).

Broadly, laparoscopic equipment and instruments are classified into equipment on a trolley or laparoscopic cart and instruments on a laparoscopic tray.

Imaging System [3–8]

Telescope (Laparoscope)

Laparoscopic surgery is unrealizable without the laparoscope. Located at the distal end of the endoscope is the objective lens which determines the viewing angle—forward, oblique, lateral, or retrograde. The angle of view of the laparoscope varies from 0° to 120° (commonly 0° and 30°).

Color codes are used to differentiate the angle of vision of the telescope: Green for 0° telescopes and red for 30° oblique view devices. It also comes with a diameter of 1.5 mm to 15 mm but commonly 5 mm and 10 mm (Fig. 2.2). The 0° telescope provides a view of 76° compared to 30° telescopes which permits a view of 152°.

There are two types of lens system designs in use in laparoscopes:

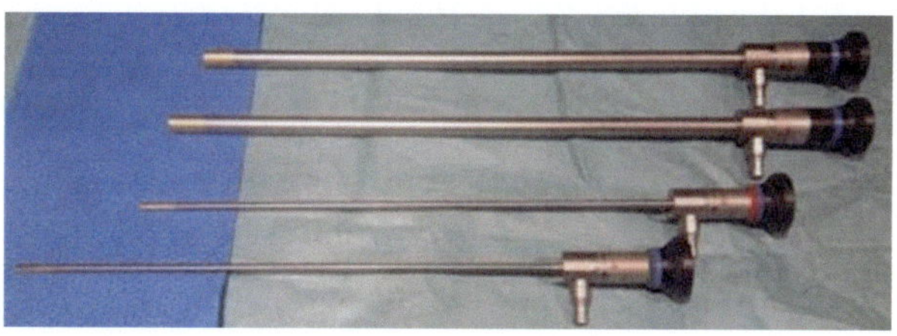

Fig. 2.2 Telescopes of different sizes

(a) *Conventional lens system*

This thin lens system telescope is used less commonly and has a series of objective lenses for the relay of image down the telescope.

(b) *Hopkins rod-lens system*

This is a reusable endo-vision system device comprising an eyepiece encased in a jacket tube made of a non-corrosive material (stainless steel) that encloses the rod-lens system. It has an in-built fiber-optic light carrier with a connection for a fiber-optic light cable. By using more glass than air, the Hopkins system has an improved light transmission. An inverted real image lens system (IRILS) located at the distal end of the telescope creates an inverted and real image of the object. Also contained in the telescope are parallel optical fiber bundles that transmit light to the abdomen. The light post is at the end of the light bundle and allows the fiber light cable to be attached to the fiber optic light bundle within the endoscope, transmitting light to the distal portion of the endoscope.

A laparoscope is held and manipulated by the assistant surgeon, surgeon (during diagnostic laparoscopy), or a robotic arm (during robotic surgery). It works with the rest of the imaging system. Complications from the use of the telescope are not common; however, measures should be taken to avoid potential visceral burn injury from heated laparoscopes and postoperative anterior abdominal port-site adhesion or herniation from port sites.

Endo-Vision Camera

The endo-vision camera provides a magnified clear view of the surgical field using a charge-coupled device CCD as a sensor. The CCD is an electronic memory that records the intensity of light as a variable charge. It comes as a single-chip or three-chip camera (and a high-definition camera). The single-chip camera uses one CCD, while the three-chip camera is built with three CCDs. In principle, the three primary colors of blue, green, and red are compressed in composite transmission in the single-chip camera with consequent >400–600 lines resolution whereas these colors are separated in the three-chip camera with a resolution range between 600 and 1000 lines and hence increased light sensitivity and color definition. A three-chip camera with a resolution of >1000 lines is a high-definition camera.

A camera head (Fig. 2.3) is mounted onto the laparoscope and the endo-vision camera unit. Any incompatibility between the camera system and monitor can lead to poor visibility and complications. For reason of efficiency, the endo-vision system should preferably be of the same manufacturer.

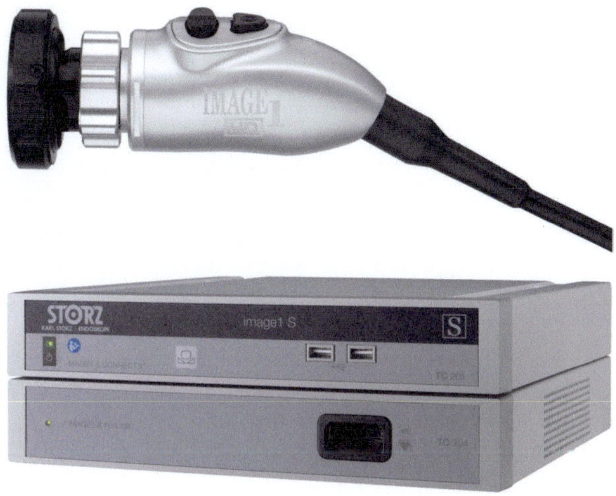

Fig. 2.3 Endo-vision camera unit with camera head (©Karl Storz SE & Co. KG)

Video Monitor [8]

This is a four-corner screen from which the laparoscopic surgeon and team visualize a magnified image of the body cavity and what is being manipulated (Fig. 2.4). It is positioned directly opposite and preferably about 3 meters from the operating surgeon on a mobile laparoscopic cart/trolley (or installed on a hanging rotating arm on the roof of the operating room). This permits all members of the operating team to view the operative field simultaneously; a second monitor could also be used by the assistant surgeon. The resultant image output depends on the following characteristics of the monitor: number of lines of resolution; scanning lines; pixels and dot pitch. The color images are formed by super-imposing color data on existing black and white pictures—black and white is monochromatic whereas the color image is a composite color signal. A medical-grade monitor is of higher quality than a normal television screen. The preferable size of the monitor for laparoscopic surgery is 20 inches or more with at least 400–600 lines resolution. It is noteworthy that there are different television systems for different regions. The Sequential Colour and Memory (SECAM) for the French; National Television System Committee (NTSC) for America; and Phase Alternation by Lines (PAL) for European countries. Table 2.1 shows the features of each.

A limitation of laparoscopic surgery is the two-dimensional image of the video monitor depicting the operating field only by monocular cues. The high definition (HD) monitors, with 1–2 million pixels per frame, wider screen, and higher contrast ratio, have improved anatomical details with visualization much better than the traditional monitors. However, a three-dimensional image is an advanced feature of monitors in robotic surgery.

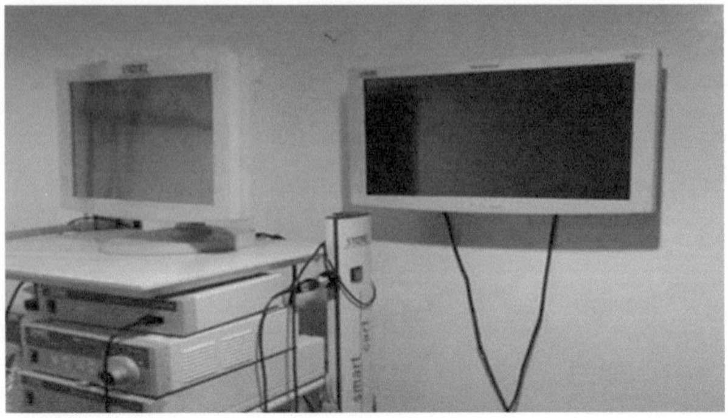

Fig. 2.4 Laparoscopic video monitors

Table 2.1 Television systems and characteristics

Systems	SECAM	NTSC	PAL
No of lines	625	525	625
Maximum visible lines	575	486	575
Field frequency cycles per second	50	60	50
Frames per second	25	30	25

Light Source [8]

Typically, a light source has a manual or automated control circuit, condensing lens, heat filter, and lamp (bulb). The common lamps in use are halogen, metal halide, xenon, and LED (Light Emission Diode) (Fig. 2.5), Table 2.2. Halogen lamps impart a yellowish tinge to light while xenon has a bluish hue. To achieve a near natural mid-day sunlight an adjustment of the light (white balancing) is done by placing a piece of white gauze at 6–8 cm from the tip of the telescope then pressing the function button on the video camera head or camera control unit CCU. This creates an optimal view for the surgeon. Intra-operatively, an adjustment to the red, blue, and green wavelengths of the LED light has been associated with the ability to identify tumor metastases expressing fluorescent proteins of different wavelengths, which greatly enhanced the signal without compromising background illumination. The development of this technology is applied for clinical use to improve the staging and treatment of malignancies including pancreatic and colorectal cancer. A 175 W light source is considered enough for routine laparoscopy however a 300 W source is needed for special/advanced interventions or the use of a mini laparoscope. It is important to note that though the light filter removes much of the heat energy generated at the source, the light delivered to the tip of the lighted laparoscope still has residual heat which if left in contact with the tissues or material for more than 20–30 s may lead to burns.

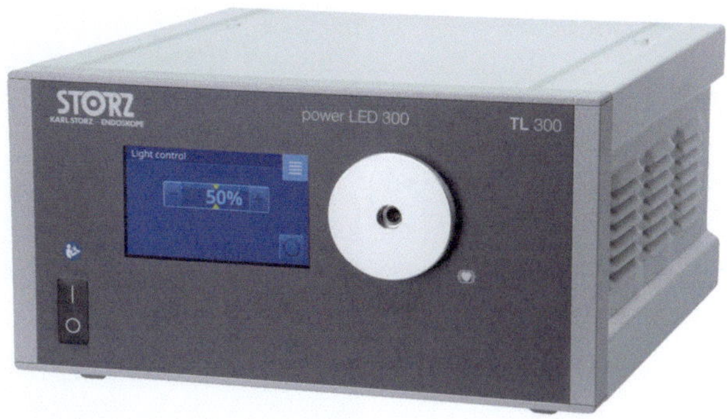

Fig. 2.5 Xenon light source (©Karl Storz SE & Co. KG)

Table 2.2 Light sources and characteristics

S/ No	Light source	Characteristics
1	Tungsten/Halogen (Bulb)	Halogen gas is compressed in a chamber of a transparent quartz bulb Cheaper, gives brilliant yellow-colored light Has been in use in the medical field for more than two decades
		Uses low voltage
		Colour temperature of 3200 Kelvin
		Average life span of 2000 hours
2	Metal Halide (Bulb)	Difficult to handle
		High-intensity discharge lamp
		Two types: iron iodide and gallium iodide
		Can generate up to 400 W units needed for three-chip cameras
3	Xenon (Bulb)	Colourless, odorless, highly unreactive gaseous non-metallic element
		Atomic number of 54
		Has two electrodes (cathode and anode) with no filament
		Temperature at cathode tip is about 20000C
		Colour temperature of 6000–6400 Kelvin
		Can generate 300W unit
		Has approximately fixed life span of about 1500 h
4	Light Emission Diode (LED—Bulb)	Cost-saving, eco-friendly Can be used with an HD camera
5	Battery-powered LED light source	Lithium battery-operated white light Light intensity of 100,000 Lux.
		Long operating life of LEDs (up to 50,000 hours) and a run time of more than 120 minutes.
		No light cable required

Note: Mid-day sunlight color temperature is 5000–6000 Kelvin

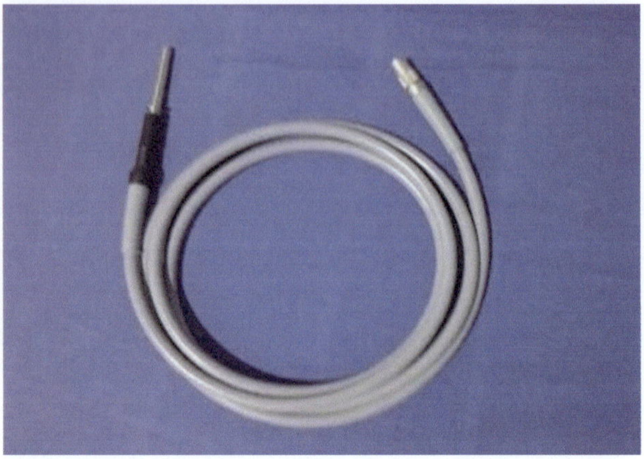

Fig. 2.6 Optic cable

Light Cable

This is a tubal structure that contains glass fiber bundles or special fluid (liquid crystal gel cable can transmit 30% more light than fiber-optic cable) for light transmission (Fig. 2.6). A plastic insulator is used as a coating. It works by the total internal reflection of light through the fiber optic cable. Light rays generate considerable heat energy most of which is filtered by a heat filter. As a precaution, the distal end of the fiber-optic cable should not be placed under the drapes or on the patient to avoid burn injury.

The optic cable should be handled carefully avoiding twisting and excessive folding of the light cable beyond the recommended arc (not less than a 15 cm radius); otherwise, this can result in damage. Other useful tips include disconnecting the cable first after operation; avoiding a direct glare of the light emanating from the cable to exclude the risk of retinal damage; and cleaning the outer plastic coat with disinfectant.

Exposure and Manipulation Equipment/Instruments

Electronic Insufflator

The electronic carbon dioxide insufflator is an automated device that is used to inflate carbon dioxide into the peritoneal cavity. The machine is designed to autoregulate according to pre-set parameters. It consists of quadro-manometric indicators for the pre-set pressure; actual pressure of gas delivered; flow rate (speed of gas flow); and the total volume of gas delivered (Fig. 2.7). Mutually independent safety circuits and optical and acoustic alarms that are built into the system also help to ensure patient safety. The newer model insufflators are designed to warm the carbon dioxide before insufflating the peritoneal cavity thus reducing heat loss and fogging of the lens.

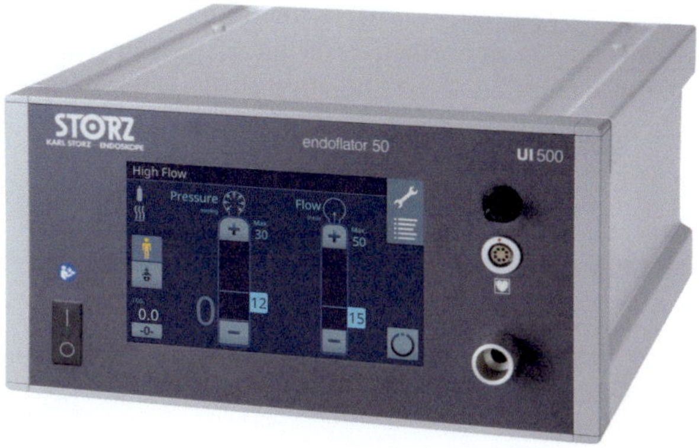

Fig. 2.7 Electronic insufflator (© KARL STORZ SE & Co. KG, Germany)

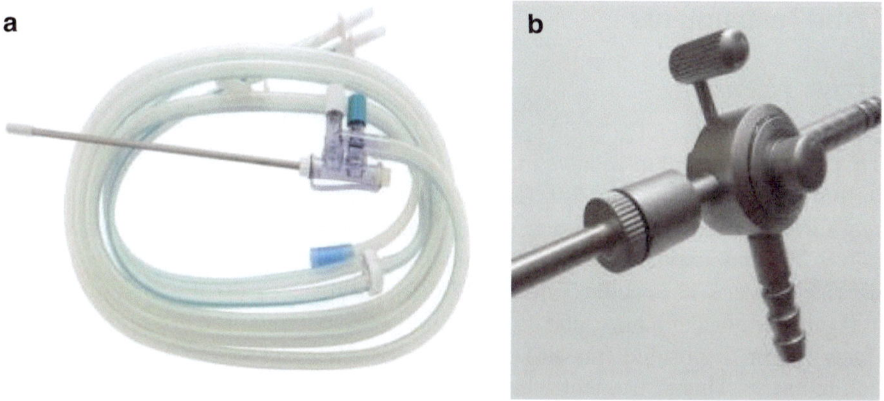

Disposable Reusable

Fig. 2.8 Laparoscopic suction irrigation system (**a**) Disposable (**b**) Reusable

It requires some training to read and interpret displayed figures for patients' benefit. There may be complications of gas embolism; gastric reflux following increased intra-abdominal pressure; effects of resultant increased intra-abdominal pressure on cardiac, renal, and liver physiology; and extra-peritoneal gas insufflation.

Suction Irrigation System

The suction irrigation system comprises a suction machine; a connecting tube; a probe (5 mm or 10 mm size) bearing a regulator Fig. 2.8. Normal saline, Ringer's Lactate, or heparinized saline are solutions that are used by most surgeons for irrigation and to clear the operation field of blood and fluid collection. The tip of the suction probe is dipped directly into the blood or collection before activating as it can frustrate the operative process due to gas depletion. When there is the presence of blood clots or more than 1500 ml of hemo-peritoneum it is advisable to use the 10 mm size probe. In addition to the role of the suction probe in the suction and irrigation of the operative site, it can also come in handy in the manipulation of tissues.

Energy Sources

These include electrical, laser, ultrasonic, and mechanical equipment. This topic is discussed in detail in the next chapter of this book.

Hand Instruments

Veress Needle

This is a device used to achieve initial access for the pneumoperitoneum before the introduction of trocars Fig. 2.9. It consists of an outer beveled-tip cannula for cutting through tissues and an inner spring-loaded blunt-tip stylet to prevent visceral injury. The inner stylet has a lateral hole towards its tip for intra-peritoneal carbon dioxide delivery. The needle comes in different length sizes: 80 mm for thin patients; 100 mm for normal adults; and 120 mm for obese patients. It can also be reusable (metallic) or disposable (plastic). A test for patency and spring action is advised before its use. This instrument is held like a dart between the thumb and index finger

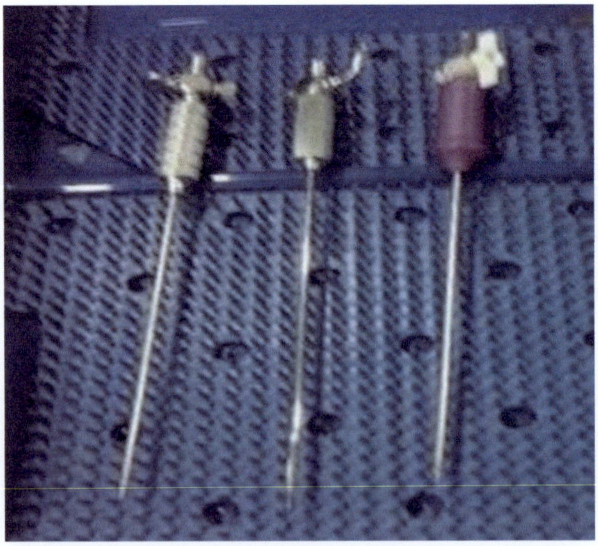

Fig. 2.9 Veress needles—reusable and disposable

when in use. The signs that confirm correct intra-peritoneal placement include: two separate "give" sounds on penetrating the single rectus sheath (at the umbilical cicatrix) and the peritoneum; hissing sound indicating negative intra-peritoneal pressure suction; hanging-drop test; suction pressure and manometric tests. This instrument is risky in unskilled hands as vascular injury, gas (carbon dioxide) embolism and intra-peritoneal visceral injury can occur.

Trocars and Cannulas

A trocar is an appliance passed through the anterior abdominal wall in laparoscopic surgery (skin, subcutaneous tissues, rectus sheath (or otherwise), extra-peritoneal fascia, and peritoneum) via a small incision. This acts as a port as other instruments are then passed through it to perform laparoscopic procedures. The term trocar is derived from the French word "Trois" meaning "three". Thus, it is made up of three components: a cannula—hollow port; an obturator—blunt/conical tip or sharp tip cylindrical tool; and a flap valve. The cannula varies in size with diameters ranging from 3 mm to 30 mm, though the commonly used are 5 mm, 10 mm, and 15 mm. The 5 mm size is used for the introduction of hand instruments; 10 mm for laparoscope; and 15 mm may be used for the introduction of larger instruments e.g. mesh fixator for ventral hernia repair. Several new disposable trocar designs incorporate unique features such as direct serial incision of the tissue under visual control (Excel Visiport), serial dilatation of the Veress needle tract, or capacity for varying sizes of instruments without gas leak (Versaport).

Disposable trocar usually has a blade incorporated into the tip of the obturator. The sharp edge trocar has a risk of injury to anterior abdominal wall vessels (e.g. inferior epigastric vessels) and internal abdominal viscera. It is safe practice to avoid too much tension and resistance during entry and to do a good anterior abdominal wall mapping always before inserting the primary (non-optical trocar) under direct laparoscopic vision. These three-piece appliances are metallic (reusable) or plastic (disposable) (Fig. 2.10). The choice of the trocar in open access technique is the Hasson cannula (Fig. 2.11).

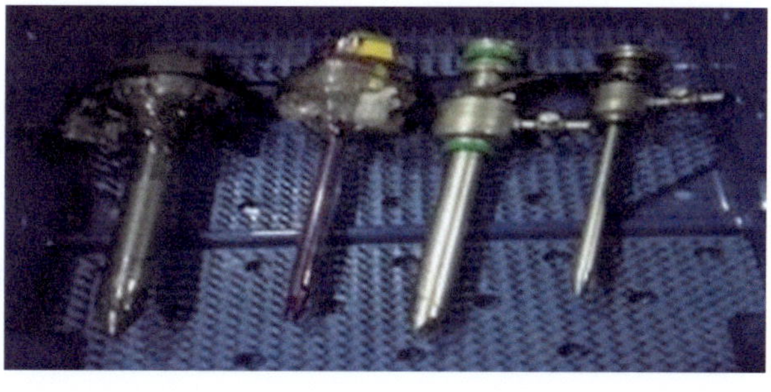

Fig. 2.10 Trocar varieties (plastic disposable and metal reusable)

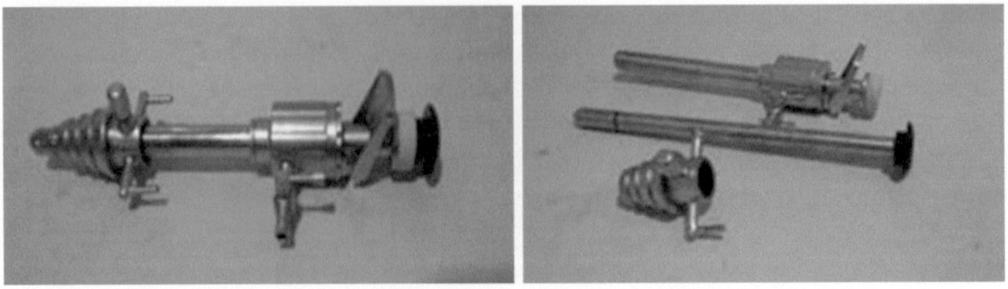

Fig. 2.11 Hasson Cannula: (**a**) assembled (**b**) dismantled

Table 2.3 Laparoscopic grasping instruments

Grasping instruments	Special features/identification	
Laparoscopic Bowel Grasping Forceps 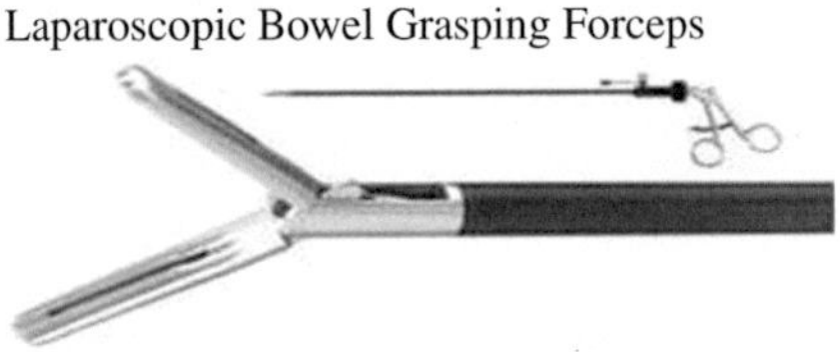	Ratcheted handle, double action fenestrated tissue jaws For grasping and manipulation the bowel	of
Laparoscopic Allis grasping forceps 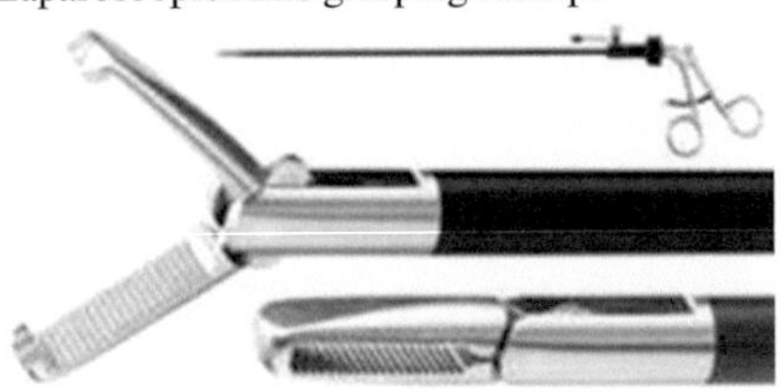	Sharp tip for grasping tough tissue	
Laparoscopic Babcock grasping forceps 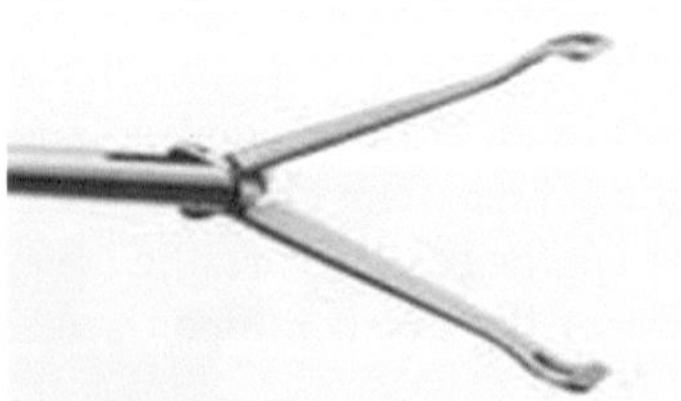	For grasping the bowel/appendix	

Working Instruments

The laparoscopic working instruments are designed for the same purpose as those used in open surgery: tissue holding (Table 2.3), dissection (Tables 2.4 and 2.5), retraction, hemostasis, tissue approximation (Table 2.6), etc. In contrast, they have a thin/slender doubly insulated shaft—that transits the anterior abdominal wall—connecting the tissue (distal) end with the instrument handle which is held and manipulated outside the peritoneal cavity. The tissue ends are adapted for different purposes and for identifying each tool. They may have single or double-action tissue-end jaws, and the shaft length is

Table 2.4 Laparoscopic dissecting instruments

Dissecting instruments	Special features/identification
Laparoscopic hook (electrode) forceps 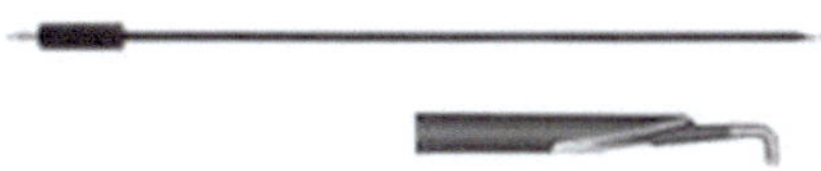	Has curved hook-like tissue end with insulated shaft, non- ratcheted monopolar powered handle For tissue dissection and separation of tissues
Laparoscopic Maryland forceps 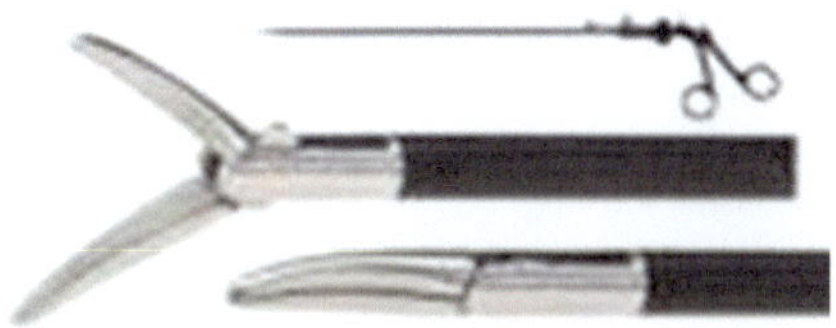	Has curved dual-action serrated jaws Insulated sheath & handle Non-ratchet handle For tissue dissection

Table 2.5 Laparoscopic scissors and biopsy forceps

Laparoscopic scissors	Special features/identification
Laparoscopic straight. Curved or hook scissors 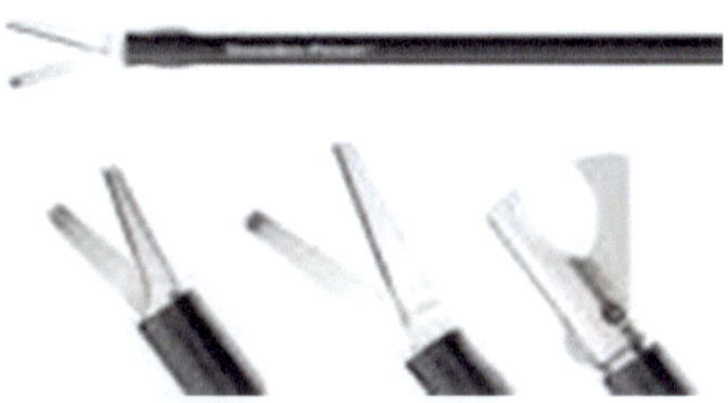	Lightweight dual or single action curved or straight tissue end Has an insulated shaft and non-ratcheted handle For cutting tissues
Laparoscopic biopsy forceps 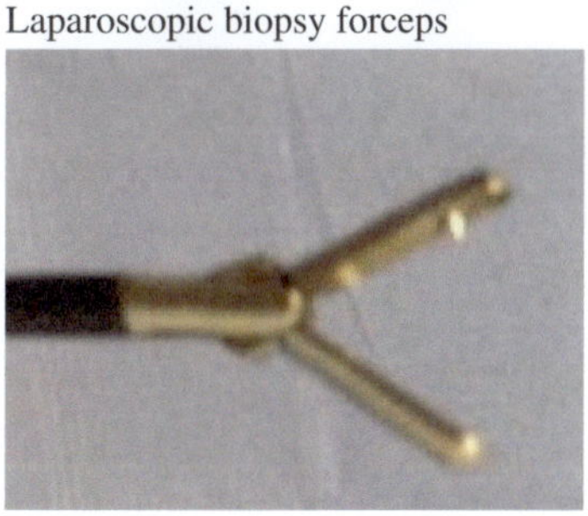	Has oval fenestrated jaws, with a spike for fastening to tissue for biopsy, single-action Non-ratchet handle w/rotation lock, mono-polar port, insulated sheath & handle For tissue biopsy

about 25 cm for pediatric surgery patients; 35 cm for adult patients, or 45 cm for bariatric patients. First-generation laparoscopic instruments lack the luxury of disassembling for cleaning; the second-generation instruments have flush ports but cannot be disassembled, whereas the third-generation can be completely disassembled for proper cleaning. These instruments function as first-class levers where the load and the effort are on opposite sides of the fulcrum with a shorter distance between load and fulcrum, hence improving efficiency. They are designed for either monopolar or bipolar energy use with an appropriate site for attachment of monopolar or bipolar cable.

Table 2.6 Laparoscopic tissue approximation instruments

Laparoscopic tissue approximation tools	Special features/identification
Laparoscopic needle holding forceps 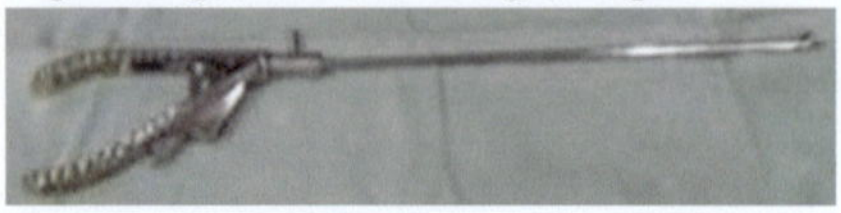	Has stout crisscrossing lines with a groove at the tissue end Has an insulated shaft and ratcheted handle For holding needle
Laparoscopic clip applicator 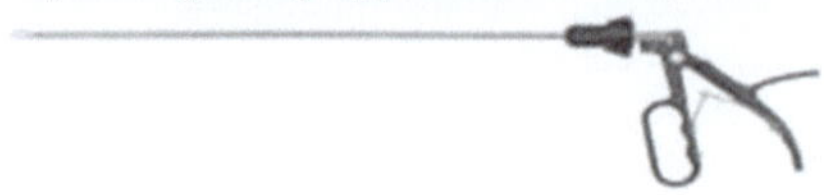	Has curved dual-action stout jaws Non-insulated sheath & handle For holding and applying clips
Laparoscopic staplers 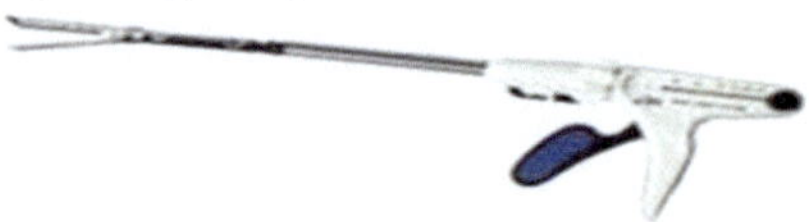	For tissue stapling Varying types

Miscellaneous Tools

These include the instruments listed in Table 2.7 with a brief description of their function.

Morcellator

This is a hand-held instrument used in general surgery, urology, and most commonly in gynecological surgery to slice resected solid tissue mass into "spiral ribbon-like pieces" for easy retrieval. It consists of a powered machine and a hand instrument. This is not advocated for malignant tissue masses resected from the site of operation. It has a high risk of adjacent visceral injury if not properly used hence the need for proper training on its use.

Laparoscopic Insulation Tester

The 9-volt battery insulation tester is a necessary piece of equipment for success in laparoscopic surgery practice. Its function is to determine the insulation integrity of the electrosurgical instrument for repair or otherwise as tiny insulation breaches on hand instruments can lead to electro-surgery injuries.

Table 2.7 Miscellaneous Laparoscopic instruments

Laparoscopic tools	Special features/identification
Laparoscopic knot pusher 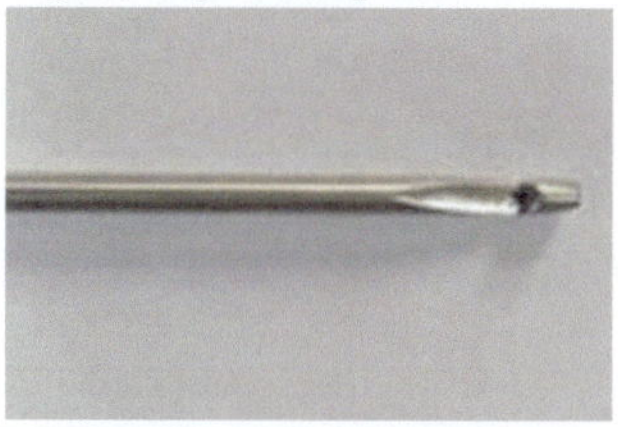	For pushing and tightening of intra-corporeal knot
Laparoscopic Aspiration Needle 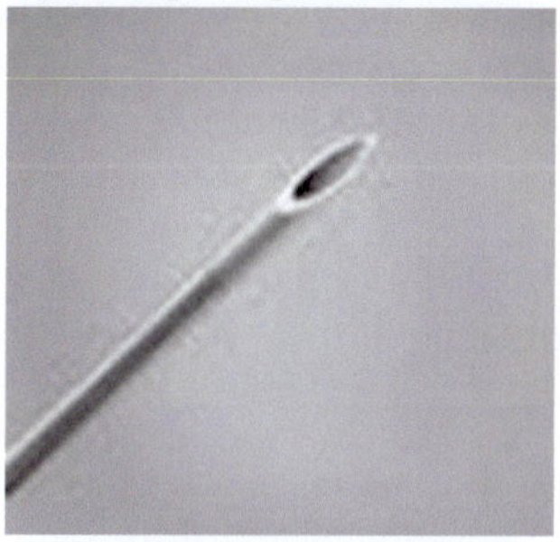	For aspiration of fluid collection
Laparoscopic Needle Introducer 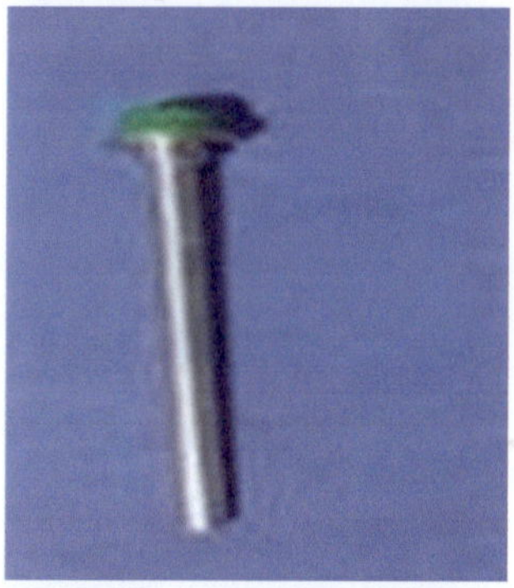	For introducing a needle into the peritoneal cavity
Reducer 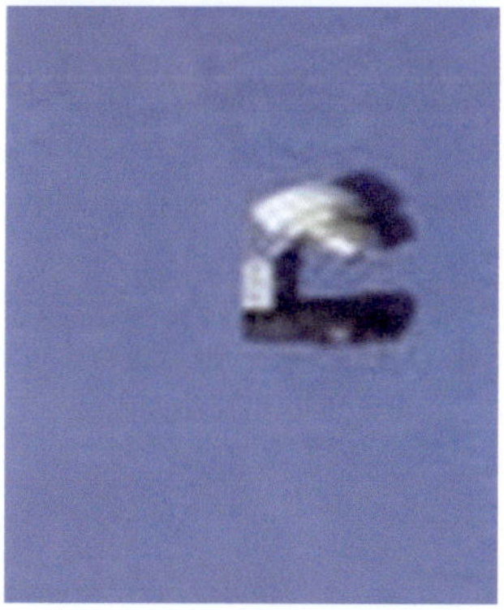	Used to adapt/reduce a large port cannula to a smaller size for the introduction of a small-hand instrument to prevent gas leakage

Recent Advances in Equipment and Instruments

Sensor-Integration to Laparoscopic Instruments Research on sensor-integration of medical tools has been ongoing, and this applies to a wide range of medical instruments [9]. Incorporation of sensors into laparoscopic instruments using 3-axial force sensing during the surgical process has been proposed, to provide force-feedback [10].

3-D Laparoscopic Imaging Systems An upgrade from the conventional 2-dimensional video imaging in traditional laparoscopy to 3-D image provides the much-needed improvement in stereoscopic view, enhancing spatial orientation and depth perception. These advantages translate to reduced task completion time, accuracy, and less surgeon fatigue [11, 12].

Future Prospects in Laparoscopic Equipment and Instruments

The future is expected to be brighter for laparoscopic equipment and instruments following ongoing research and dynamic improvement in technology with the intent to reduce invasiveness, enhance surgical precision and improve patient recovery times.

Smart Surgical Tools The current era of artificial intelligence and augmented reality may impact the future design of laparoscopic equipment and instruments to an advantage.

Hybrid Laparoscopic Procedures The future is likely to be shaped by ongoing research focused on integrating the advantages of robotic tools and surgery (improved imaging and flexible equipment) into laparoscopic instruments and procedures for improvement in general surgery, urological, gastrointestinal, cardiothoracic, and gynecological surgeries [13].

Incorporation of Artificial Intelligence and Robotic Surgical Systems Incorporation of artificial intelligence into robotic surgical systems is estimated to improve surgical perception and navigation, surgical planning, and control strategies [14].

Other Developments Computer-aided diagnostics, 3-D image enhancement and automation of instruments, miniaturized and flexible instruments, tele-mentored robotic surgery, and autonomous surgical robots [15–18].

References

1. Jaffary SA, Shamim MS, Raza SJ, Dastgir A. Instrument failure: a preventable cause of conversion in laparoscopic cholecystectomy. Pak J Surg. 2007;23(2):92–5.
2. Paracchini S, Bustos B, Aviles R, Bourdel N, Canis M, Rabischong B, Slim K, Botchorishvili R. Equipment failures in laparoscopic surgery: causes and consequences. J Visc Surg. 2021;158(6):476–80.
3. Courdier S, Garbin O, Hummel M, Thoma V, Ball E, Favre R, Wattiez A. Equipment failure: causes and consequences in endoscopic gynecologic surgery. J Minim Invasive Gynecol. 2009;16(1):28–33.
4. Soper NJ. Chapter 2: Access to Abdomen. In: Scott-Conner CE, editor. SAGES manual—fundamentals of laparoscopy, thoracoscopy, and endoscopy. 2nd ed; 2006. p. 23.
5. Siu J, Hill AG, MacCormick AD. Systematic review of reusable versus disposable laparoscopic instruments: costs and safety. ANZ J Surg. 2017;87(1–2):28–33.
6. Mishra RK. Textbook of practical laparoscopic surgery. 3rd ed. New Delhi: Jaypee Brothers Medical Publishers (P) Ltd; 2013. p. 3–7.
7. Oak S, Praelkar SV, Agarwal P, editors. Equipment and instrumentations. In: Colour Atlas of paediatric laparoscopic surgery. New Delhi: Jaypee Brothers Medical Publishers Ltd; 2003. p. 5.
8. Metildi CA, Kaushal S, Lee C, Hardamon CR, Snyder CS, Luiken GA, Talamini MA, Hoffman RM, Bouvet M. An LED light source and novel fluorophore combinations improve fluorescence laparoscopic detection of metastatic pancreatic cancer in orthotopic mouse models. J Am Coll Surg. 2012;214(6):997–1007e2.
9. Park J, Seo B, Jeong Y, Park I. A review of recent advancements in sensor-integrated medical tools. Adv Sci. 2024;11(20):2307427.
10. Li Y, Gaozhang W, Hu J, Cao D, Dasgupta P, Liu H. Optical-waveguide based 3-axial tactile sensor for minimally invasive surgical instruments. IEEE Robot Automat Lett. 2024;9(2):1604–11.
11. Arezzo A, Vettoretto N, Francis NK, Bonino MA, Curtis NJ, Amparore D, Arolfo S, Barberio M, Boni L, Brodie R, Bouvy N. The use of 3D laparoscopic imaging systems in surgery: EAES consensus development conference 2018. Surg Endosc. 2019;33:3251–74.
12. Sui C, Wu J, Wang Z, Ma G, Liu YH. A real-time 3D laparoscopic imaging system: design, method, and validation. IEEE Trans Biomed Eng. 2020;67(9):2683–95.
13. Cheema MJ, Hassan MM, Asim A, Nathaniel E, Shafeeq MI, Tayyab MA, Valiyakath CR, Abdallah S, Usman A. Innovations in hybrid laparoscopic surgery: integrating advanced technologies for multidisciplinary cases. Cureus. 2024;16(6):e63219.
14. Liu Y, Wu X, Sang Y, Zhao C, Wang Y, Shi B, Fan Y. Evolution of surgical robot systems enhanced by artificial intelligence: a review. Adv Intell Syst. 2024;6(5):2300268.
15. Subido ED, Pacis DM, Bugtai NT. Recent technological advancements in laparoscopic surgical instruments. In AIP Conference Proceedings 2017; Bali AIP Publishing. 2018; 1933 (1): 0400071–0400077. https://doi.org/10.1063/1.5023977.
16. Arezzo A, Vettoretto N, Francis NK, Bonino MA, Curtis NJ, Amparore D, Arolfo S, Barberio M, Boni L, Brodie R, Bouvy N. The use of 3D laparoscopic imaging systems in surgery: EAES consensus development conference 2018. Surg Endosc. 2019;33:3251–74. https://doi.org/10.1007/s00464-018-06612-x.
17. Mosafer S, Najarian S, Hajizadeh S, Simforoosh N. Design motorized hand-held flexible instrument for Minimally Invasive Surgery (MIS). In: 2009 IEEE symposium on industrial electronics & applications, vol. 2. IEEE; 2009. p. 934–7.
18. Attanasio A, Scaglioni B, De Momi E, Fiorini P, Valdastri P. Autonomy in surgical robotics. Annu Rev Contr Robot Autonom Syst. 2021;4(1):651–79.

Chapter 3
Energy Sources in Laparoscopic Surgery

Emeka Ray-Offor and Mukhtar Ahmad

Introduction

Laparoscopy involves closed-cavity precision surgery with minimal tissue damage and reduced blood loss. Energy sources are invariably needed to aid dissection and hemostasis. The different energy sources include electricity, ultrasound, laser, argon gas, microwaves, or radiofrequency waves; however, the fundamental principle involves tissue necrosis and hemostasis by heating [1]. The unique properties of the energy source, the surgeon's preference, and availability are determinants of choice. For blood vessel sealing, an energy device's effectiveness depends on the size of the blood vessel.

Different devices have proven merits but have the potential for serious complications. Mastery of the surgeon's preferred device is demanded, as optimal patient outcomes depend on the applicator and the appliance. A complete understanding of the equipment, energy source physics, potential complications, and limitations is necessary for safe surgery. Monopolar electrosurgery devices are the most common devices in use [2]. Hence, deserves more emphasis on their use and complications in this chapter while highlighting other newer technologies.

E. Ray-Offor (✉)
College of Health Sciences, University of Port Harcourt, Choba, Rivers State, Nigeria

Minimal Access Surgery Program, University of Port Harcourt Teaching Hospital (UPTH), Port Harcourt, Rivers State, Nigeria

Department of Surgery, UPTH, Port Harcourt, Rivers State, Nigeria

Oak Endoscopy Centre and Radiodiagnostics, Port Harcourt, Rivers State, Nigeria
e-mail: emeka.ray-offor@uniport.edu.ng

M. Ahmad
University Hospitals Dorset NHS Foundation Trust, Poole, UK

E. Ray-Offor, R. J. Rosenthal (eds.), *Principles and Practice of Laparoscopic Surgery*, https://doi.org/10.1007/978-3-031-96321-6_3

Relevant Physics [3, 4]

Current This is the flow rate of charge around a circuit. It is measured in amperes (A). There are two types—alternating or direct (unidirectional) current.

Resistance (Impedance) This is the ability to resist the flow of electric current. A good conductor has low resistance while a poor one has a high resistance. The unit of resistance is ohms (Ω).

Voltage This is the work of moving current from one point to another. This is measured in volts (V)

$$\textit{Ohm's Law}\quad \mathrm{V} = \mathrm{I} \times \mathrm{R}$$

(V-voltage, I-Current, R-Resistance, V-Volt)

$$\textit{Current density} = \left(\mathrm{I} / \mathrm{A}\right)$$

(I = current, A = area).

Concerning current density, smaller-sized active electrodes provide a higher current density resulting in a concentrated heating effect at the tissue contact site. Similarly, a large-sized return electrode during monopolar electrosurgery disperses the current return to the electrosurgical unit and minimizes heat production at this return site.

Electrosurgery

Electrosurgery describes the passage of high-frequency electrical current through the tissue to create a desired clinical tissue effect [2]. This involves alternating current in the range of 500,000 to 2 million Hz (AM radiofrequency) in surgery (Fig. 3.1). Energy conversion from electrical through kinetic to thermal energy is accomplished. Applying this current to the body tissue generates a rapid alternating polarization effect on electrons resulting in heat generation for controlled tissue deformation

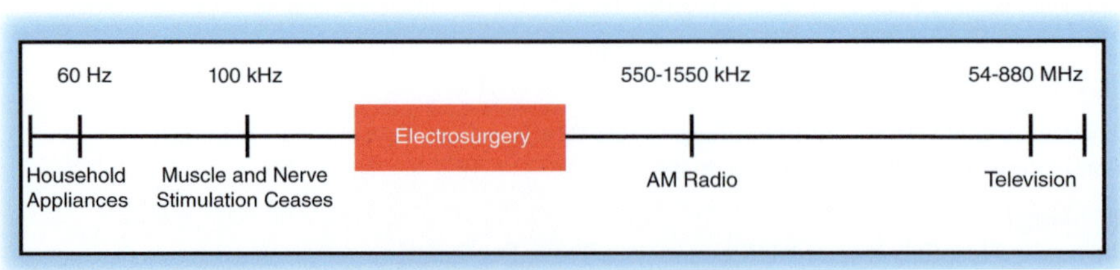

Fig. 3.1 Electromagnetic spectrum

relevant to surgery. The alternating current frequency of 500, 000 Hz does not cause depolarization of the neuromuscular membrane or ventricular defibrillation, unlike household current at 60 Hz. Electrocautery is often interchangeably used for electrosurgery however this is incorrect as electrocautery only involves the direct transfer of heat energy from a metallic object for tissue desiccation or fulguration.

Tissue Effect [2]

Electric current flows through the path of least resistance. In the body, this is directly proportional to the water content of the tissue. Body tissue in descending order of conductance is as follows: blood, nerve, muscle, adipose, and bone. The thermal energy generated raises body temperature. At 60–95 °C there is denaturation of protein and rupture of hydrogen crosslink with tissue **desiccation.** On cooling there is deformation and permanent coaptation of tissue to form a coagulum which achieves **coagulation** leading to haemostasis. At 100 °C there is cell rupture and **vaporization** of water content. This controlled effect has a **cutting** effect on tissue in close approximation to the active electrode. A short activation duration of the active electrode in contact with tissue is recommended as very long activation will produce wider and deeper tissue damage. Meanwhile, an absence of the desired tissue effect is associated with very short activation.

Electrosurgical Unit

An electrosurgical unit is needed, which converts alternating current from the frequency for household appliances to radio frequency. The modern electrosurgical unit (ESU) (Fig. 3.2) has an isolated circuit. The active electrode delivers the current and returns to the ESU through the dispersive electrode.

The ESU can alter the duty cycle. A continuous sine wave current (100% duty cycle) is generated for the **cut mode**, A pulsed higher voltage current that flows in less than 20% of the duty cycle is generated in the **coagulation mode**. In the **blending mode,** a higher frequency sine wave current is generated as for cut mode but in pulsed frequency. This mode leads to the fulguration of tissue. There are two types of circuits in electrosurgery devices-monopolar and bipolar type.

Monopolar Electrosurgery

This is the most used energy source due to its cost, ready availability, and diverse tissue effects [5]. Monopolar devices can be used for blunt dissection, coagulation of vessels, contact coagulation on the surface of tissues, and non-contact fulguration.

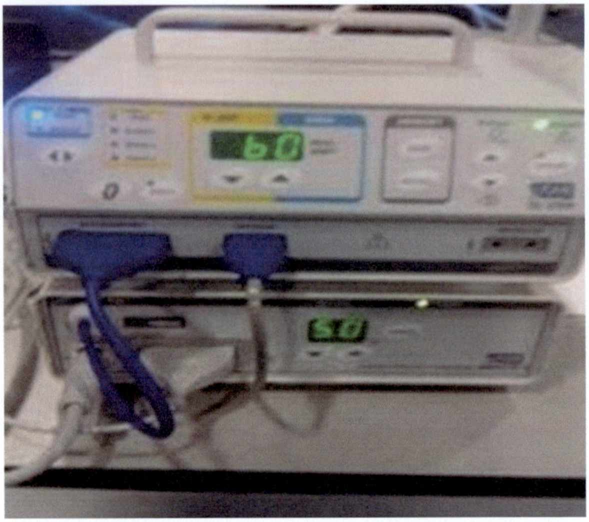

Fig. 3.2 Electrosurgery unit

However, they cannot seal vessels ≥2 mm in diameter; require high power settings; and conduct current through the patient's body. Though specific devices are designed for electrocoagulation, some laparoscopic hand instruments are also designed to be powered via a port on the insulated handle for electrosurgical function.

Mechanism of Electrosurgical Injury [5]

The second most common cause of complications in laparoscopic surgery next to access and trocar placement is thermal injury from electrosurgery (ES). The risk of thermal injury is highest in monopolar ES, and the mechanisms are herein highlighted.

Active Electrode Injury

The active electrode's unintentional activation or direct extension may result in iatrogenic injury. Some useful precautions include activating the unit only when the tip is in view and close to the target tissue; deactivating the unit before the tip leaves the surgical site; placing the active electrode device in a holster when not in use excluding other foot pedal-activated instruments in the same holster. Also, the electrosurgery cable should be disconnected from the active electrode device when not in use, and rubber sleeves for overactive electrodes should be avoided.

Dispersive Electrode Injury

The dispersive electrode returns current to the ESU. A correct and secure application of this plate forestalls current concentration and resultant injury. The contact with the patient must be uniform over a large surface area of skin which is clean, dry, and free of hair. In positioning a dispersive electrode (neutral plate) the following areas should be avoided: bony prominences; metal implants or prosthesis; scar tissue; hairy areas; adjacent to leads/electrodes; pressure areas/points; skin discoloration/injury, limbs with circulatory compromise. Avoid cutting the size of the plate.

Current Diversion

Monopolar ES involves controlled application of current for desired tissue effect. This alternating current may be diverted in several ways from the desired circuit resulting in thermal injury.

Insulation Failure

Laparoscopic hand instruments have a pin connector for cable attachment to ESU on the handle; and a slender insulated shaft to internally conduct current to the working tip when the circuit is activated. Insulation failure may result from scratches on the shaft leading to current diversion on activation of current flow. Depending on the zone involved, thermal injury may not be apparent during surgery (Fig. 3.3). When an injury occurs in Zone I this is easily seen by the surgeon while Zone II injury can also be seen but after careful inspection intraoperatively. Further up, the appearance of demodulated current-induced fasciculations will suggest a Zone 3 injury. The surgeon and other personnel are at risk of injury from Zone 4-related faults.

Direct Coupling

This occurs when one conductive source makes contact or arcs with another (e.g. active electrode tip touches another metal instrument like a hemostat or grasper). Direct coupling is demonstrated in open surgery by touching a hemostat handle with the tip of the activated diathermy pencil to achieve hemostasis on the tissue. An inadvertent arcing of current in a closed cavity laparoscopic surgery may result in bowel injury.

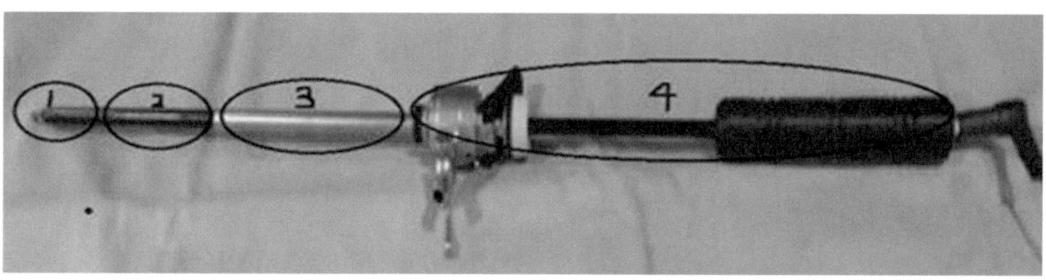

Fig. 3.3 Zones of thermal injury in laparoscopic surgery

Capacitive Coupling

Capacitance is stored in electrical charge when an insulator separates two conductors. In laparoscopic surgery, the cannula and metal instrument when activated can create a capacitive effect. The charge is stored in the capacitor until either the generator is deactivated or the pathway to complete the circuit is achieved. The capacitive coupling current completes the circuit by finding a pathway to a dispersive electrode. The generation of electrical current by capacitance is greatest with high voltage coagulation current and more likely through 5 mm than 11 mm cannula. Also, eschar with the high resistance to current flow, increases the risk of capacitive. An equation for capacitance coupling effect is related to cannula length (L), the radius of cannula (b), the radius of the active electrode (a), and the dielectric constant of insulator (k) is:

$$C = L / 2k\,\text{In}\left(b / a\right)$$

Antenna Coupling

The leads and electrical cables adjacent to activated monopolar cable may result in coupling of current which can migrate to a distant site on the body a long way from the operating field-antenna effect. An example is the arborizing effect of antenna coupling from entangled leads from a blood pressure cuff adjacent to a monopolar cable on the drapes. The latter which is in the view over the patient results in upper arm thermal injury on activation of the ESU.

Tissue Injury-Pedicle Effect

Sequel to current flow and increased current density created by a smaller radius at the pedicle of a structure, a marked tissue effect may result in the pedicle rather than the distal point of contact with an active electrode. This may result in an undesired thermal injury.

Surgeon Burns/Surgical Glove Injuries

The incidence of burn injury to the surgeon from surgical gloves is uncommon in laparoscopic surgery compared to open surgery. Generally, the handles of most laparoscopy hand instruments that have a connecting terminal by design are made of materials with poor conductance ability. Surgical glove injuries result from high voltage from coagulation or blend mode breaking the insulating capacity of a glove. The risk is increased by prolonged application and the effect of saline sweat in reducing glove resistance.

Smoke-Related Injury

The heat with vaporization from monopolar energy can generate bioaerosol of blood fragments. The most obvious adverse effect is interference with laparoscopic visualization. There is the need to intermittently let out the smoke from the inserted ports to improve visualization. Sparking and arcing can generate smoke which comprises toxic vapor and gases e.g. benzene, hydrogen cyanide, and formaldehyde. These chemicals are irritants and may result in methemoglobin and carboxyhemoglobin in laparoscopic surgery. The use of closed-system smoke evacuators mitigates any smoke-related health issues to the surgeon.

Explosion and Fire

Explosions and fire are rare occurrences in the operating room. The use of air as distension media in laparoscopy is not advisable as this supports combustion, unlike carbon dioxide. The risk of explosion is marked with unprepared bowel as hydrogen-air mixtures between 4 and 7%, methane 5–15%, and nitrous oxide which are potentially explosive are present. The use of mannitol for bowel prep promotes the production of methane.

Safety Tips

Electrosurgical Unit

- Inspect for any damage
- No fluids on top of ESU
- Do not use in the presence of flammable material e.g. alcohol, or nitrous oxide.
- Use the lowest power setting possible
- Confirm/communicate power settings before starting and verify any changes during the case
- Use brief activation not prolonged activation.
- Audible activation and indicator alarms needed
- Move the foot pedal out of the way
- Use the tip of the instrument for dissection and try to always keep it in view.

Precautions with Cardiac Rhythm Management Devices (CRMD) [6]

- Position the ES tool and patient return electrode so that the current path is not through or near CRMD

- Avoid proximity of ES field to pulse generator or leads
- Use short, intermittent, and irregular energy bursts at the lowest possible setting
- Use bipolar or ultrasonic energy if feasible
- Have temporary pacing and defibrillation equipment available before, during, and after the procedure
- Continuous ECG and peripheral pulse monitoring regardless of anesthesia type
- Post-operative interrogation and restoration of CRMD function

Argon Beam Coagulator

Argon beam coagulator is an advancement in monopolar electrosurgical technology. The active electrode of this device is not in direct contact with the tissues. Argon, a non-combustible, chemically inert gas is introduced into the body between the active electrode and target tissue. Applying electric current, this gas becomes ionized forming a plasma cloud between the active electrode and tissue with electric arcs formed. The penetration depth is limited to a few millimeters minimizing the risk of perforation [7]. There is quick and efficient coagulation, less tissue damage, reduced charring, and less smoke, and consequently good visibility of the operating area. There is no risk of tissue adhesion in use as the active electrode is not in direct contact with tissue, embolism is a possible complication, especially in liver surgery.

Bipolar Electrosurgery

Conventional Bipolar Systems

Bipolar electrosurgical devices use radiofrequency alternating current which passes from the active electrode to the closely applied dispersive electrode interspaced by target tissue. Heat is generated evenly with the risk of inadvertent leakage or spread lower compared to monopolar devices [8]. However, conventional bipolar devices have no cutting of fulguration effect but achieve coagulation with less lateral thermal spread. The major disadvantages of conventional bipolar instruments include the surgeon-dependent force of compression to tissues and the duration of activation [9]. These may influence the completeness of vessel sealing and lateral thermal damage. The devices require more time coagulating with char formation and sticking electrodes to tissue. Tearing of tissues on separation of the electrode may result in bleeding. The newer generation bipolar devices have remedied these limitations.

Advanced Bipolar Systems with Integrated Impedance and/or Temperature Monitoring

These bipolar devices are designed to overcome some of the perceived deficiencies of conventional bipolar systems. They can seal vessels up to 7 mm with a constant temperature of approximately 100 °C minimizing tissue sticking. Also, a blade within the jaw simultaneously cuts sealed vessels. An example is ENSEAL (Ethicon Endo-Surgery US) which integrates a polymer compound within the jaw and uses positive temperature coefficient (PTC) technology to modulate energy flow. It enables coagulation without cutting when only hemostasis is required (Fig. 3.4).

Another example is the LigaSure™ (Medtronic). This is a vessel-sealing system comprised of an isolated output generator, a connecting cord, a pedal footswitch, and a hand instrument (Fig. 3.5) with a vessel-sealing technology that provides a controlled time to achieve complete and permanent tissue fusion with minimal sticking, charring, or thermal spread to adjacent tissue. The device has smart functions including a vessel sealing re-grasp indicator which alerts the user in situations where a full seal cycle has not been achieved; instant response technology; a memory button to recall prior intensity and power settings used and adjustable activation tone volume. Other advanced bipolar systems include the Plasmakinetic system (Gyrus), Marseal™(KLS Martin Germany), Codman (Integra Germany), and ALAN. Although newer advanced bipolar and ultrasonic energy devices seem appealing and safer than conventional monopolar and bipolar devices, there is insufficient evidence to conclude on superiority of one of these vessel sealing technologies over another [10].

Fig. 3.4 ENSeal tissue sealer

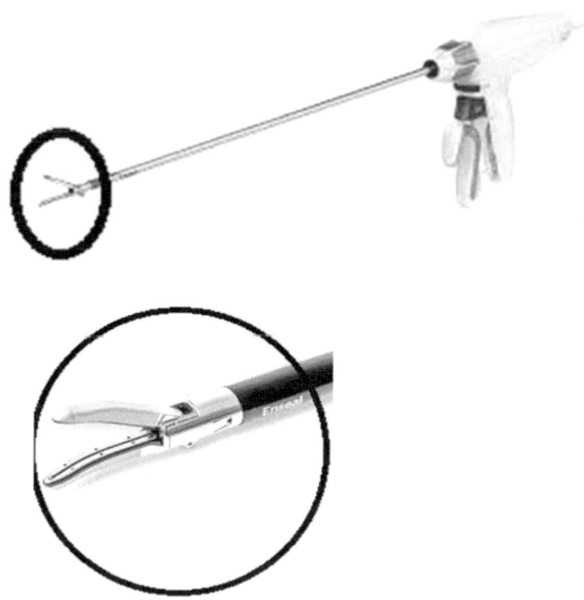

Fig. 3.5 LigaSure Maryland laparoscopic instrument

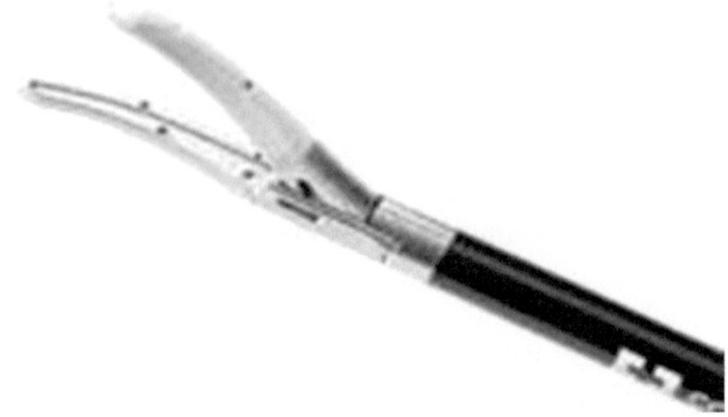

Ultrasonic Energy

Energy systems integrated with the lower frequency of the ultrasonic spectrum of electromagnetic waveforms can facilitate surgery without the risks associated with ES instrumentation. Modern ultrasonic surgical devices are multifunctional instruments capable of performing tissue plane dissection, coaptation, coagulation, and transection during laparoscopic or open surgical procedures. They are marketed as single-use instruments that require a dedicated controller unit for generating and adjusting energy output.

Harmonics® (Ethicon EndoSurgery OH US)

This Harmonic scalpel uses ultrasound technology to denature proteins in vessel walls and tissues up to 5 mm thick leading to coagulation [11]. A harmonic scalpel uses vibrations/mechanical energy converted to heat energy to cut and coagulate. This device comprises a generator unit and a handpiece (shears). The jaws of the shears used to clasp tissue comprise a vibrating rod and a clasping arm (Fig. 3.6). The rod vibrates at 55,500 Hz or 55,500 cycles per second (20,000–60,000 Hz) [11]. This high-frequency vibration of tissue molecules leads to stress and friction in tissue clasped between the jaws of the shears or in direct contact with the tip of the vibrating rod to generate heat and cause protein denaturation. No smoke is created, only atomized droplets which are rapidly absorbed on surfaces. It features improved safety properties as only the tissue in contact with the vibrating shears is cut, unlike electro-surgery and laser appliances. The complications are much less compared to other ES tools. An inadvertent injury occasioned by the wrong positioning of the vibrating shears is a potential problem. To avoid this, the mobile vibrating rod of the activated shears should be positioned away from normal tissues and in the direct view of the surgeon. However, the residual heat of ultrasonic devices is much higher than monopolar devices and the risk of collateral injury is higher.

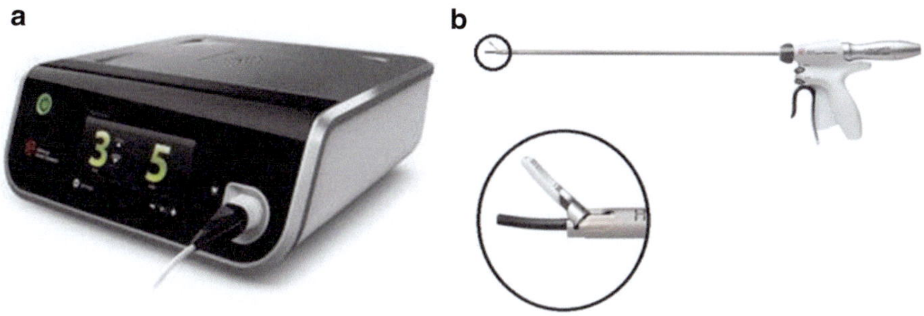

Fig. 3.6 (**a**) Harmonic generator (**b**) Harmonic scalpel

Fig. 3.7 Thunderbeat (Olympus Japan)

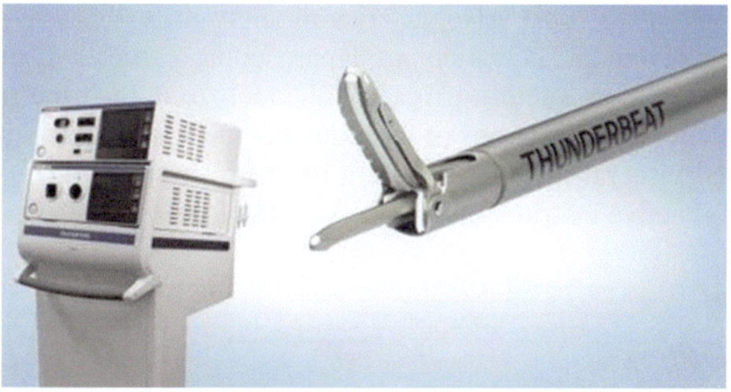

Thunderbeat® (Olympus)

This ultrasonic energy device (Fig. 3.7) combined with bipolar technology is endowed with intelligent tissue monitoring (ITM) which offers precise dissection close to vital structures and minimal thermal spread [11]. This device can convert ultrasonic through mechanical to heat energy like the Harmonic scalpel but has an additional temperature control technology which can reduce complications. The intelligent tissue monitoring works by detecting sudden pressure changes on the probe; transmitting the information to the generator; immediately stopping the energy supply with audible feedback; and commencing the cooling phase. The energy output will automatically be stopped when the tissue transection is complete thereby decreasing the residual probe temperature by 26.9% and reducing the risk of accidental tissue damage [12]. It cuts faster and can seal vessels up to 7 mm. The Thunderbeat also has a standalone bipolar mode that can be used for coagulation without the cutting effect. This makes it a versatile device with easy switching between the 'cut and seal' and 'seal' modes.

Lasers

This acronym means light amplification by the stimulated emission of radiation. Different types of lasers depend on the medium employed: argon laser; neodymium yttrium aluminum garnet (Nd-YAG) laser; carbon-dioxide laser; neon laser; holmium laser; and erbium laser [11]. Laser machines generate a monochromatic coherent beam of light (same wavelength and same phase in time and space). The photon energy of light waves absorbed by the body tissues is converted to kinetic and thermal energy for cutting or coagulation. The laser beam diverges from 10° to 15° as it leaves the delivery catheter, so the power density decreases with the distance from the catheter to the tissue. The effect of the laser beam changes from cutting to coagulation as the delivery catheter is backed away from the tissue. Laser energy may be delivered continuously with the potential for wider tissue surface area affectation. Also, a series of short pulses has the potential for localized tissue involvement. A variety of laparoscopic catheter systems are available and may incorporate suction-irrigation channels to deliver the laser to the surgical site. The major complications of laser devices are the past pointing of the beam and accidental visceral injury. There is a need for protective eye spectacles and avoidance of reflective instruments while using the laser.

Others

Radiofrequency Ablation

Radiofrequency ablation (RFA) works by delivering heat energy (typically 60–100 °C) to laparoscopically targeted specific tissues through percutaneously inserted needles in a catheter [13]. It involves the use of radiofrequency energy to generate thermal energy, which destroys or ablates abnormal or diseased tissues while preserving surrounding healthy structures. This is particularly useful in the selective destruction of lesions such as liver tumors (primary and metastatic), small renal tumors, uterine fibroids, pancreatic tumors, and endometriomas.

Microwave Ablation

Microwave ablation (MWA) uses electromagnetic waves to selectively destroy lesions in a similar way to RFA. Its applications are also like RFA.

Hydro Dissection

Hydrodissection uses a jet of water to separate tissues. An example of its application is separating the gallbladder from its liver bed [14].

References

1. Sankaranarayanan G, Resapu RR, Jones DB, Schwaitzberg S, De S. Common uses and cited complications of energy in surgery. Surg Endosc. 2013;27(9):3056–72.
2. Wu MP, Ou CS, Chen SL, Yen EY, Rowbotham R. Complications and recommended practices for electrosurgery in laparoscopy. Am J Surg. 2000;179(1):67–73.
3. Alkatout I, Schollmeyer T, Hawaldar NA, Sharma N, Mettler L. Principles and safety measures of electrosurgery in laparoscopy. JSLS. 2012;16(1):130–9.
4. Massarweh N, Cosgriff N, Slakey D. Electrosurgery: history, principles, and current and future uses. Am Coll Surg. 2006;202:520–53.
5. Voyles CR, Tucker RD. Education and engineering solutions for potential problems with laparoscopic monopolar electrosurgery. Am J Surg. 1992;164(1):57–62.
6. Zaidan JR, American Society of Anaesthesiologists Task Force. Practice advisory or perioperative management of patients with CRMDs. Anesthesiology. 2005;103:186–98.
7. Nezhat C, Kho KA, Morozov V. Use of neutral argon plasma in the laparoscopic treatment of endometriosis. JSLS. 2009;13(4):479–83.
8. Sutton PA, Awad S, Perkins AC, Lobo DN. Comparison of lateral thermal spread using monopolar and bipolar diathermy, the harmonic scalpel, and the Ligasure. Br J Surg. 2010;97:428–33.
9. Zorzato PC, Ferrari FA, Garzon S, et al. Advanced bipolar vessel sealing devices vs conventional bipolar energy in minimally invasive hysterectomy: a systematic review and meta-analysis. Arch Gynecol Obstet. 2024;309(4):1165–74.
10. Abi Antoun M, Etrusco A, Chiantera V, Laganà AS, Feghali E, Khazzaka A, Stabile G, Della Corte L, Dellino M, Sleiman Z. Outcomes of conventional and advanced energy devices in laparoscopic surgery: a systematic review. Minim Invasive Ther Allied Technol. 2024;33(1):1–12.
11. Jaiswal A, Huang KG. Energy devices in gynecological laparoscopy—archaic to modern era. Gynecol Minim Invasive Ther. 2017;6(4):147–51.
12. Olympus Thunderbeat: double your energy, enhance safety and speed. https://www.olympus.se/company/en/news/press-releases/double-your-energyenhance-safety-and-speed.html. Accessed online 13 Jan 2025.
13. Yu S, Silverberg K, Bhagavath B, Shobeiri SA, Propst A, Eisenstein D. Post-market safety of laparoscopic ultrasound-guided radiofrequency ablation. JSLS. 2020;24(4):e2020.00050.
14. Ananth S, Umemoto KK, Vyas D. Hydrodissection in laparoscopic cholecystectomies for gangrenous gallbladders. Int J Gen Med. 2022;15:7735–8. Published 2022 Oct 10

Chapter 4
Care and Maintenance of Laparoscopy Instruments

Johnson Ogundare

Introduction

The increasing prevalence of minimally invasive surgery underscores the importance of proper care and maintenance of laparoscopic instruments for surgical care facilities. These sophisticated instruments represent a significant financial investment and require adherence to specific handling protocols to ensure longevity and optimal performance. The Joint Commission has advocated that every patient who has chosen minimally invasive surgery (laparoscopy or robotic-assisted surgery) should experience the benefits and not be harmed [1]. Surgical team members must understand the basic care and maintenance of laparoscopic instruments for patient safety and safe surgery outcomes. However, Sterile Processing (SP) professionals play a crucial role in healthcare by ensuring medical and surgical instruments are properly cleaned, decontaminated, sterilized, and distributed [2, 3]. The prevention of infection for all patients undergoing surgical intervention is a primary goal for all team members, especially in today's dynamic healthcare environment (Fig. 4.1). An essential prevention practice for reducing the risk of a surgical site infection is proper reprocessing of surgical instruments. As laparoscopic instruments (Fig. 4.2) vary in size, complexity, fragility, sensitivity to cleaning agents, immersibility, and other properties that affect the choice of cleaning method, the device manufacturer is in part responsible for ensuring that a device can be effectively cleaned and sterilized by providing written reprocessing instructions.

The guideline for disinfection and sterilization in healthcare facilities from the Center for Disease Control and Prevention (CDC) notes that failure to disinfect and sterilize laparoscopic instruments effectively carries not only the risk associated with a breach of host barriers but also the risk for person-to-person transmission as

J. Ogundare (✉)
Society for Nurses in Endoscopy and Minimally Invasive Surgery-Nigeria (SNEMIS-NG), Ibadan, Oyo State, Nigeria
e-mail: Johnson.ogundare@snemis.com

E. Ray-Offor, R. J. Rosenthal (eds.), *Principles and Practice of Laparoscopic Surgery*, https://doi.org/10.1007/978-3-031-96321-6_4

Fig. 4.1 Intraoperative care environment

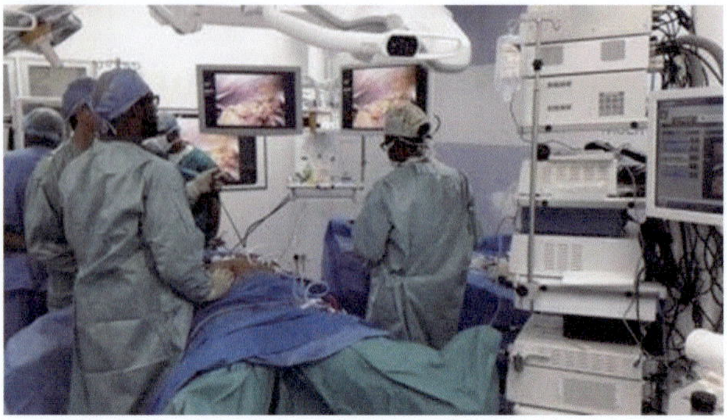

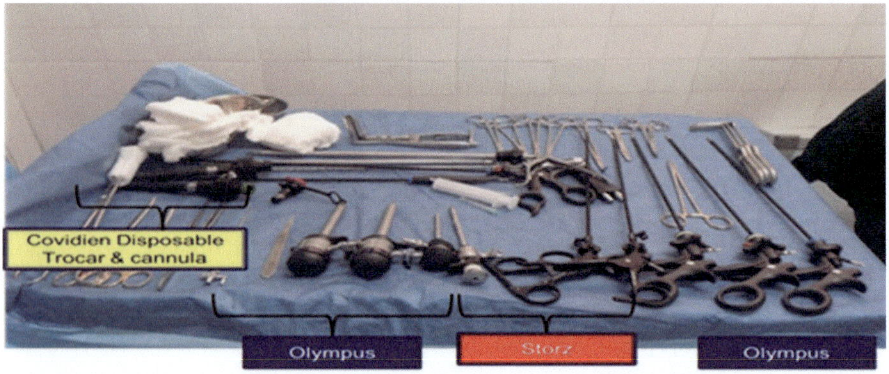

Fig. 4.2 Laparoscopic instruments

well as transmission of environmental pathogens [4]. Furthermore, thorough cleaning is required before disinfection and sterilization because inorganic and organic materials that remain on the surfaces of instruments interfere with the effectiveness of these processes.

The latest Association of periOperative Registered Nurses (AORN) "Guideline for Sterilization" offers critical updates to improve the laparoscopic surgical team approach to selecting sterilization methods, designing sterile processing areas, and transporting sterile items to offsite locations. Additionally, it addresses the sterilization of items produced through additive manufacturing. The guideline further clarifies immediate-use steam sterilization (IUSS) and short-cycle sterilization while emphasizing water quality, monitoring, and planning recommendations. Following these guidelines supports high standards of safety and effectiveness in sterilization processes [5]. Furthermore, the revised guideline recommends that items created through additive manufacturing (such as 3D printing) be sterilized according to the manufacturer's instructions for use (IFU), covering the specific device, packaging, and sterilization equipment. This addition addresses the lack of clear regulations for hospitals producing devices onsite by offering guidance on essential processes and requirements [5]. This chapter reviews the key considerations in the basic care of laparoscopy instruments and the selection and use of detergents/ disinfectants for instrument cleaning. It also outlines the steps of the instrument cleaning process.

Basic Definitions

Instructions for Use (IFU) A step-by-step user's guide on the care and maintenance of equipment as outlined by original equipment manufacturers to ensure the safe use of surgical products.

Laparoscopy A surgical approach with minimal invasiveness.

Guidelines Systematically developed recommendations designed to assist perioperative professionals in the proper handling, cleaning, sterilization, and storage of surgical instruments.

Sterilization A process resulting in the complete elimination or destruction of all microbial life.

High-Level Disinfection (HLD) A physical or chemical process that ensures the destruction of all microorganisms except for high levels of bacterial spores.

Low-Level Disinfection A process that can eliminate/destroy most bacteria, some viruses, and some fungi. It is not effective on resistant organisms like tubercle bacilli or bacteria spores.

Minimum Effective Concentration (MEC) It is the lowest concentration of active ingredient necessary to meet the label claim of a reusable high-level disinfectant.

Biofilm An extracellular matrix on a device in contact with a wet surface that harbors complex micro-organisms.

Spaulding Classification of Medical Devices

This is a system to group the cleaning, disinfection, and sterilization needs for equipment used in the clinical care of patients. Devices are grouped thus:

Critical These are devices that meet intact mucous membranes, sterile tissue, or the vascular system. Most of these are purchased in sterile packs e.g. ligating clips and needles.

Semi-critical These are devices that meet intact mucous membranes, and non-intact skin but do not ordinarily penetrate sterile tissue. They should receive at least high-level disinfection e.g. laparoscopes, trocars, hand instruments, etc.

Non-critical These are devices that do not ordinarily touch patients or touch only intact skin. These may be cleaned by low-level disinfection ('wipe down') e.g. diathermy cables.

Cleaning, Maintenance & Sterilization in Laparoscopic Surgery

The cleaning and/or microbicidal process appropriate for a device depends on several factors, including:

- The device manufacturer's written instructions. Device labeling should identify the specific methods of cleaning and sterilization that have been validated by the manufacturer. This written instruction as provided by the manufacturer includes details like compatibility with specific chemical agents or sterilization methods. These should always be followed.
- The necessary level of microbial kill; for example, a higher assurance of lethality is needed for items that may encounter blood, body tissues, or body fluids than for items that will only meet unbroken skin.
- The design of the device; for example, items that have sharp points or edges capable of puncturing or abrading the skin should be subjected to a decontamination process that includes disinfection or sterilization.
- Other characteristics of the device; for example, whether the device can tolerate high temperatures or whether it is fully immersible and immersion time.

The AORN guidelines for cleaning and care of surgical instruments provide detailed recommendations for cleaning surgical instruments, which include point-of-use treatment, transportation, decontamination, inspection, and routine care of reusable devices like surgical tools. They also address selecting suitable cleaning agents (such as detergents, enzymatic cleaners, and disinfectants), choosing appropriate decontamination equipment, monitoring water quality, and using personal protective equipment (PPE) during instrument care to maintain safety and efficacy [5].

Stages in HLD/Sterilization

From the beginning, all personnel handling contaminated instruments and equipment must wear appropriate personal protective equipment (PPE) and be vaccinated against hepatitis B virus. Personal protective equipment helps shield reprocessing staff from exposure to bloodborne pathogens and other potentially infectious materials. The PPE appropriate for the anticipated exposure must be worn, as splashes, splatters, and skin contact can be reasonably anticipated when handling contaminated instruments (Fig. 4.3). Appropriate PPE for these types of exposures include, but are not limited to:

1. Fluid-resistant gown
2. Heavy-duty gloves
3. Mask
4. Eye protection.

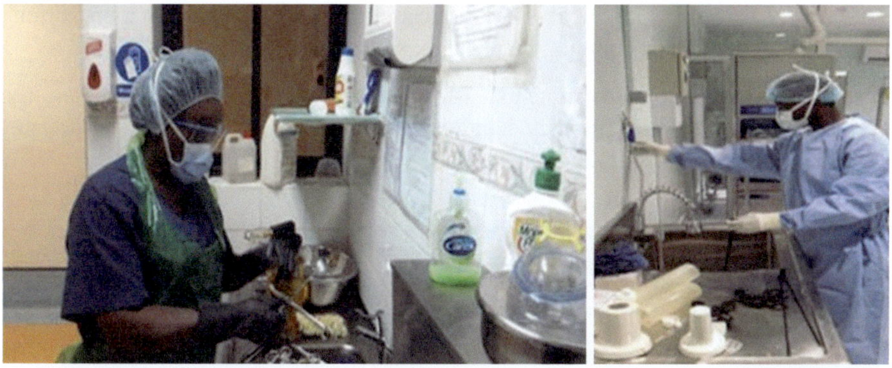

Fig. 4.3 Personal protective equipment (PPE)

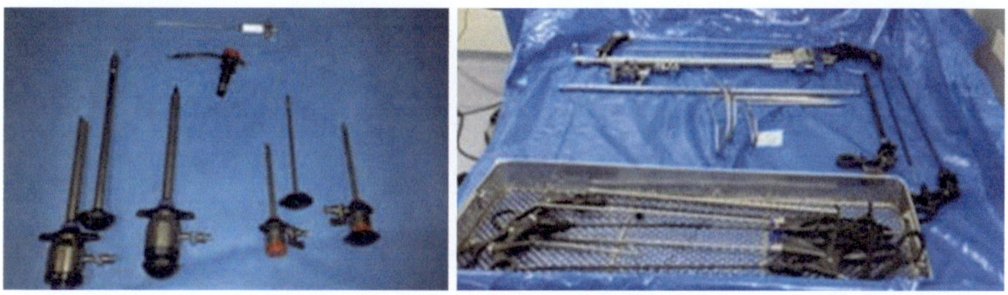

Fig. 4.4 Assembling instruments for reprocessing

To effectively prevent infection from biofilms on laparoscopic instruments, it is crucial to implement a thorough point-of-use cleaning protocol. The scrub personnel should regularly wipe visibly soiled instruments with sterile water, as opposed to normal saline, throughout the procedure. Furthermore, instruments featuring hollow designs should be promptly flushed following laparoscopic procedures before proceeding to decontamination and reprocessing. Consistent wiping and flushing of surgical instruments during both open surgery and laparoscopic procedures is advised to mitigate the risk of surgical site infections (SSIs), particularly those associated with multidrug-resistant organisms (MDROs). This approach is essential for minimizing biofilm accumulation and ensuring patient safety [5].

The various stages in the care of laparoscopy instruments are as follows: assembling and dissembling; precleaning; cleaning and rinsing; drying; sterilization/high-level disinfection and storage.

Assembling and Disassembling

The instruments are carefully assembled (Fig. 4.4), taking care to separate telescopes to avoid damage. Optical cables also need careful handling in a loop without twist.

Trocar and Cannula It is necessary to disassemble port devices into their various parts namely the trocar, cannula, diaphragm, and rubber shod/lids (Fig. 4.5).

Laparoscopic Hand Instruments: Most laparoscopic hand instruments are designed into three parts namely handle, shaft, and insert. The handles are unscrewed, and the inserts are uncoupled to separate hollow shafts (Fig. 4.6).

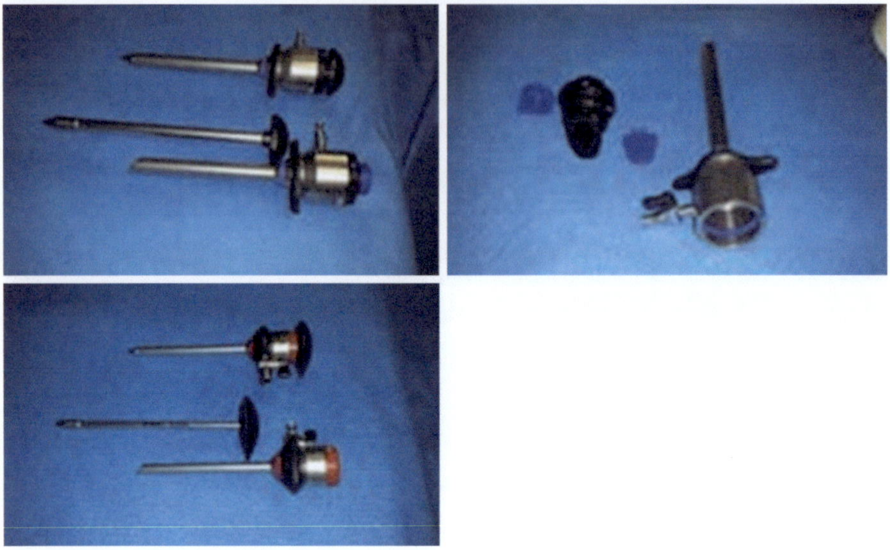

Fig. 4.5 Dissembling of port device

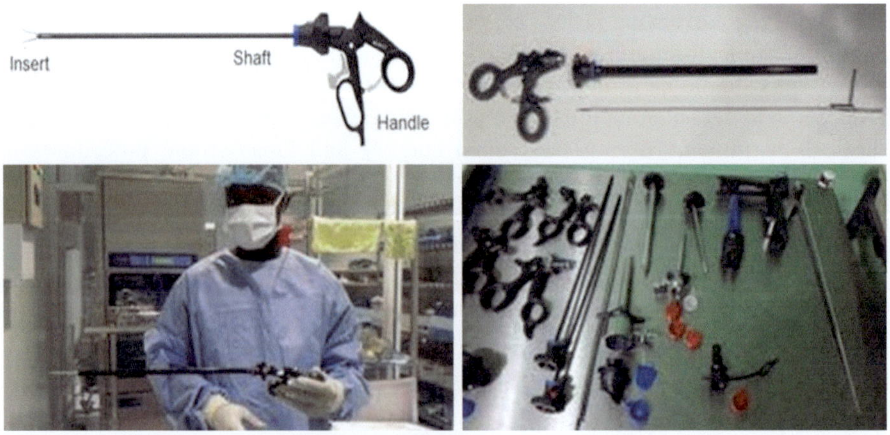

Fig. 4.6 Dissembling laparoscopy hand instrument

Precleaning

Any method of reprocessing is adversely affected by the number, types, and inherent resistance of microorganisms and the amount of bioburden including biofilms, on the items to be reprocessed. Soil and other materials may shield microorganisms from contact with instruments or combine with and inactivate the sterilant or disinfectant. Therefore, precleaning instruments and items to be sterilized lowers the bioburden to the lowest possible level. This is recommended as soon as possible after they are used. A wet gauze or an instrument wipe is used to wipe off blood and gross secretions from dissembled instruments. These are soaked and washed in an enzymatic solution (Fig. 4.7). The enzymatic solutions (detergents) and disinfecting agents available today are specially formulated to meet specific cleaning needs from the most basic cleaning functions to proper high-level disinfection and sterilization. Variable factors include ingredients, chemical composition, foaming properties, chelating ability or performance, and free rinsing ability; thus, detergents are not interchangeable and differ from each other in many ways by the manufacturer. The detergent or disinfectant agent used to clean surgical instruments is a key factor in instrument reprocessing, as well as safe patient care. Because there are various types of detergents available today, all personnel involved in the care and cleaning of surgical instruments must be knowledgeable about these agents and the proper instrument-cleaning process.

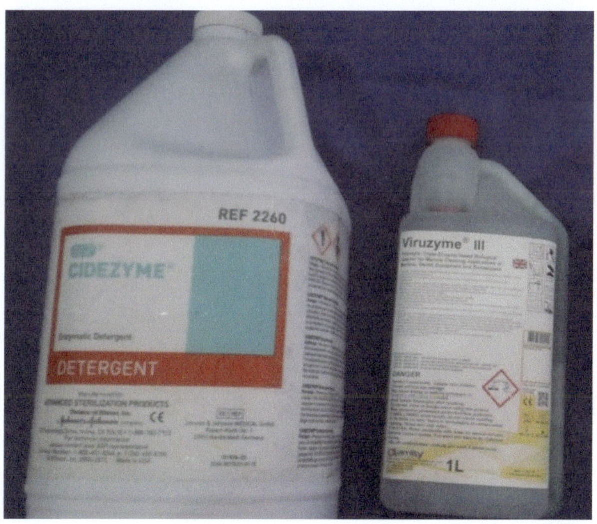

Fig. 4.7 Pre-cleaning agents

Cleaning

Effective sterilization or high-level disinfection can only occur after the items have been thoroughly cleaned. Therefore, a key step in reprocessing reusable medical devices is thorough cleaning with rinsing. Since the cleaning process is not microbicidal, i.e. it primarily removes rather than kills microorganisms, a subsequent disinfection or sterilization process may be necessary to ensure that an item is safe for handling. The cleaning process can be accomplished manually, mechanically, or by combining both methods. Manual brushing of the lumen of the shaft (Fig. 4.8) and insert (jaws), particularly the inner surface is done under a running tap water or with a high pressurized instruments -cleaning gun (if available). A careful rinse in water and drying is crucial before the next stage of instrument reprocessing. An automated washer (Fig. 4.9) can be used but requires visual inspection before autoclaving. Likewise, an ultrasonic cleaning machine mechanically cleans instruments.

- Check the insert for bent or misaligned business tips (Fig. 4.10) to prevent the instrument from dislodging into the patient, which may lead to the issue of retained foreign bodies) [6].
- Lubricate the connector between the handle and the shaft to maintain unlimited rotation.

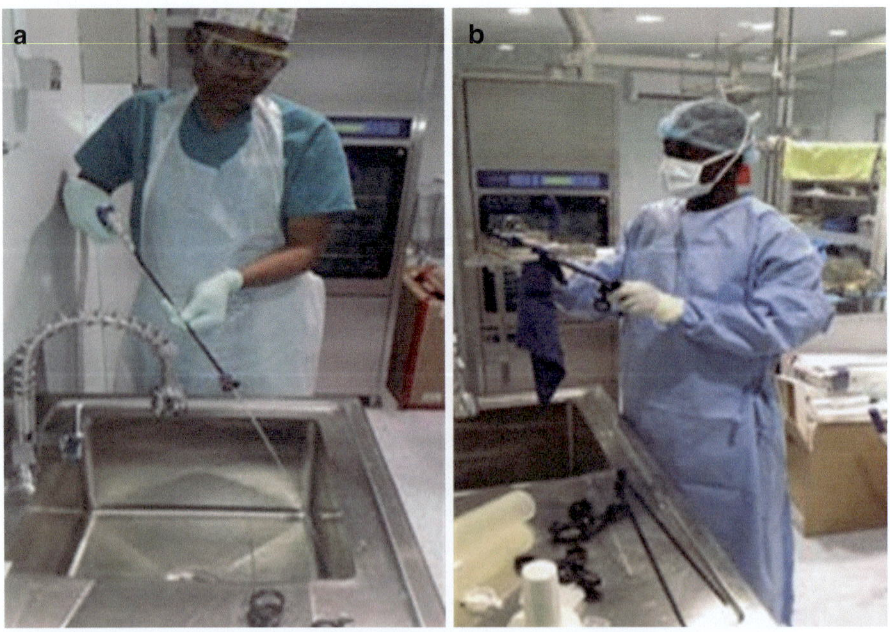

Fig. 4.8 (**a**, **b**) Cleaning laparoscopy hand instruments

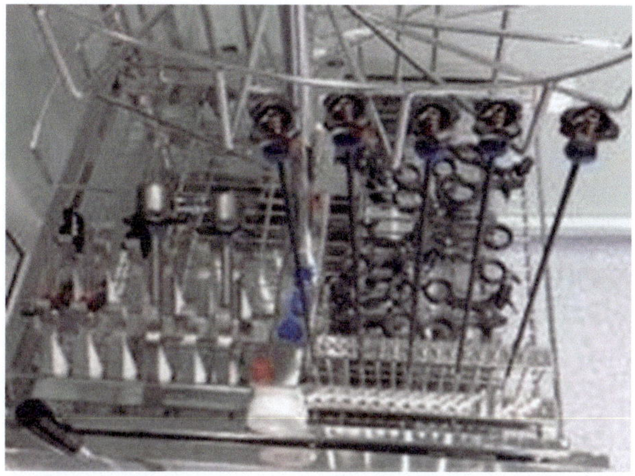

Fig. 4.9 Loading cart for automated washer

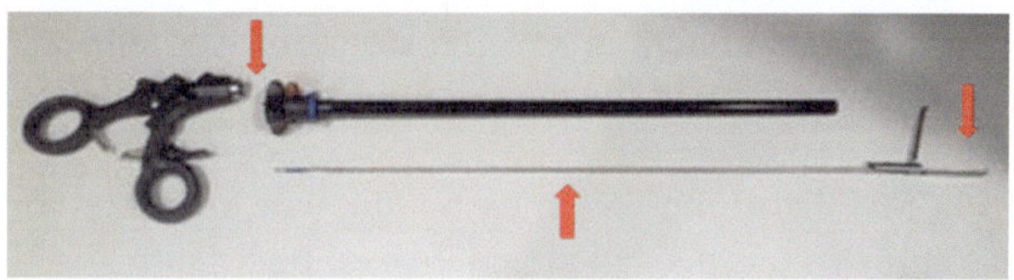

Fig. 4.10 Quality check for working instruments

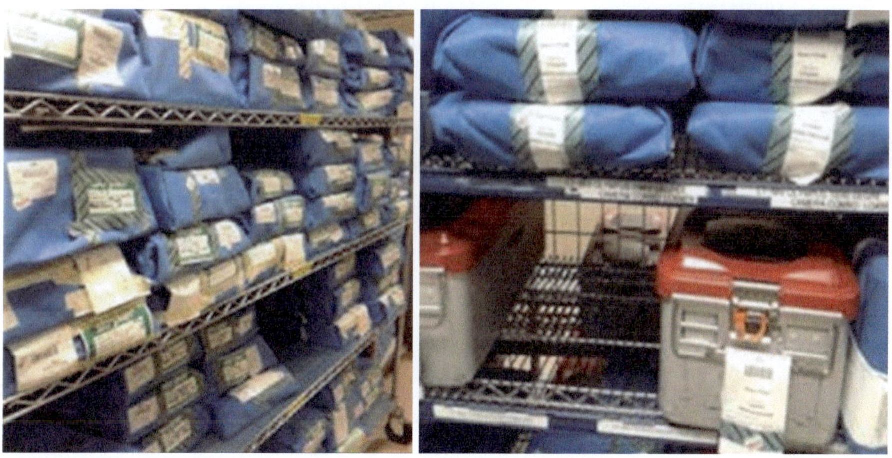

Fig. 4.11 Storage room

High-Level Disinfection/Sterilization

Laparoscopy instruments and endoscopes can be processed with chemicals for high-level disinfection (HLD). The common chemicals for HLD or immediate-use sterilization include orthophthalaldehyde OPA (Fig. 4.11) or glutaraldehyde.

Glutaraldehyde has long been in use in a 2% concentration. The personnel who perform high-level disinfection should follow the manufacturer's instructions for use and precautions to help ensure patients and personnel are not exposed to the chemicals in the high-level disinfectant solution. A process should be in place to ensure rinsing and drying of items [7]. In addition, after disinfection, items should be inspected for damage or contamination.

Sterilization

There are varying methods of sterilization with proven efficacy.

Steam Sterilization (Autoclaving) This is the best option for reusable laparoscopy hand instruments and autoclavable telescopes. The main properties of autoclaving are heat temperatures up to 137 °C, high humidity, and high pressures about 300 kPa. It is crucial to check instruments for autoclavability from instructions for use before selecting the temperature for steam sterilization.

Gas Sterilization This may be ethylene oxide or formaldehyde sterilization. An aeration time is needed after sterilization.

Plasma Sterilization (STERRAD®) It utilizes hydrogen peroxide at a high frequency to create plasma. There is no water, steam, wastewater, or exhaust gas while using STERRAD devices.

Peracetic Acid-Based Sterilization (STERIS) This also offers plasma sterilization. It is crucial to always pre-check your device compatibility for this sterilization method. Any device not labeled as applicable by the manufacturer should not be processed using STERIS.

Storage

A Central Surgical Services Department CSSD is recommended for sterile packaged endoscopes and laparoscopy instruments equipped with a clean and proper storage environment, temperature (18–25 °C); relative humidity not greater than 70%, and at least 4 air exchanges per hour. These conditions prevent cross-contamination or damage during storage. It is important to shelve all the sterile instruments applying "FIFO" (First-In –First-Out) since contamination of sterile equipment/instruments is event-related.

Care of Camera Head, Light Guide Cable, and Telescopes

Handling and Care of Camera Heads

Many camera heads available in the market are either autoclavable or non-autoclavable medical products (Fig. 4.12). It is advisable to read the manufacturer's instructions for use about the appropriate care method of care before, during, and after use [8]. For example, Olympus camera heads products with golden tape or plates are autoclavable.

It is very important to note that camera heads **SHOULD NOT** be soaked in any solution in the name of cleaning, as this act has been responsible for several camera heads' damage. The gold standard is to "**SLEEVE**" and not "**Soak**" in water. Different types of sterile pre-packed camera sleeves (covers) are used during laparoscopic procedures for this safety purpose.

Handling of Light Guide Cable

Most light guide cables are made up of fiber-optic glass bundles hence delicate and easy to mishandle if appropriate precautions are not taken. See (Fig. 4.13a–c). It is important to hold circularly.

Handling and Cleaning of Telescopes (Laparoscopes)

Endoscopes are very expensive and delicate instruments so are not the same in terms of methods of cleaning and autoclaving. To reduce the risk of the endoscope being dropped, considering the detergent property of most cleaning agents which makes cleaning solution slippery, it is imperative to always hold the laparoscope

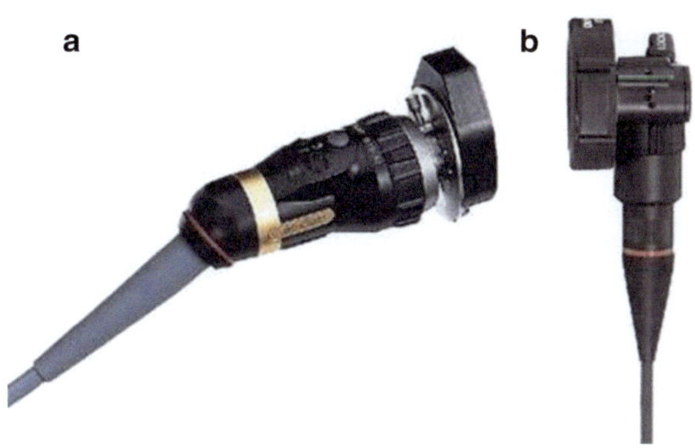

Fig. 4.12 Autoclavable and Non-autoclavable Camera Heads (**a**) Autoclavable (**b**) Non-autoclavable

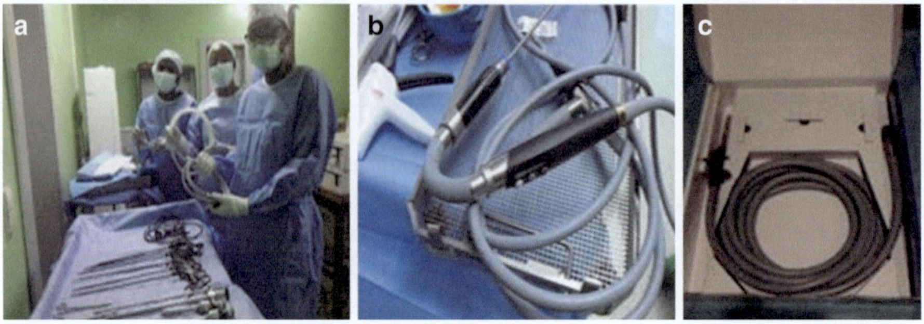

Fig. 4.13 (**a–c**) Care of Light guide cable (**a**) Fold in a circular manner (**b**) DO NOT KINK! (**c**) diameter > 15 cm

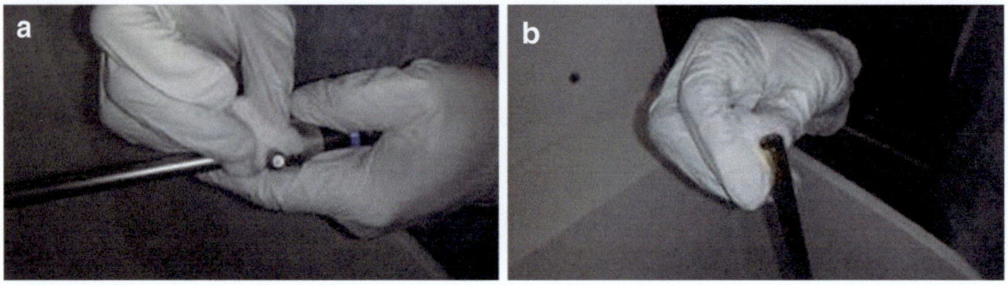

Fig. 4.14 (**a**) Ocular Lens in the palm (**b**) Objective lens

with the ocular lens facing the palmar surface and not by grasping the shaft of the endoscope (Fig. 4.14). Check the objective, ocular lens, and light funnel for damage.

Pre-cleaning the Endoscope

Immediately after the patient's procedure, use an enzymatic detergent solution to initialize the cleaning process and complete the following steps:

1. If using an automated washer, place the laparoscope in a stainless-steel instrument basket and run the cleaning cycle according to instructions. If not, manually clean the rigid scope (laparoscope) by paying more attention to the ocular lens, light funnel, and objective lens; wipe the surfaces with a lint-free gauze dampened with enzymatic detergent or use an enzymatic detergent sponge. Always check the manufacturer's instructions before applying any enzymatic pre-treatment spray to the endoscopes. Also, using saline solutions can harm endoscopes by damaging the metal and glue cement that holds the lenses in place.

2. Safely transport the endoscope with a lid or a transport bag to keep it moist during transport.
3. Ensure no instruments or equipment are lying on top of the telescope on transit to CSSD
4. Terminal reprocessing takes place in CSSD.

Inspection for Damage and Visual Quality

There is the need to ascertain that the image is clear and sharp, without any distortion, discoloration, or haziness observed, this may have occurred due to a broken optical lens or misaligned optics. Furthermore, improper cleaning, rinsing, and moisture within the endoscope may distort image clarity and sharpness.

Packaging for Sterilization

Not all telescopes are autoclavable. Autoclaving can wash off the glue cement at the distal tip and light guide connector. Any tiny weakness of laser welded or cemented connections will cause water leakage into the system during autoclaving; humidity/water will flood the telescope system. As an example, Olympus gold tapped-tip telescopes are autoclavable (Fig. 4.15).

The packaging protocols and style may vary from one hospital facility to another depending on the availability and cost of the recommended autoclavable (sterilization) materials. Wrap in cloth or paper or sterilizing foil or use a sterilization container. Rigid endoscopes may be wrapped separately or containerized with other instruments according to the facility's infection control policy or manufacturer's instructions for use (Fig. 4.16). Endoscopes added to a tray with other instruments should be protected so no other instrument can rest on the endoscope. Always consult the manufacturer's instructions for the best packaging options.

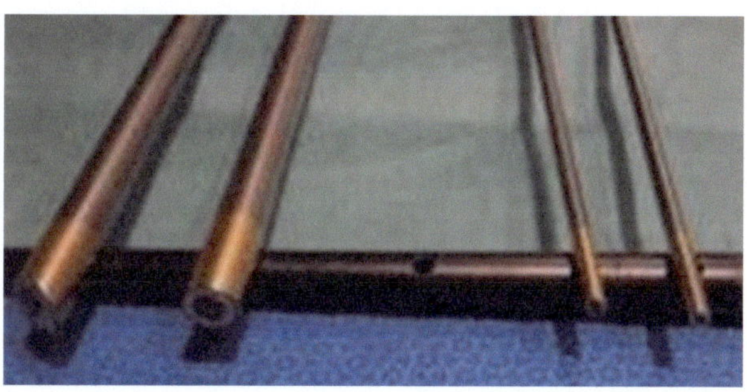

Fig. 4.15 Autoclavable Telescope, 0 and 30 degrees

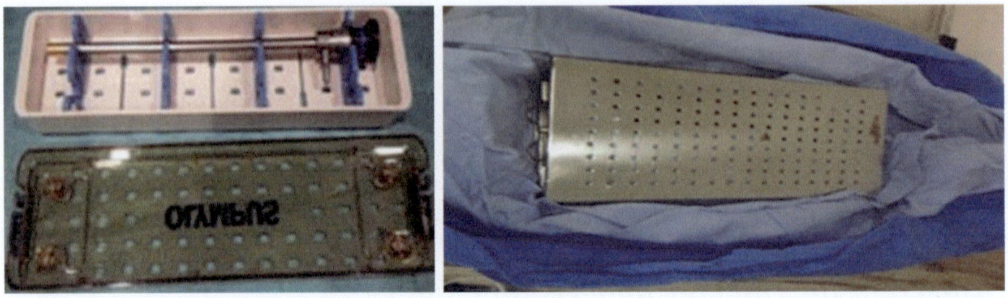

Fig. 4.16 Endoscope sterilizing containers

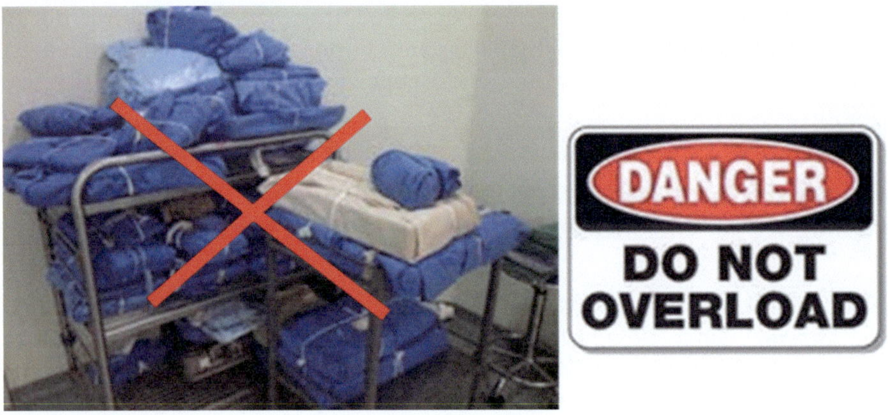

Fig. 4.17 Transportation of Instruments and endoscopes

Transport and Sterilization

It is imperative to prevent equipment damage from preventable situations such as falls associated with the high cost of repair/replacement. Thus, it is highly recommended not to overload the CSSD instruments' cart or trolley for the safety of both the equipment and CSSD personnel (Fig. 4.17). Already packaged instruments should be transported safely from the reprocessing room to the appropriate sterilization unit (CSSD). It is important to follow sterile reprocessing departmental or the AORN- and AAMI-recommended policy and procedures on surgical instruments safety and sterilization.

Instructions for Use (IFU)

Proper maintenance of endoscopic instruments requires careful handling and should follow the guidelines provided by the manufacturer [6]. Surgical staff should be encouraged to speak up when recommended guidelines and IFU are not being followed [9]. The FDA's guidance for manufacturers is a key document that outlines recommendations for formulating and validating reprocessing instructions for reusable medical devices. It also addresses the content and review of various premarket submissions, including 510(k), PMA, HDE, de novo, and IDE applications related to these instructions. The document underscores the critical responsibility of manufacturers to ensure these instructions allow for the safe use of the devices as intended. The surgical team and sterile processing staff are integral to the proper care and maintenance of both reusable and single-use laparoscopic instruments. Their role in following the manufacturer's instructions for use is crucial, as it ensures the devices are maintained in optimal condition.

References

1. The Joint Commission. Potential risks of robotic surgery. 2021. https://www.jointcommission.org/resources/news-andmultimedia/newsletters/newsletters/quick-safety/quick-safety-issue-3-potential-risks-of-robotic-surgery/potential-risks-of-robotic-surgery/. Accessed 11 Nov 2024.
2. Association for the Advancement of Medical Instrumentation [AAMI]. Comprehensive guide to steam sterilization and sterility assurance in health care facilities. AAMI; 2017.
3. Healthcare Sterile Processing Association [HSPA]. Homepage. Healthcare Sterile Processing Association website; 2020. https://myhspa.org/ Accessed 11th Nov 2024
4. Centers for Disease Control and Prevention [CDC]. (2020). Guidelines for disinfection and sterilization in healthcare facilities.
5. Association of periOperative Registered Nurses [AORN]. Guidelines for perioperative practice. AORN; 2023.
6. Lata K, Panwar A, Kriplani I, Kriplani A. Intraoperative dislodgment and retrieval of broken parts of laparoscopic instruments: arduous exercise and lessons gleaned. J Obstet Gynaecol India. 2021;71(2):201–4. https://doi.org/10.1007/s13224-020-01379-5.7.
7. Link T. Guidelines in practice: instrument cleaning. AORN J. 2021;114(3):241–51. https://doi.org/10.1002/aorn.13495.
8. Gomez T, Yanai J. Instrument care and maintenance for optimal performance. J Clin Steriliz Healthc. 2020.
9. Association of periOperative Registered Nurses [AORN]. Using equipment according to the manufacturer's instructions for use. AORN J. 2024;120(5):307–9. https://doi.org/10.1002/aorn.14243.

Chapter 5
Ergonomics in Laparoscopic Surgery

Patrick O. Igwe

Introduction

The term *ergonomics* is derived from the Greek words "ergon" meaning work, and "nomos" meaning natural law. It is the application of knowledge from human sciences to match jobs, systems, products, and environments to people's physical and mental capabilities to promote safety, health, and well-being while performing tasks effectively [1, 2]. As new technology and products arise, ergonomics has become increasingly important in the healthcare industry. Ergonomic guidelines should be exploited to enhance the man-machine interface and work efficiency to reduce the risk of injury and ensure employees' health. The use of the term in laparoscopy can be redefined. A laparoscopic surgeon uses tools to carry out surgical procedures. How well or awkwardly this is done with these tools has a substantial impact on the length of the procedure and the overall outcome. The "relationship" between laparoscopic surgeon and their use of tools also determines how much effort is expended by the surgeon. Ergonomic principles should be applied in the operating room (OR) to make the best possible use of the surgical instruments [1–4].

In laparoscopic surgery, the senses of vision, touch, and position are working under normal conditions and with a large performance reserve so that standard surgical instruments, although not perfect, serve us well. The surgeon has an indirect binocular view of the operative field on a two-dimensional video monitor with poor depth perception and can only touch the intra-abdominal tissues with long instruments through ports fixed in positions. Thus, the visual axis is decoupli from the

P. O. Igwe (✉)
Faculty of Clinical Sciences, University of Port Harcourt, Port Harcourt, Rivers State, Nigeria

Colorectal/Minimal Access Surgery Unit, Department of Surgery, University of Port Harcourt Teaching Hospital (UPTH), Port Harcourt, Rivers State, Nigeria

E. Ray-Offor, R. J. Rosenthal (eds.), *Principles and Practice of Laparoscopic Surgery*, https://doi.org/10.1007/978-3-031-96321-6_5

motor axis [5, 6]. The surgeon's senses work much harder to achieve the same goals compared to those for open surgeries. The proper design of the instruments and the operating room layout become precarious to avoid exhaustion and human blunders. Hence, the interface between man and machine to improve performance denotes the definition of ergonomics. [7, 8].

Ergonomic Adjustments for Safe Laparoscopic Surgery Outcome

The objective of proper posture is comfort, efficiency of movement, and reduction of the risk of musculoskeletal injuries to the surgeon. The surgeon's neck and back should be kept in a comfortable and upright position facing the monitor. Back posture tends to be straighter in laparoscopic surgery and over 15% of surgeons still report recurrent back pain and stiffness following laparoscopic operations. Although these symptoms may be due to the adoption of a more static posture, they arise from increased concentration and the frequent need to look in one direction at the monitor while handling instruments or foot pedals in another direction [9, 10]. Ergonomic assessment of the tasks of Endosurgery helps in the design of instruments and in decreasing the mismatch of human capabilities and technology. It requires the study of constraints of working between narrowed fixed ports and understanding of how processes of gripping and dividing tissues are determined by its mechanical property [11]. During laparoscopic surgery, the ability to achieve this ideal posture is determined by adequately answering the following questions:

- What is the height of the operating room table?
- Is the position of the visual display (e.g., monitor) adequate?
- Are foot pedal positions comfortable?
- What are the selected hand instruments?
- Are the ports properly placed?
- What is the Surgeon and team position?

Height of Operating Table

A proper adjustment of the height of the operating table is very important in laparoscopic surgery. Ideally, the angle between the lower and upper arm should be between 90° and 120° when performing manual work. The operating table should be raised or lowered in such a position that the surgeon will be able to work within this ideal "window." In setting the position of the table for laparoscopic procedures, the table height should be adjusted so that laparoscopic instrument handles (after the instruments have been inserted into the ports) are roughly at, or slightly below, the level of the surgeon's elbows (between 90° and 120°). Mathematically, [12–14]

$$\text{Height of table} = 0.49 \times \text{height of Surgeon in cm.}$$

Laparoscopic instruments are much longer than their open counterparts, so lowering the table substantially may be difficult in some cases, and one may need to stand on one or more lifts to achieve the proper table height.

Foot Pedals

These are frequently used during laparoscopic surgery to activate instruments such as the diathermy, ultrasonic shears, bipolar devices, or other similar tissue instruments. Foot pedals, often wrongly positioned, demand difficult and unnatural postures and should be avoided [12–14]. Ideally, foot pedals should be placed near the foot and aligned in the same direction as the instruments, toward the area or region of the procedure and the principal laparoscopic monitor. Such positioning will permit the surgeon to activate the pedal without twisting any part of the body, especially the leg. If the surgeon is standing on a lifting stage, the pedal must be placed at the same level off the ground. A foot pedal with an integrated footrest is preferable, so the surgeon does not have to hold the foot in the air or move it back and forth on the floor. If there are two pedals (for different devices), the surgeon must be careful not to confuse them while working in a dark environment [12–14].

Positioning of Video Monitor

The positioning of the monitor should be vertical because the surgeon views the surgical field through this visual display for lengthy periods during laparoscopic surgery. This position of the monitor will affect neck and back posture during surgical procedures. The display monitor should be placed directly in front of the surgeon, 15°–40 °C below eye level for maximum comfort in co-axial alignment. This means the surgeon, the target point, and the monitor are in a straight line. A separate monitor is recommended for the assistant to reduce neck strain. For optimal picture quality, it is recommended that video monitors should be at five times the diagonal length of the monitor. Video display devices mounted on flexible booms permit the surgeon to alter the vertical position of the monitor to obtain the ideal angle between eye level and the monitor [13, 14].

Laparoscopic Hand Instruments

The instruments for laparoscopic surgery are lengthy because they must reach inside the inflated but closed abdomen. Unlike open surgery, the surgeon works distantly from the target organ. The instruments are passed through narrow ports that are in fixed positions. Given these restrictions, it is not surprising that these instruments are more awkward and difficult to use than open instruments. Various attributes of the laparoscopic instruments account for their handling characteristics, including decreased mechanical efficiency, increased length, movement about a fulcrum on the body wall that is the port, and the design of the handle. In general terms, the surgeon needs to squeeze more, bend the wrists too, and hold their arms higher when using laparoscopic instruments compared to open instruments. These factors, together, can produce substantial hand and shoulder weariness and discomfort during laparoscopic surgery [11–14].

There is no single laparoscopic instrument design that is substantially superior to others, therefore, each surgeon needs to choose the design(s) that best achieves the following desired objectives:

(i) Allow the laparoscopic surgeon to keep both wrists in a neutral position.
(ii) Allow the laparoscopic surgeon to keep both arms at the sides of their body.
(iii) Evade pressure points on the hands and legs.
(iv) Permits fine manipulation with a precision grip.

When continuous grasping force to tissues is needed, seek an instrument incorporating a locking or ratchet mechanism to maintain the force. "Palming" an instrument (removing the thumb from the ring and placing the palm against the handle) can reduce the amount of wrist flexion and increase the surgeon's power when grasping tissues for a longer period or when an especially forceful grip is required. When even larger forces must be applied to tissue, such as during stapling, seek instruments that provide a power grip handle with large smooth, and better contact surfaces [11–14].

Many laparoscopic instruments are designed with a pistol grip-type handle or an axial (in-line) handle. The pistol grip allows the hand to remain at an angle to the instrument shaft and can lessen the ulnar deviation and movement needed to use the axial handles. Nevertheless, the axial handles allow the use of a fine grasp and rotation of the instrument in the hand which can be useful in fine manipulation and suturing. The most important or unique features to look for in laparoscopic instruments are these:

(a) Instrument handles that are smooth and broad surfaced to avoid pressure points and finger entrapment.
(b) an internal mechanism that is smooth, precise, and allows good tactile feedback from the tip of the instrument to the handle.
(c) Easy and intuitive access for the fingers to any additional controls that govern shaft rotation, jaw locking, or electrocautery or suction activation.
(d) Sturdy insulation of the instrument shaft to the base of the jaws to avoid stray electrocautery injury during use.
(e) An electrosurgery unit connector pin that keeps the electrosurgery unit out of the way of the surgeon's hand when using the instrument.
(f) Instruments that require substantial force to use (staplers, clip appliers, heavy graspers) should have a broad and smooth pistol-type hand that permits the surgeon to use a power-grasp hand position [13, 14].

Ergonomic Adjustments for Safe Laparoscopic Surgery Outcome

Good surgical technique for performing laparoscopic surgery requires the proper placement of the access ports and the efficient and safe use of the instruments to accomplish tissue dissection, division, sealing, and approximation. The siting of the access ports is paramount because they determine the reach, and the working angle of the instruments passed through them. A manipulation angle range of 45°–75° in the horizontal plane, the acceptable range of angles between the instruments inserted through the different ports, or with equal azimuth angles (the elevation angles range in the vertical plane) is recommended. Ideally, the surgeon maintains similar elevation angles for each instrument that the surgeon holds. The manipulation angle (MA) is the angle between two working instruments, and the Azimuth angle (AA) is the angle between the telescope and a working instrument [14]. The elevation angle (EA) is the angle between the body of the patient and a working instrument. In contralateral port positioning, MA should be 60°, AA should be 30° and EA should be 30°. Instruments should be inserted so that at least half of the instrument is inside the patient. This will give the type one lever. If the instrument is utilized while inserted less than half of its length, excessive motion at the shoulder will be required, which is likely to result in surgeon. This gives the wrong lever type [14].

There is no report in the literature to strongly support the use of one type of laparoscopic instrument handle design over another. Laparoscopic suturing is generally best performed with axial/in-line instruments because they allow the surgeon to finely grasp the needle holder and facilitate rotation of the instrument with simple wrist motions. Laparoscopic needle drivers and forceps should integrate a locking mechanism to hold the needle, thus removing the need for the surgeon's constant application of force. Several excellent reviews of the suturing technique have been reported. Furthermore, ergonomic principles should always be adopted when choosing instruments and port locations. Triangulation and the baseball-diamond concept (Fig. 5.1) play a major role in reducing the clashing of instruments and an optimal surgical technique [14].

Surgeon and Team Position

Surgeon and team positions differ with surgery and preference. For example, American laparoscopic surgeons are comfortable performing laparoscopic cholecystectomy positioned to the left side of the patient on the operating table facing the target site. A more favored position for French surgeons is standing between the patient's abducted lower limbs on the operating table [14].

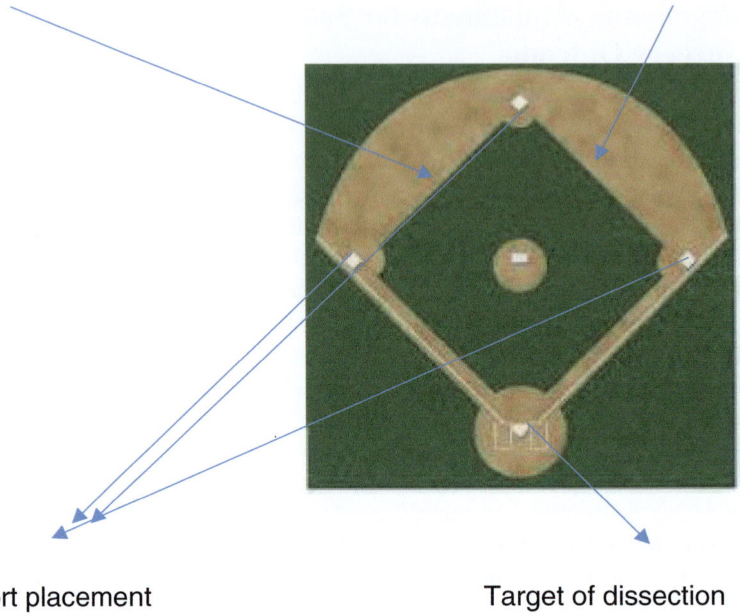

Fig. 5.1 Baseball diamond concept

Advances in Laparoscopic Surgery

Single-Incision Laparoscopic Surgery

This is considered in a port placement to achieve the best ergonomics for good surgical improvement or ease of use, especially the outcome.

Robotic Surgery

This is currently gaining ground in some middle and low-income countries. Ergonomics is the role of the game.

Artificial Intelligence (AI)

AI is being used to assess data on different performances and outcomes. Soon, AI will play a major role in laparoscopic ergonomics.

Simulators

Using simulators will enable a beginner to understand and note new techniques and methods to surmount challenges faced in clinical practice,

Key Points

- Adjust the operating table height so that the instrument handles are inserted into the abdomen at your elbow height.
- Place the visual display (monitor) directly in front of you and 15°–40° below the line of sight.
- Choose laparoscopic instruments that minimize wrist flexion and rotation and ulnar deviation [6].
- Choose instruments with comfortable and efficient handles matched to the tasks performed (e.g., power grip for grasping chores or fine grip for suturing).
- Loosening/resting of hands intermittently helps to ward off fatigue.
- If foot pedals must be used, place them close to the foot and use a footrest.
- Where possible, use large operating rooms with integrated and moveable storage systems that decrease clutter and turnaround times [6].
- In using floor-based equipment carts, carefully position all equipment so that movement in the room is not obstructed and devices required for only one portion of the case can be easily moved to the field when needed [11–14].
- Similarly, the cables and tubes associated with laparoscopic cases must be carefully grouped and secured, in the operative field and on the floor, to minimize the hazard they represent and permit operating room personnel and surgeons' flow.
- Team training for the laparoscopic operating room members or staff is critical [4].
- Learn to minimize the risk of slips and mistakes and learn from them when they occur [14].

References

1. Berguer R. Surgery and ergonomics. Arch Surg. 1999;134:1011–6.
2. Berguer R, Forkey D, Smith W. Ergonomic problems associated with laparoscopic surgery. Surg Endosc. 1999;13:466–8.
3. Berguer R, Rab GT, Abu-Ghaida H, Alarcon A, Chung J. A comparison of surgeons' posture during laparoscopic and open surgical procedures. Surg Endosc. 1997;11:139–42.
4. Corrigan J, Kohn LT, Donaldson MS. To err is human: building a safer health system. Washington, DC: National Academy Press; 2000. p. 287.
5. Emam TA, Hanna G, Cuschieri A. Ergonomic principles of task alignment, visual display, and direction of execution of laparoscopic bowel suturing. Surg Endosc. 2002;16:267–71.

6. Cuschieri A, Szabo Z. Tissue approximation in endoscopic surgery: suturing and knotting techniques. Oxford: Isis Medical Media; 1995.
7. Emam TA, Hanna GB, Kimber C, Dunkley P, Cuschieri A. Effect of intracorporeal extracorporeal instrument length ratio on endoscopic task performance and surgeon movements. Arch Surg. 2000;135:62–5; discussion 66
8. Hanna GB, Shimi S, Cuschieri A. Optimal port locations for endoscopic intracorporeal knotting. Surg Endosc. 1997;11:397–401.
9. Hanna GB, Shimi SM, Cuschieri A. Task performance in endoscopic surgery is influenced by the location of the image display. Ann Surg. 1998;227:481–4.
10. Kenyon TA, Lenker MP, Bax TW, Swanstrom LL. Cost and benefit of the trained laparoscopic team. A comparative study of a designated nursing team vs a nontrained team. Surg Endosc. 1997;11:812–4.
11. Patkin M, Isabel L. Ergonomics, engineering and surgery of endosurgical dissection. J Rl Coll Surg Edinb. 1995;40:120–32.
12. Salvendy G. Handbook of human factors and ergonomics, vol. xxii. New York: Wiley; 1997. p. 2137.
13. Szabo Z, Hunter J, Berci G, Sackier J, Cuschieri A. Analysis of surgical movements during suturing in laparoscopy. Endosc Surg Allied Technol. 1994;2:55–61.
14. Mishra RK. Ergonomics in laparoscopy. In: Mishra RK, editor. Textbook of practical laparoscopic surgery. 3rd ed. Jaypee Brothers Medical Publishers (P) Ltd; 2013.

Chapter 6
Physiology of Pneumoperitoneum and Anesthesia

Job G. Otokwala and Sotonye Fyneface-Ogan

Introduction

Laparoscopic surgery is rapidly expanding in scope and patient characteristics and occasionally it is offered ambulatory. This poses challenges to the perioperative team and the need to ensure safety and excellent outcome is imperative as a defined goal of the procedure. While attempts are made to improve the infrastructure required to offer surgical convenience, a proper understanding of the complex interactions between the mechanical effects of pneumoperitoneum in gas laparoscopy is needed. The associated biochemical milieu and place of anesthetic techniques and positioning reflect the need for a better understanding of the basic underlying physiology of pneumoperitoneum and the safe delivery of anesthesia. This chapter evaluates the physiology of pneumoperitoneum and the various anesthetic options and possible complications following the initiation of anesthesia.

J. G. Otokwala (✉)
Faculty of Clinical Sciences, University of Port Harcourt, Choba, Rivers State, Nigeria

Department of Anesthesia, University of Port Harcourt Teaching Hospital (UPTH), Port Harcourt, Rivers State, Nigeria
e-mail: job.otokwala@uniport.edu.ng

S. Fyneface-Ogan
Department of Anesthesia, University of Port Harcourt Teaching Hospital (UPTH), Port Harcourt, Rivers State, Nigeria

Department of Anesthesia, Faculty of Clinical Sciences, University of Port Harcourt, Choba, Rivers State, Nigeria

E. Ray-Offor, R. J. Rosenthal (eds.), *Principles and Practice of Laparoscopic Surgery*, https://doi.org/10.1007/978-3-031-96321-6_6

Pneumoperitoneum and Body Systems

Gas laparoscopy requires the insufflation of gas, commonly carbon dioxide at a regulated pressure into the peritoneal cavity. The use of carbon dioxide has been found to induce mechanical, metabolic, and immune effects with clinical implications [1]. The interactions of these modifications of the peritoneal or extraperitoneal space with anesthesia could influence patient outcomes. Mechanical effects of pneumoperitoneum from the increase in intra-abdominal pressure affect various organs and systems in the body. A combination of the mechanical effects and the adopted positioning of the patient could exaggerate physiological variables and portend danger for high-risk populations. The organs and systems affected are:

Cardiovascular System

Critical determinants of cardiovascular function are the intra-abdominal pressure (IAP) and patient position. Pneumoperitoneum at a pressure that is greater than 15 mmHg compresses the inferior vena cava, the aorta, and renal arteries causing increases in mean arterial pressure (MAP), and systemic vascular resistance (SVR). These events result in decreases in the splanchnic blood flow, renal blood flow, venous return, and reduction in cardiac output. See (Fig. 6.1). Initially, owing to auto-transfusion of pooled blood from the splanchnic circulation, there is an increase

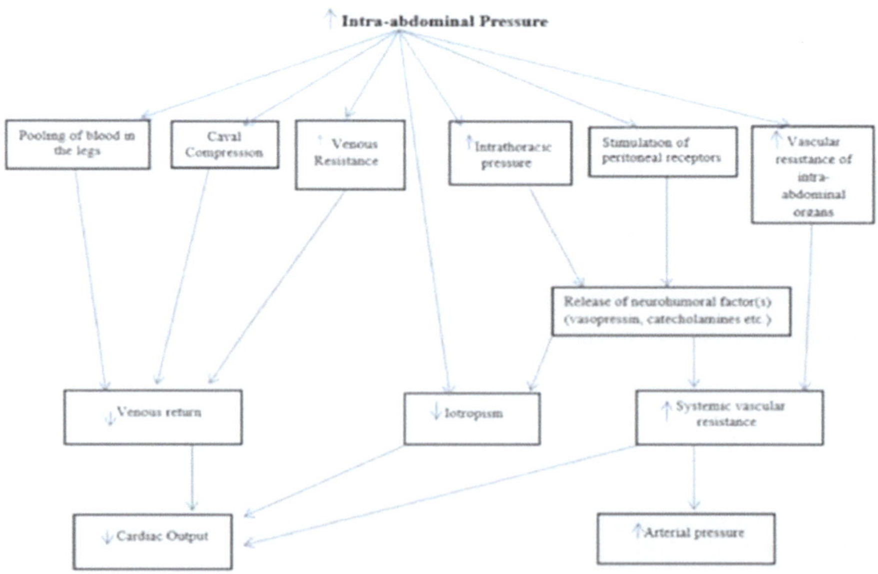

Fig. 6.1 Different mechanisms leading to decreased cardiac output during pneumoperitoneum

in the circulating blood volume, increasing venous return and cardiac output. The SVR is increased not only because of the direct effects of the IAP but also due to an increase in the release of circulating neuro-humoral factors from the renin-aldosterone system, the catecholamines, especially epinephrine, and norepinephrine. Gas insufflation also stimulates the peritoneal stretched receptors to provoke a vasovagal reflex which can result in sinus bradycardia, nodal rhythm, and asystole because of excessive vagal stimulation. The vagal output is higher at the beginning of the insufflation because of the rapid stretching of the peritoneum. Cases of intra-operative cardiac arrest following sudden elevation of intra-abdominal pressure have been reported [2]. The cephalad displacement of the diaphragm from the pneumoperitoneum and compression of the pulmonary parenchyma could also increase pulmonary vascular resistance. The change in SVR is generally greater than the reduction in cardiac output, maintaining or even increasing systemic blood pressure. The increasing SVR, systolic and diastolic blood pressures, and tachycardia result in a large increase in myocardial workload. Consequently, myocardial ischemia may result. Further increases in IAP may decrease cardiac output with a subsequent fall in blood pressure, an effect more pronounced in patients who are hypovolemic or have cardiovascular disease.

Healthy individuals will tolerate laparoscopy well, while individuals with underlying cardiopulmonary or renal diseases may not tolerate prolonged insufflation. Additionally, patient positioning, for example, steep Trendelenburg in prostatectomy, can exacerbate cardiovascular alterations in laparoscopy. It has been observed that microcirculation is significantly compromised as the intra-abdominal pressure rises to 15 mmHg. Most procedures are undertaken at about 12–15 mmHg of IAP in adults. An increase above 15 mmHg will tilt towards the causation of abdominal compartment syndrome with its attendant consequences [3].

Respiratory System

The supine position generally reduces the functional residual capacity (FRC) of patients. This respiratory parameter is further worsened in Trendelenburg's position. The combination of positioning in the Trendelenburg state and pneumoperitoneum provokes a ventilation/perfusion (V/Q) mismatch.

The pneumoperitoneum and the Trendelenburg position shift the diaphragm cephalad further decreasing FRC, possibly to values less than the closing volume. This effect could lead to airway collapse, atelectasis, further V/Q mismatch, potential hypoxemia, and hypercarbia. It has been shown that there is an increase in airway resistance and a reduction in compliance which potentiates the risk of barotrauma with positive pressure ventilation. This physiological change is worse in chronic obstructive airway disease and morbidly obese patients who usually have limited lung compliance. Peak airway and plateau pressures also increase up to 50% and 81%, respectively during laparoscopic surgery [4]. It is important to note that end-tidal CO_2 value may not be reliably determined as it is frequently underestimated. Periodic arterial blood gas measurement is essential during the procedure and when abnormally high values are obtained, pneumoperitoneum or pneumo-retroperitoneum should be relieved immediately. Once the partial pressure of arterial CO_2 value has fallen to the acceptable range, CO_2 insufflation could be resumed and the laparoscopic procedure continued.

Gastrointestinal System

The patients undergoing anesthesia for laparoscopic surgery are frequently prone to regurgitation of gastric contents with an associated risk of pulmonary aspiration following increased IAP. This is encountered in clinical states such as the obese and other patients with large intra-abdominal mass frequently described as having ‘full stomach’. It is essential to observe the fasting guidelines and administer antacids and prokinetics.

Neurological System

With the increase in abdominal pressure, the intracranial pressure (ICP) also increases leading to a fall in cerebral perfusion pressure (CPP). The resultant increase in intra-thoracic pressure from an increase in IAP also reduces the intracerebral venous drainage leading to an increase in ICP. A fall in the perfusion pressure in the presence of markedly reduced cardiac output could result in areas of poor cerebral perfusion and ischemia. Cerebral edema at the immediate post-laparoscopy period has been reported to affect emergence. The CO_2 absorbed during insufflation equally acts as a weak anesthetic and can cause unconsciousness, an effect that could lead to a delay in returning to normal cognitive function after the surgery. Carbon dioxide narcosis could also lead to transient visual disturbances, headache, reduction of reasoning ability, and a ‘sense of air hunger’ or dyspnea.

Metabolic Response

Raised levels of cytokines have been observed following a marked increase in intra-abdominal pressure [5]. Cortisol, C-reactive protein, tumor necrosis factor-α, interleukin-6, interleukin-10, granulocytic elastase, catecholamines, and leukocytes are some of the factors that could be released during laparoscopy. The release of these immune factors is transient. As opposed to open surgical procedures, minimally accessed surgery is associated with attenuated responses to the activation of cytokines and other inflammatory factors. A rare but potentially fatal complication of gas insufflation is gas embolism. This event occurs mostly when the Veress needle is used in the closed technique gas insufflation method where the insufflating gas is inadvertently instilled directly into a blood vessel or by gas reflux into open vessels. Immediate resuscitation and prompt deflation of the abdomen and aspiration of air with the patient in the left lateral position through a central line, if it is in, will suffice. It has been observed that prolonged surgery in lithotomy, semi-lithotomy, or lateral decubitus position tends to cause an increase in the intra-compartment pressures in an otherwise healthy limb and in the absence of underlying systemic risk factor(s)-Well leg compartment syndrome [6].

Renal System

Raised IAP causes reduced blood flow to the kidneys and reduces renal function and urine output due to an increase in renal vascular resistance and a decrease in glomerular filtration rate. Renal injury and dysfunction are usually either from a steep decrease in cardiac output or a direct effect on the afferent and efferent renal veins. An adequate fluid balance should be maintained.

Physiological Effect of Positioning

The Trendelenburg (the body is laid supine or flat on the back with the feet higher than the head by 15–30°) and reverse Trendelenburg (the body is laid supine or flat on the back with the head higher than the feet by 15–30°) positions have effects on the normal physiology of the patient (Table 6.1). In the Trendelenburg position, the abdominal contents shift cephalad exert pressure on the diaphragm, and reduce the vital capacity, the functional residual capacity, and an increased tendency for tracheal tube migration. Prolonged procedures in Trendelenburg result in airway edema and raised intracranial pressure in which intravenous mannitol is indicated. In the cardiovascular system, there is a transient increase in venous return leading to a rise in cardiac output. This increase

Table 6.1 Physiological effects of positioning

Variable	Trendelenburg	Reverse Trendelenburg
Cardiovascular system		
Vascular resistance	↑	↓
Cardiac output	↑	↓
Blood pressure	↔	↓
Respiratory system		
Lung volumes	↓	↔
V/Q mismatch	↑	↔
Atelectasis	↑	↔

in venous return could be detrimental in patients with cardiac disease. The reverse Trendelenburg position causes a redistribution of blood flow towards the periphery and resultant hypotension.

The pneumoperitoneum also tends to compress the lower limb vasculature to impede venous return. The resultant effect is a decrease in the cardiac output and hence, hypotension. The cardiac index is said to decrease by about 50% of the pre-procedure values. The combination of these factors and an increase in intrathoracic pressure from pneumoperitoneum can cause an exaggerated decrease in mean arterial blood pressure and hypotension. Underhydration should be avoided in this group of patients.

Anesthetic Management

Pre-operative Assessment

A pre-operative evaluation of the patient for laparoscopic surgery is essential for achieving a better outcome of anesthesia. Detailed evaluation of the patient is directed towards the cardio-respiratory systems as the potential complications are exaggerated in these systems [7]. Any concurrent disease like a pre-existing raised ICP (for example, hydrocephalus, intracranial masses, head injury) ischemic or valvular heart disease, or unstable hemodynamic system should be a contraindication for anesthesia to laparoscopic surgery. A detailed review by the attending anesthetist should be carried out a day before surgery or early on the day of the procedure to assess any comorbid state, obtain medication history, conduct a proper clinical examination of other systems, and obtain consent for anesthesia. The goal of anesthesia is to provide a relaxed surgical field, with the protection of the airway in an environment of raised intra-abdominal pressure and awkward positioning. The relative loss in the gastro-esophageal reflex makes airway protection mandatory, and the routine use of prokinetics and proton pump inhibitors before the initiation of anesthesia is also advocated [8].

Premedication

Most patients for laparoscopic surgeries do not require premedication. Anxious patients may need anxiolytics either through the enteral or parenteral route. Type-2 histamine receptor blockers (H2-receptor blockers) or proton pump inhibitors such as omeprazole may be administered to patients predisposed to having an increased risk of regurgitation and aspiration. Following the risk of developing arrhythmias from peritoneal stretching, atropine may be administered. It is noteworthy that only medications necessary should be administered.

Anesthetic Techniques

The choice of anesthetic technique aims at achieving a rapid recovery with minimal residual effects, and good quality pain control with minimal post-operative nausea and vomiting. The options available for laparoscopy include general, regional, and local infiltrative anesthesia. The use of other methods such as transversus abdominis plane block (TAP), as well as the use of the laryngeal mask airway has been described [9].

General Anesthesia

This is a traditionally most acceptable technique and offers the advantage of having a definitive airway and controlled ventilation. Confirming the correct placement of and preventing migration of the tracheal tube (by firmly securing the tube) is essential to maintaining airway patency [10]. The tracheal tube tends to migrate with the patient in the Trendelenburg position. The use of muscle relaxants provides more room for flexibility and hence a better view of the surgical field. During maintenance of anesthesia, minute ventilation can be increased (achieved by large tidal volumes of 6–8 ml/kg) to attain values of 30–40 mmHg of end-tidal CO_2. Occasionally permissive hypercapnia is allowed in pediatric or thoracic surgeries. The increase in the tidal volume helps to prevent micro-atelectasis and hypoxemia. However, the disadvantage of this increase is a consequent increase in intrathoracic pressure and its effect on the cardiac output. The use of positive end-expiratory pressure (PEEP) increases the intra-operative FRC and reduces hypoxemia and postoperative atelectasis.

Induction agents: Post-operative recovery can be fast-tracked with induction agents such as propofol, etomidate, midazolam/ fentanyl/sulfentanyl, and maintenance of anesthesia with sevo/isoflurane will facilitate quick recovery [11]. The hangover effect of these agents is minimal. Laparoscopic surgery is a major risk factor for postoperative nausea and vomiting, so a potent anti-emetic is usually administered intraoperatively. The use of intravenous dexamethasone not only functions as only prophylactic anti-emetic but is indicated in postoperative pain management due to its anti-inflammatory properties. Other antiemetics such as 5-HT3 antagonists(ondansetron) are equally effective in reducing the incidence of postoperative nausea and vomiting.

Epidural Anesthesia

Several authors have described the successful use of epidural anesthesia for laparoscopy [12]. The argument to support it has been its usefulness in post-operative analgesia and in patients with comorbid states that are unstable for general anesthesia. The authors attempted the use of epidural anesthesia for laparoscopic ovarian cystectomy and observed the extent of discomfort that the patients experienced. Shoulder pain from sub-diaphragmatic irritation and the effect of pneumoperitoneum on the diaphragm in a conscious patient can cause severe discomfort. Low levels of gaseous insufflation may be helpful to ameliorate discomfort. Some workers had reported the use of diclofenac injections in addition to opioids to attenuate the shoulder pain (incidence varies 25–45%) [13]. The choice of epidural anesthesia must be determined from a platform of safety. Some of the advantages of epidural anesthesia for laparoscopic surgery include the decreased incidence of postoperative nausea and vomiting, rapid and excellent recovery, prevention of complications of the use of general anesthesia such as sore throat and airway trauma, and less need for opioids. However, this type of anesthesia is not devoid of its disadvantages. Some of these disadvantages include the inability to achieve a T2-T4 block if required. This high block could lead to severe myocardial depression, bradycardia, and impaired venous return.

Single Shot Spinal Anesthesia

The safety of spinal anesthesia has been demonstrated to provide a faster onset and shorter recovery times, a reduced incidence of postoperative nausea and vomiting (PONV), significant postoperative analgesia, and the sparing of airway manipulations. The major drawbacks of regional anesthesia are the high incidence of shoulder pain, hypotension (could be as high as 21%), and abdominal discomfort [4]. The associated hypotension can be further worsened by the Trendelenburg positioning and increased abdominal pressure. However, this can be circumvented if liberal preloading with fluid, minimizing head tilt, reducing the insufflation pressure, and the use of vasopressors are carried out. A lower intra-abdominal pressure of about 10–12 mmHg has been advocated to contribute to the safe use of regional anesthesia [14].

Combined Spinal-Epidural Technique

This subset of epidural anesthesia offers a better platform for laparoscopic procedures than either epidural or single-shot spinal technique. Combined spinal-epidural (CSE) anesthesia has the advantages of rapid onset of anesthesia compared to epidural alone and reduced intra-thecal doses of local anesthetic required compared to spinal anesthesia. It is not clear if shoulder pain or abdominal discomforts can be ameliorated with the CSE. The addition of opioids can reduce the prevalence of shoulder discomfort. CSE has the benefit of post-operative analgesic use and topping up analgesia for a prolonged procedure. The choice of regional anesthesia as the sole technique with the patient in Trendelenburg's position and breathing spontaneously is fraught with anxiety and should be reconsidered when deciding on the choice of anesthesia. This is irrespective of the advantages it confers.

Transversus Abdominus Plane Block (TAP)

As an adjunct to general anesthesia to provide peri-operative analgesia, transversus abdominus plane block (TAP block) has been described [15]. The TAP block, first described in 2001, is the administration of a local anesthetic into the anatomical plane between the internal oblique and transversus abdominis muscles, where the thoracoabdominal nerves (T6-L1) contribute to the main sensory supply of the skin, muscles, and parietal peritoneum of the anterior abdominal wall. These nerves branch and communicate extensively with each other in the transversus abdominis plane. TAP blocks are said to be quite safe. With the TAP block technique, it is possible to avoid airway management as well as hemodynamic instability that might be associated with the induction of general anesthesia. It is also a viable anesthetic plan for any patient who might need minimal airway instrumentation or neuraxial intervention.

However, complications that could be associated with the block could include intra-peritoneal injection, bowel hematoma, transient femoral nerve palsy, visceral organ injury as well as local anesthetic toxicity. Precautions should be taken to minimize risks including using a small gauge short bevel blunt needle.

The potency and efficacy of TAP block as a single technique are doubtful as there is a dearth of literature as regards this technique of anesthesia.

Post-laparoscopic Surgery Pain Management

It is well known that laparoscopic surgery confers benefits such as reduced postoperative pain and short hospital stays. Good post-operative analgesia should be administered [16]. The post-operative analgesic needs after laparoscopic surgery are usually minimal. As part of multimodal analgesics, non-steroidal anti-inflammatory agents (NSAIDs) or COX-2 selective inhibitors and acetaminophen (Paracetamol) are given preoperatively or intraoperatively. Intravenous dexamethasone if not given already as antiemetic, is recommended as part of first-line medication for pain management in laparoscopic. Opioids are reserved as second-line analgesics if other analgesics cannot adequately manage the pain due to their side effects [17].

The Infiltration of the port site with long-acting local anesthetic ideally before incision is recommended for pain management [17] Also, intraperitoneal local anesthesia infiltration has been shown to offer additional analgesic benefits above basic analgesia or wound local anesthetic infiltration. Regional techniques are equally utilized in laparoscopic surgery pain management. The type of regional block depends on the expertise of the anesthetist, the expected severity of pain, and the length of hospital stay (day case or in-patient). Regional blocks that could provide postoperative analgesia include the Erector spinae plane block (ESP) and Transabdominal plane block (TAP). The increased risk of local anesthetic systemic toxicity and the required expertise make these blocks less preferable to intraperitoneal and port site infiltrations.

Other surgical techniques that can reduce the severity of postoperative pain include; low-pressure peritoneum, active aspiration of remaining pneumoperitoneum, and irrigation with normal saline.

References

1. Joshi GP. Anesthesia for laparoscopic surgery. Can J Anaesth. 2002;49(Supp 1):6–7.
2. De Keulenaer BL, De Waele JJ, Powell B, Malbrain ML. What is normal intra-abdominal pressure and how is it affected by positioning, body mass, and positive end-expiratory pressure? Intensive Care Med. 2009;35:969–76.
3. Hayden P, Cowman S. Anaesthesia for laparoscopic surgery. Contin Educ Anaesth Crit Care Pain. 2011;11:177–80.
4. Sotunmbi PT, Otokwala JG. Anesthesia for gasless laparoscopy: our experience. Afr J Med Sci. 2009;38:217–20.
5. Jayashree S. Anil K1 Anaesthesia in laparoscopic surgery. New Delhi: Jaypee Brothers; 2006. p. 5–6.
6. Ray-Offor E, Fyneface-Ogan S. Sedation, analgesia and patient monitoring. In: Ray-Offor E, editor. Flexible gastrointestinal endoscopy—basic principles. 1st ed. TND Press Ltd; 2017. p. 69–79.
7. Ivankovich AD, Miletich Dl Albrecht RF, Heyman HJ, Bonnet RF. Cardiovascular effects of intraperitoneal insufflation with carbon dioxide and nitrous oxide in the dog. Anesthesiology. 1975;42:281287.
8. Ishizaki Y, Bandai Y, Shimomura K, Abe H, Ohtomo Y, Idezuki Y. Safe intra-abdominal pressure of CO2 pneumoperitoneum during laparoscopic surgery. Surgery. 1993;114:549–54.
9. Slodzinski M, Merritt WT. Anesthesia for gastrointestinal surgery. In: Longnecker DE, editor. Anesthesiology. New York: The McGraw-Hill Companies; 2008. p. 1314–38.
10. Wilcox S, Vandam LD. Alas, poor Trendelenburg and his position! A critique of its uses and effectiveness. Anesth Analg. 1988;67:574–8.
11. Olufolabi AJ, Charlton GA, Sparges PM. Effect of head position on tracheal tube position in children. Anesth Analg. 2004;59:1069–72.
12. Sukhminder JSB, Ashish K. Anaesthesia for laparoscopic surgery: general vs regional anesthesia. J Minim Access Surg. 2016;12:4–9.
13. Tiwari S, Chauhan A, Chatterjee P, Alam MT. Laparoscopic cholecystectomy under spinal anesthesia. A prospective randomized study. I Minim Access Surg. 2013;9:65–71.
14. Goyal S, Goyal S, Singla S. Laparoscopic cholecystectomy under spinal anesthesia with low-pressure pneumoperitoneum-prospective study of 150 cases. Arch Clin Exp Surg. 2012;1(4):224–8.
15. Cunningham A. Laparoscopic surgery-anaesthetic implications. Surg Endosc. 1994;8:1272–84.
16. Onajin-Obembe BOI. Day case laparoscopic gynaecological procedure-current trends in Anaesthetic management. Nig J Clin Pract. 2009;12:311–8.
17. Barazanchi AWH, Kehlet H, et al. Evidence-based management of pain after laparoscopic cholecystectomy: a PROSPECT review update. Br J Anaesth. 2018;121(4):787–803.

Chapter 7
Access, Creation of Pneumoperitoneum and Trocar Placement in Laparoscopic Surgery

Chukwuemeka C. Osuagwu and Emeka Ray-Offor

Introduction

Creating peritoneal access for the pneumoperitoneum is the first and one of the most critical steps in laparoscopic surgery. The key consideration in the site of choice for peritoneal access and instruments is a clear appreciation of the anatomy and physics of the abdominal wall. Previous abdominal surgery, suspected /known adhesion, and obesity can modify peritoneal access technique. Although various techniques and devices are available for peritoneal access, there is an unresolved controversy about a single method suitable for all cases. The access technique may be individualized in each case after a proper preoperative evaluation and with the requisite surgical skill [1]. Hence, all laparoscopic surgeons must gain broad experience in all the different ways and sites for creating pneumoperitoneum to ensure patient safety and optimal outcomes.

Peritoneal access for the pneumoperitoneum is one of the common causes of complications associated with laparoscopic surgery. It is reported that >50% of complications result from events related to the insertion of the primary port [2]. These minor and major complications can occur before the main laparoscopic dissection commences. The incidence of these access-related injuries has remained

C. C. Osuagwu
Department of Surgery, Al Quwayiyiah General Hospital, Riyadh Region, Saudi Arabia

E. Ray-Offor (✉)
College of Health Sciences, University of Port Harcourt, Choba, Rivers State, Nigeria

Minimal Access Surgery Program, University of Port Harcourt Teaching Hospital (UPTH), Port Harcourt, Rivers State, Nigeria

Department of Surgery, UPTH, Port Harcourt, Rivers State, Nigeria

Oak Endoscopy Centre and Radiodiagnostics, Port Harcourt, Rivers State, Nigeria
e-mail: emeka.ray-offor@uniport.edu.ng

E. Ray-Offor, R. J. Rosenthal (eds.), *Principles and Practice of Laparoscopic Surgery*, https://doi.org/10.1007/978-3-031-96321-6_7

constant over the past quarter of a century [3]. They may lead to delay in commencing the surgery properly, conversion to laparotomy, and adverse outcomes such as morbidities and mortality if unrecognized. Therefore, caution in using instruments for creating peritoneal access cannot be overemphasized. It is important to note that most if not all complications are preventable with proper adherence to good technique and practice.

Primary Peritoneal Access Points

The points of primary peritoneal access in laparoscopy include the umbilicus, the periumbilical area, Palmer's point (3 cm below the left costal margin at the midclavicular line), Lee-Huang point (midway between the xiphoid process and umbilicus), and either flank [4–6]. The periumbilical area is favored and may be supra, infra-umbilical, or through the umbilical cicatrix. Palmer's point is used in a scarred abdomen from a midline incision, the presence of abdominal mesh or umbilical hernia repair, pelvic and abdominal adhesions, and obesity. Gastric decompression is recommended before the use of the route. Palmer's point is avoided in left hypochondria scar; inability to decompress the stomach, splenomegaly; portal hypertension; and gastric and distal pancreatic tumors [5]. When the periumbilical area and Palmer's point are encumbered, the flank or right subcostal area may be used.

Other rare spots for pneumoperitoneal access include the ninth or tenth intercostal space anterior axillary line above the lower corresponding rib [7]. In females, transuterine Veress needle carbon dioxide (CO_2) insufflation and trans-cul-de-sac CO_2 insufflation are performed through the uterine cavity and fundus or the posterior fornix respectively [8, 9]. Females with previous pelvic inflammatory disease (PID) and pelvic surgery may not be good candidates for the genital tract routes.

With innovations in minimally invasive surgery, Laparoendoscopic single-site surgery (LESS) is performed using an umbilical access site and is associated with improved post-operative pain outcomes [10]. Transvaginal natural orifice transluminal endoscopic surgery is another innovative technique in which the vagina is used as an entry point into the peritoneal cavity (vNOTES). A meta-analysis demonstrated non-inferiority of vNOTES hysterectomy compared to multiport conventional multiport laparoscopic hysterectomy in terms of early postoperative outcomes [11].

Techniques for Peritoneal Access

Access in laparoscopy is guided by the strategic, safe placement of the instrument that will permit the creation of pneumoperitoneum. The patient is usually positioned supine, skin routinely prepped, and sterile drapes placed to expose the anterior axillary line for a broad surgical field to facilitate additional port placements (Fig. 7.1).

The techniques are closed or open-access methods.

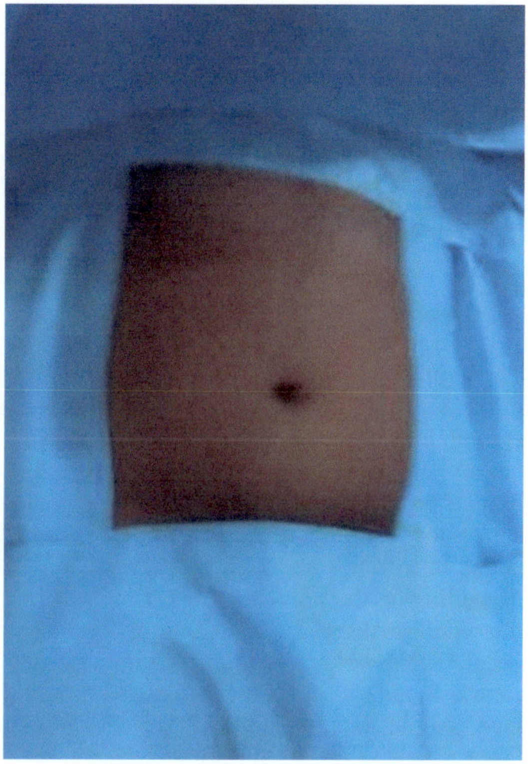

Fig. 7.1 Abdominal draping for access and port placement in laparoscopic Surgery

Closed Access

Closed access techniques involve the insertion of devices to create pneumoperitoneum through the abdominal wall via small snugly fitting incisions. It includes the use of a Veress needle, optical trocars (OT), and direct(blind) trocar insertion (DTI).

Veress Needle Access Technique

This technique remains the most popular access technique for the creation of pneumoperitoneum. Though widely used yet is associated with slow insufflation rates and potentially life-threatening complications thus will be described at length in this chapter.

The Veress needle was popularized by Raoul Palmer in 1947 following a documented literature of its use in 250 cases [3]. The report suggested that it is safe for the creation of initial pneumoperitoneal access. It consists of an outer cannula with a distal sharp beveled tip and an inner, spring-loaded, distal, blunt-tipped obturator (Fig. 7.2). The obturator, which projects beyond the bevel-tipped cannula, has a side hole close to the apex that allows the delivery of carbon dioxide.

Fig. 7.2 Veress needle

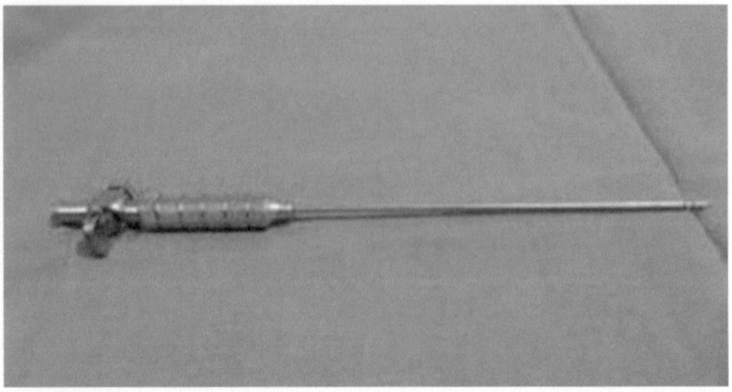

The proximal end of the Veress needle has an orifice for connection to the carbon dioxide insufflation tubing and a lever to open or close the channel for conveying carbon dioxide from the tubing to the tip of the Veress needle. The Veress needle has a blunt distal end which on meeting resistance such as fascia and peritoneum retracts to expose the beveled cutting tip that pierces the resisting tissue. The spring-loaded, blunt, central obturator springs back when the resistance is overcome. In a good state, it should have a smooth spring mechanism. This is tested by pulling on the proximal end and observing the retraction of the obturator and the recoil of the spring-like action. An alternative test is to press the tip of the needle against a tray or kidney dish and observe the retraction and return of the central obturator. The central cannula should not be obstructed, and the locking lever should move smoothly. The patency of the Veress needle could be tested using a syringe filled with water or air.

Handling and Insertion of Veress Needle

Veress needle could be inserted by pushing a predetermined length of the Veress needle through a small skin incision. At the periumbilical area, the distance between the anterior abdominal wall and intraperitoneal viscera is about 1–2 cm. This distance could be increased by pulling the anterior abdominal wall up by hand or with the use of towel clips applied to the skin. The needle is held like a dart, guard-protected to the predetermined length (Fig. 7.3), Then perpendicular-controlled thrust is made through a 0.5–1 cm skin incision on the anterior abdominal wall into the peritoneal cavity. Since the position of the umbilicus concerning the aortic bifurcation varies according to the patient's body mass index, the angle of insertion of the Veress needle at the umbilicus should be adjusted accordingly—from 45° in women of normal body mass to 90° in women with obesity [9]. The aim is to enter the peritoneal cavity and stay between the anterior abdominal wall and the viscera.

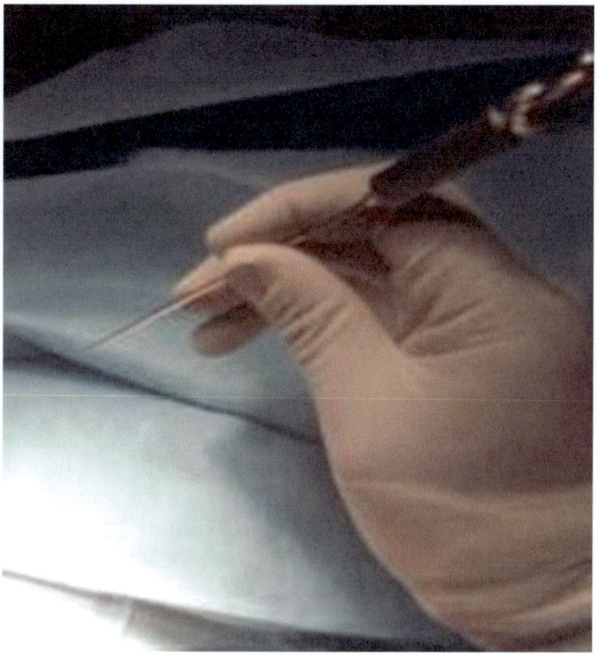

Fig. 7.3 Handling the Veress needle

Confirmation Test for Peritoneal Access [12]

The confirmatory tests for correct intra-peritoneal placement of the Veress needle include:

(a) Click test: At an umbilical peritoneal access site, the double-click sound is made during the insertion of the Veress needle. The first click is heard on the penetration of the fascia/rectus sheath. The anterior and posterior sheaths fuse in the periumbilical area. A second click is made on the penetration of the peritoneum. If less than two clicks or more than two clicks are heard it suggests defective placement. In the left upper quadrant, three clicks are elicited as the needle traverses the aponeuroses of the external and internal oblique muscles, and the peritoneum.
(b) Hanging drop test: After entry into the peritoneum using a Veress needle access technique, the valve on the extra-abdominal part of the needle is opened and some drops of water applied to the top of the extra-abdominal part of the Veress needle. A column of water is created in the Veress needle with a visible drop seen at the top. If the drop of water is sucked into the Veress needle on lifting the anterior abdominal wall, this indicates there is no resistance or obstruction from extraperitoneal placement or encumbrance from the bowel or omentum at the tip of the Veress needle. The drop of water is drained towards the lower pressure in the peritoneal cavity.

(c) Aspiration test: The Veress needle is aspirated at first to check for the presence of fluid, feces, or blood. Then 5mls of water is injected with a 5mls syringe through the needle. The absence of resistance on pushing down the plunger on the syringe suggests intraperitoneal placement. Thereafter, attempts are made to aspirate the water. If none is recovered, it means the water has dissipated in the peritoneal cavity. If some water is recovered, then the tip of the needle is probably in an extraperitoneal space or resting in a pocket of adhesions.

Extraperitoneal placement and visceral injuries can occur in the presence of positive tests. Thus, failure to perform these tests does not imply inferior care.

(d) Serial intra-abdominal gas pressure measurement.: The pressure is noted on the creation of the Veress needle access. This initial reading is noted before insufflation commences through a Veress needle after opening the valve. The initial flow rate of CO_2 is set at 1 L/min. The next four, successive, pressure readings from the quadro- manometric gauge in the first 5 seconds are noted. If the readings are less than 10 mmHg, it rules out the preperitoneal placement of the Veress needle, but not other forms of wrong placement such as bowel penetration.

Efficacy, Safety, and Adverse Outcomes

Veress needle is effective in creating pneumoperitoneum, but it may require multiple attempts to achieve pneumoperitoneal access. After the creation of the pneumoperitoneum, the Veress needle is removed, and a trocar is inserted blindly into the insufflated peritoneum through the slightly widened tract. The snug fit around the trocar is associated with minimal leakage of CO_2 into the subcutaneous plane or the air. Hence, the absence of a leak will maintain the intraperitoneal working space, above and around the viscera, for laparoscopic procedures. Complications with Veress needle access increase with many attempts to establish pneumoperitoneal access from 0.8% to 16% in the first attempts to 16.3%–37.5% and 44.4%–64% in the second and third attempts, respectively [12, 13]. Peritoneal placement is successful on the first attempt in 85.5–86.9% of cases; however, the chances of success decline rapidly to 8.5–11.6% of cases with two attempts and less than 5% with three attempts [12, 13]. Therefore, three attempts are allowed when using the Veress needle for the closed-access technique. The injuries could be minor, such as extraperitoneal insufflations, anterior abdominal vessel injuries, and omental vessel injuries and insufflations. Other minor complications include stomach, small and large bowel, urinary bladder, liver, and spleen injuries, which could be repaired with advanced laparoscopic skills. Major complications are retroperitoneal major vessel injuries, which may need a conversion to laparotomy.

Optical Trocar Access

An optical trocar has a removable obturator with a central hollow cannula. The tip of the obturator has a transparent tip that transmits light from a zero-degree telescope (Fig. 7.4). The advantage is that the layers of the abdomen, the subcutaneous fat; fascia, multiple layers of muscle; extraperitoneal fat; peritoneum, and greater omentum or bowel are seen. The trocar is advanced until the peritoneum retracts to the base of the transparent obturator. The bowel and omentum are identified, and intraperitoneal placement is confirmed. The optical trocar access technique is effective in creating pneumoperitoneum. It is reported to be six times faster than the time it takes to create open access [14]. The other advantage is that peritoneal inspection can commence immediately with that trocar.

Optical trocar access is associated with intraperitoneal injuries and other complications of pneumoperitoneal access; however, these may be recognized readily. The visceral injury rate may be reduced by insufflating the abdomen with a Veress needle to lift the anterior abdominal wall off the viscera before using the optical trocar. It is important to note that there is a paucity of literature comparing optical trocar access with other access techniques.

Direct Trocar Insertion

Direct trocar insertion is performed by inserting a trocar directly through a small 1–2 cm incision in the skin. The trocar is pushed through the abdominal wall into the peritoneal cavity and insufflation of the peritoneal cavity is commenced. This use of the same device for creating pneumoperitoneum and inspection of the peritoneal cavity and laparoscopic dissection is potentially faster. This is supported by studies on laparoscopic cholecystectomy and diagnostic laparoscopy in obese females, in which direct trocar insertion was found to be about two times faster than the Veress needle in creating pneumoperitoneal access [15, 16]. It reduces the

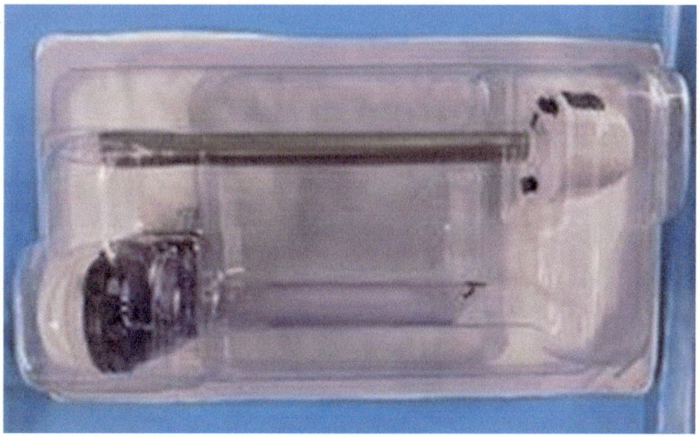

Fig. 7.4 Optical trocar

number of "blind steps" from 3 with the Veress needle (insertion, insufflation, and first trocar introduction), to just one, the trocar introduction. It is effective and safe in the hands of surgeons who have trained and practiced it. Therefore, it is an option that competes favorably with the other access techniques for pneumoperitoneum in laparoscopy.

In comparison, Veress needle access, direct trocar insertion (DTI), and optical trocar insertion have similar major complication rates, but they differ in the minor complication rate. Veress is reported to have a higher minor complication rate compared to direct trocar insertion (DTI) but optical trocar insertion may have a lower visceral injury rate [15]. However, few of the injuries caused by optical trocar will lead to clinical interventions in the patient.

Open Access

This access technique was developed in 1971 by Dr. Harrit Hasson [17]. Open access involves making 1-2 cm incisions through the anterior abdominal wall into the peritoneal cavity, then an appropriate trocar size is inserted under direct vision (Fig. 7.5). This is also called the Hasson technique. The advantages of this procedure are that, with appropriate practice, it takes no longer, and can be used in all possible situations, including previous surgery. Though the open technique is attractive it is associated with increased gas leakage [18]. Visceral injuries do occur during open Hasson as it does not necessarily allow good visualization of the peritoneal cavity at the point of entry particularly in obese patients, because the incision is only 10 mm long. A systematic review that compared open technique versus closed needle/trocar insertion, suggested a trend towards reduced risk of major intra-abdominal complications and minor complications alongside decreased conversion to laparotomy in favor of open technique [19]. However, an earlier review suggested that neither closed nor open technique is safer [20].

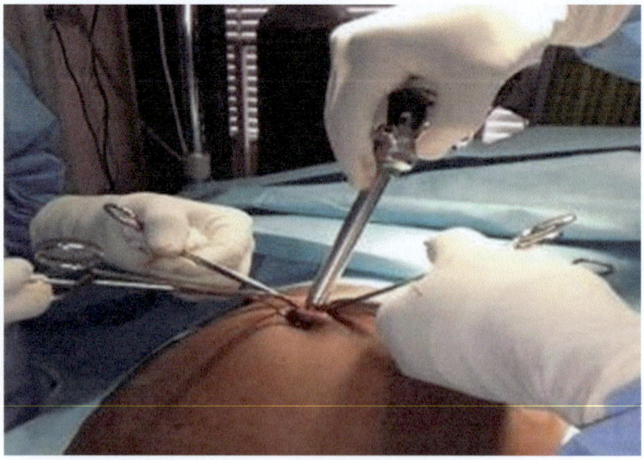

Fig. 7.5 Open access technique

In summary, there is very little to choose between both techniques. Since the closed and open techniques are effective and safe [21]. It is wise for a laparoscopic surgeon to acquire competence in two techniques at the very least, and practice the technique he finds comfortable.

Confirmation of Access

The confirmation of the intraperitoneal placement during insertion of optical trocar, direct trocar insertion, and open access is by visualization of the bowel or omentum.

Peritoneal Insufflation

Peritoneal insufflation is commenced with a flow rate of about 1 liter per minute. The preset pressure ranges from 10 mmHg to 15 mmHg. The purpose of insufflations is to create a working space above the intra-abdominal and retroperitoneal viscera. The pressure should not exceed the venous pressure in the inferior vena cava. It is important to have adequate paralysis of the anterior abdominal muscles. If the preset pressure is achieved and the abdominal working space is still suboptimal, consider inadequate paralysis, and leakage of carbon dioxide through the ports or port site. Distended bowel and retroperitoneal hematoma/edema should be excluded as well.

Five parameters are displayed on the quadro-manometric insufflations device. These may be displayed as digital parameters or dials in older machines.

(i) The preset pressure which is the target pressure of 10–15 mmHg for optimum working space
(ii) The actual intraperitoneal pressure rises gradually from zero to the preset pressure.
(iii) The flow rate of carbon dioxide per minute through the trocar or the Veress needle.
(iv) The actual volume of carbon dioxide used during the surgery.
(v) Additionally, the fullness of the carbon dioxide cylinder is seen from the number of green bars.

The understanding of the quadro-manometric display can prevent injuries to the patient. Extra peritoneal placement of the trocar is revealed by baseline pressures higher than 10 mmHg, and rapid rise in pressure with very little volume of $CO_{2\ \mathrm{insufflation}}$. The empty cylinder is revealed by a red light on the cylinder display, cessation of insufflation or zero flow rate, and an inactive insufflation button. A closed insufflation at the port on a trocar is revealed by high actual pressure, zero flow rate, and loss of intraperitoneal working space. After a while the insufflators will suck out the air in the body cavity or tubing and insufflations will cease. Also, this occurs when pressure is put on the abdominal wall during laparoscopic procedures. A leakage from the port site is suggested by low actual intraperitoneal pressure despite the normal flow rate and a considerable volume of carbon dioxide gas used. An intravascular trocar or Veress needle placement will be revealed by high actual pressures (pressure in the vessel) loss of working space or failure of the abdomen to distend despite normal flow rate with continued use of CO_2. The patient may develop tachycardia and hypotension from air embolism.

Access in Virgin Versus Previous Abdominal Surgery Scar

The creation of peritoneal access in an unscarred abdominal wall is a joy for the surgeon. The ports are placed at sites that will allow rapid progress of dissection with optimum surgical performance. The primary port is often placed at the periumbilical area using an open or closed access technique. An abdomen with a previous scar carries a risk of ventral intrabdominal adhesion. This risk is about 50% in patients with longitudinal laparotomy scars. Therefore, Veress needle access should be avoided in areas close to laparotomy scars, and ventral hernias to avoid iatrogenic injuries to intraperitoneal structures adherent to these areas. The abdomen with a previous midline scar will require primary port placement away from the scar to avoid enterotomies. Many surgeons favor open access, or Palmer's point.

Trocar Placement

Generally, trocar placement is guided by the site of the surgery, the target, the size and type of instruments to be used, and the extent of the surgery. Upper abdominal surgeries like laparoscopic Nissen fundoplication and laparoscopic Heller's myotomy with Dor's fundoplication will require four to five upper abdominal ports with or without an epigastric port for a self-retaining liver retractor (Fig. 7.6). Conventional laparoscopic cholecystectomy will require four ports. Often there are two 11 mm ports for the camera and a dissector/suturing port. Other ports are 5 mm. The camera port is placed in the middle with the working and retracting ports on either side of the camera port. They are placed like a triangle. Ports should be about 10 cm from each other and never on the same line to avoid clashing or clashing of instruments.

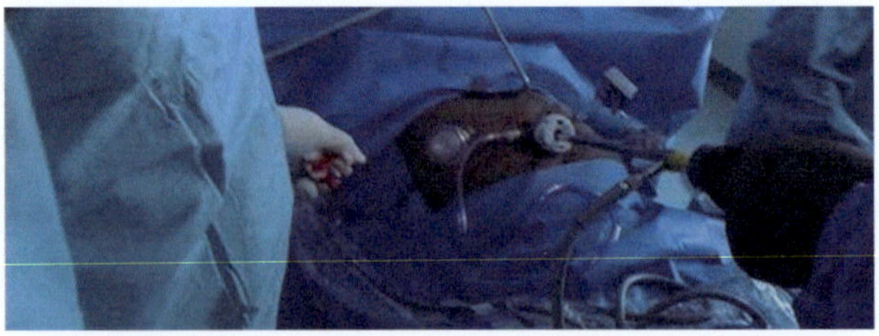

Fig. 7.6 Port placement in laparoscopic upper abdominal surgery

Following the Veress needle access technique, the primary trocar is inserted after adequate pneumoperitoneum is achieved, the Veress needle is removed, and the incision is extended to accommodate the size of the trocar used. Alternatively, a self-expanding Veress needle device permits the insufflation of the abdomen before removal of the Veress needle and subsequent dilatation of the sleeve by inserting a blunt obturator with a twisting motion. Evidence from RCT reports a lower relative risk of trocar site bleeding and overall complications with blunt laparoscopic cannulas than with bladed trocars. Hence a transition to blunt trocars for secondary cannulation of the abdominal wall under direct visualization is thus strongly recommended [22].

It is best to insert the port perpendicularly through the abdominal wall. This allows the ports to be tilted in any direction without tearing the anterior abdominal wall muscle. The tearing of the peritoneum and muscles leads to increased extraperitoneal leakage with consequent increased absorption of carbon dioxide and high-end tidal carbon dioxide readings. The midportion of the port should be in the anterior abdominal wall, a fulcrum, to allow satisfactory movement of the instrument in the abdominal cavity. The laparoscopic hand instruments should have half of their length inside and half outside like a type 1 lever. The Z-route is thought to prevent port site hernia, but it is technically difficult to create satisfactorily.

Tips to Avoid Complications and Practical Solutions for Complications

- Forceful uncontrolled entry of port occurs when the skin incision is too small. Hence, if the insertion of a trocar is a struggle, widen the incision.
- Port site gas leaks occur often in open access. The skin and muscle incision are wider than the ports. Skin suture could be used to create a snug fit around the trocar.
- Inspect the intraperitoneal area immediately underneath the port to assess for hematoma, bruising, or bleeding. Any suspicious area should be exposed and inspected to determine if there is visceral injury. Visceral injuries could be controlled laparoscopically or by conversion to laparotomy.
- There is no limit to the number of ports to be used in laparoscopy. If the progress in surgery is difficult, consider moving the camera and instrument to another port and placing more ports to enhance vision and retraction.
- Port site hernia is caused by failure to close port sites that are larger than 5 mm. All port sites wider than 5 mm should be closed or converted to 5 mm by delayed absorbable sutures such as PDS.
- When the surgery is over, inspect the port sites from the peritoneal aspect after removing a port to check for port site bleed.
- In the post-op period, if the patient's clinical course changes from the expected, then relook the patient. This may be performed laparoscopic or open. It is better to exclude intraperitoneal complications from the list of differentials.

References

1. Taye MK, Fazal SA, Pegu D, Saikia D. Open versus closed laparoscopy: yet an unresolved controversy. J Clin Diagn Res. 2016;10(2):DCD4-7.
2. Soper NJ, Swanström LL, Eubanks S, editors. Mastery of endoscopic and laparoscopic surgery. 2nd ed. Lippincott Williams & Wilkins; 2004. p. 3–13.
3. Bianchi G, Martorana E, Ghaith A, Pirola GM, Rani M, Bove P, Porpiglia F, Manferrari F, Micali S. Laparoscopic access overview: is there a safest entry method? Actas Urológicas Españolas (English Edition). 2016;40(6):386–92.
4. Palmer R. Safety in laparoscopy. J Reprod Med. 1974;13:1–5.
5. Thepsuwan J, Huang K-G, Wilamarta M, et al. Principles of safe abdominal entry in laparoscopic gynecologic surgery. Gynecol Minimal Invasive Ther. 2013;2(4):105–7.
6. Lee CL, Huang KG, Jain S, Wang CJ, Yen CF, Soong YK. A new portal for gynecologic laparoscopy. J Am Assoc Gynecol Laparosc. 2001;8:147–50.
7. Agarwala N, Liu CY. Safe entry technique during laparoscopy: left upper quadrant entry using the ninth intercostal space: a review of 918 procedures. J Minim Invasive Gynecol. 2005;12:55–61.
8. Ott J, Jaeger-Lansky A, Poschalko G, et al. Entry techniques in gynecologic laparoscopy—a review. Gynecol Surg. 2012;9:139–46.
9. Vilos GA, Ternamian A, Laberge PY, Vilos AG, AbuRafea B, Scattolon S, Leyland N. Guideline no. 412: laparoscopic entry for Gynaecological surgery. J Obstet Gynaecol Can. 2021;43(3):376–389.e1. https://doi.org/10.1016/j.jogc.2020.12.012. Epub 2020 Dec 26. Erratum in: J Obstet Gynaecol Can 2021; 43(9):1120–1121
10. Aprea G, Rocca A, Salzano A, Sivero L, Scarpaleggia M, Ocelli P, Amato M, Bianco T, Serra R, Amato B. Laparoscopic single site (LESS) and classic video-laparoscopic cholecystectomy in the elderly: a single centre experience. Int J Surg. 2016;33(Suppl 1):S1–3.
11. Michener CM, Lampert E, Yao M, Harnegie MP, Chalif J, Chambers LM. Meta-analysis of Laparoendoscopic single-site and vaginal natural orifice transluminal endoscopic hysterectomy compared with multiport hysterectomy: real benefits or diminishing returns? J Minim Invasive Gynecol. 2021;28(3):698–709.e1.
12. Teoh B, Sen R, Abbott J. An evaluation of four tests used to ascertain Veres needle placement at closed laparoscopy. J Minim Invasive Gynecol. 2005;12:153–8.
13. Richardson RF, Sutton CJG. Complications of first entry: a prospective laparoscopic audit. Gynaecol Endosc. 1999;8:327–34.
14. Tanaka C, Fujiwara M, Kanda M, Murotani K, Iwata N, Hayashi M, Kobayashi D, Yamada S, Kodera Y. Optical trocar access for initial trocar placement in laparoscopic gastrointestinal surgery: a propensity score-matching analysis. Asian J Endosc Surg. 2019;12(1):37–42.
15. Kaul R, Sharma G, Azad TP, Bhat S, Kumar B, Prashar N, Gorkha V. A randomised comparative study between direct trocar insertion Verus Veress needle technique for creating Pneumoperitoneum in laparoscopic cholecystectomy. Int J Res Med. 2016;5(2):16–21.
16. Ikechebelu JI, Eleje GU, Joe-Ikechebelu NN, Okafor CD, Okpala BC, Ugwu EO, Nwachukwu CE, Okoro CC, Okam PC. Randomized control trial on effectiveness and safety of direct trocar versus Veress needle entry techniques in obese women during a diagnostic laparoscopy. Arch Gynecol Obstet. 2021;304(3):815–22.
17. Hasson HM. A modified instrument and method for laparoscopy. Am J Obstet Gynecol. 1971;110(6):886–7.
18. Chotai NR, Choksi BB, Damor S, Bhedi A. Intraperitoneal access by closed method (Veress needle) versus open (Hasson's) method in laparoscopic surgery to create pneumoperitoneum. Int Surg J. 2017;4(8):2786–90.
19. Merlin TL, Hiller JE, Maddern GJ, Jamieson GG, Brown AR, Kolbe A. Systematic review of the safety and effectiveness of methods used to establish pneumoperitoneum in laparoscopic surgery. Br J Surg. 2003;90(6):668–79.

20. Rosen DM, Lam AM, Chapman M, Carlton M, Cario GM. Methods of creating pneumoperitoneum: a review of techniques and complications. Obstet Gynecol Surv. 1998;53(3):167–74.
21. Molloy D, Kaloo PD, Cooper M, Nguyen TV. Laparoscopic entry: a literature review and analysis of techniques and complications of primary port entry. Aust N Z J Obstet Gynaecol. 2002;42(3):246–54.
22. Antoniou SA, Antoniou GA, Koch OO, Pointner R, Granderath FA. Blunt versus bladed trocars in laparoscopic surgery: a systematic review and meta-analysis of randomized trials. Surg Endosc. 2013;27(7):2312–20.

Chapter 8
Laparoscopic Suturing and Tissue Approximation

Rex F. O. A. Ijah and Usman M. Bello

Introduction

Laparoscopic suturing and tissue approximation are necessary skills that every laparoscopic surgeon requires, especially for a successful advanced laparoscopic practice. Laparoscopic knots used today appear to be a modification of knots used by weavers, hangmen, seamen, and fishermen [1, 2]. Significant differences between conventional open surgical procedures and laparoscopic surgery contribute to the challenges with laparoscopic suturing. These differences include lack of direct manual contact with tissues; depth perception; restricted instrument mobility; and limitation of laparoscopic view to a portion of the body cavity. The prerequisite for laparoscopic suturing includes good visual perception and hand-eye coordination; unimpaired motor skill; satisfactory video magnification and imaging system; increasing efficiency; and good tissue handling [3]. Essential endosurgery skills are acquired through enthusiastic training in dry and wet laboratories.

This chapter discusses laparoscopic suturing and tissue approximation highlighting basic principles, techniques, and types of laparoscopic knots for the beginner and a subtle refresher for the practicing laparoscopic surgeon.

R. F. O. A. Ijah (✉)
Department of Surgery, Rivers State University (RSU)/Rivers State University Teaching Hospital (RSUTH), Port Harcourt, Rivers State, Nigeria

U. M. Bello
Bayero University Kano, Kano, Nigeria

Aminu Kano Teaching Hospital, Kano, Kano State, Nigeria

E. Ray-Offor, R. J. Rosenthal (eds.), *Principles and Practice of Laparoscopic Surgery*, https://doi.org/10.1007/978-3-031-96321-6_8

Table 8.1 Qualities of an ideal suture[1]

Sterile
Inert
Non-capillary
Non-allergenic
Non-carcinogenic
Good knot security
Resistance to infection
Adequate tensile strength
Consistent uniform diameter
Absorbability when desirable
Flexibility and ease of handling
Smooth passage through the tissue

[1]Source of data

Basic Definitions

Suture A suture is used to appose and ligate bleeding vessels. It is also a stitch or series of stitches made to secure the apposition of the edges of a surgical or traumatic wound. The qualities of an ideal suture are seen in Table 8.1.

Knotting This method of tissue approximation fastens or secures the suture by tying or interweaving. An ideal knot can hold the tissue edges together, resisting reverse slippage with the correct tension. Three basic stages identified in the suturing process are tying the knot (configuration), working or drawing the knot (shaping), and snuggling or locking the knot (securing) [1]. A secured knot is correctly configured, drawn to shape, and locked tightly.

Components of a Knot [2]

Bight—mid-portion of a length of suture as opposed to the ends.
Elbow—two crossing parts created by an extra twist in a loop.
Turn—part of the suture immediately behind or passing through the object.
Standing end—long end of the suture not involved in making the knot.
Standing part—section between the knot and the standing end.
Working end—tail (or live end, running end, active end) of suture used in making the knot.
Working part—section between working end and knot.
Loop—complete circle formed by passing the working end over itself.

Basic Instrumentation for Suturing

The video imaging system and the hand instruments are the basic equipment and instruments needed for endo-suturing. Chapter 2 discussed the video imaging system and general laparoscopy instruments; this chapter highlights some specific instruments.

Endoski Needle

The straight-in design and curved needles are used in laparoscopic surgery. Unique among these is the Endoski needle (Fig. 8.1), which is J-shaped. It combines the unique positive characteristics of curved and straight needles in one. The proximal straight part of the needle is about 1.5 times the length of the distal curved portion.

Laparoscopic Knot Pusher

It slides down an extracorporeal knot to the site of action in the peritoneal cavity (Fig. 8.2).

Needle Holder

See in Chap. 2

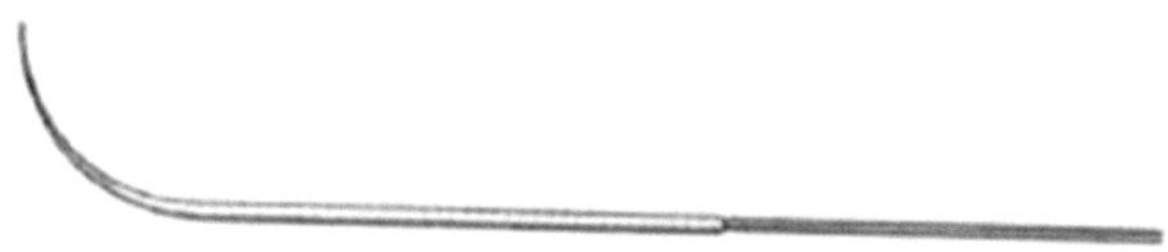

Fig. 8.1 Endoski needle

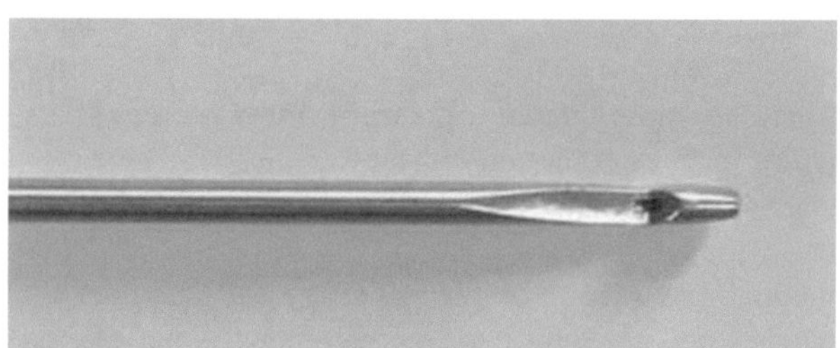

Fig. 8.2 Laparoscopic Knot Pusher

Suture Materials

This is the same as used in open surgery but is not discussed here. Appropriate surgery textbooks have these details.

Types of Knots

There are different types of knots in laparoscopic surgery. These can be tied within or outside the body cavity. When knots are tied within the body cavity, they are referred to as intra-corporeal, but when tied outside the body cavity, they are extra-corporeal.

Intra-corporeal Knots [1, 4]

These are knots wholly applied within the body cavity. They are commonly used for tissue approximation as continuous or interrupted stitches. In most instances, they are preferred to extra-corporeal knots. These include:

Square (Reef) Knot: It has two opposite half knots and is safe for securing small blood vessels.

Ligature Knot: An initial double knot crowned with a single half knot ensuring more security than a reef knot used for the same purpose.

Double Knot: It has two double half knots.

Mayo Knot: Two identical granny-like half knots crowned with a third and opposite half knot.

Surgeon's Knot: It is formed by throwing a double half knot, then crowned with two single half knots. It is commonly used for intra-corporeal interrupted suturing.

Others: Tumbled Square Knot, Dundee Jamming Knot, Aberdeen Termination Knot, etc.

Extra-corporeal Knots [1, 5]

There are more than 25 different extra-corporeal knots used by surgeons worldwide [1, 5]. In endoscopic surgery, they are used for ligation of a vessel or tubular structure; interrupted suturing; or trans-fixation of large vascular pedicles. The knot is tied externally, then drawn down (slipped down) to the target site with the knot pusher while maintaining traction on the standing part. There are certain instances when extracorporeal knots are indicated in preference to intra-corporeal knots. They include suturing in restricted access areas; ligation of large vessels; and approximation of the edges of defects requiring some degree of tension. Some popular extracorporeal knots are the Roeder Knot, Meltzer Knot, and Modified Tayside Knot.

Principles of Knot Tying

Certain guiding principles should be followed to ensure a safe, quick, and easy knot application. The type of knot used to a good extent depends on the material used; the depth and location of the incision and the stress to be contained by the wound postoperatively. Generally, the simplest knot for the material is the most desirable to approximate and not strangulate the tissue. There is the need to factor in the amount of tension exerted on the wound and make allowance for postoperative edema. This is to prevent suture breakage or tissue cut-through. Also important is limiting friction or sawing between strands which weakens sutures. Knot tying is performed maintaining traction at one end of the strand after the first loop, to avoid loosening the throw, and the final throw is made as nearly horizontal as possible. In securing a knot, the laparoscopic surgeon may need to change position concerning the patient. The knot should be as small as possible with the ends cut short to avoid excess foreign body reaction. A properly tied knot is firm without slippage and needs no extra throws for further strength.

Extracorporeal Knots

Suture material, size, and length are key considerations for sutures used in extracorporeal knots. It is better to use multifilament sutures (e.g. polyglactin) as stiff hydrophobic monofilament (e.g. Nylon) though associated with less friction, has a greater tendency to spill—change its form and rearrange its part during pulling (capsizing). The slip knot should be selected based on the ligature material, as some knots do not provide enough holding strength with all sutures. The suture length and size 2/0 sutures are most used. This length enables easy suturing. However, it is notable that the holding strength of the suture material is directly proportional to its caliber or size (size 0 or 1 suture has more holding strength than 2/0).

Intracorporeal Knots

The knot quality and ease of application depend on good vision and magnification. As the operation is entirely within the closed abdominal cavity and often limited space, an economy of movement in suturing is needed to avoid instrument crossing.

An efficient process is dependent on developing correct knot-tying choreography, clearly defining beforehand the dominant and the assisting instruments in the knotting process, and tying close to the tail. The jaws of instruments should be kept closed except during grasping. Suture length is often magnified to 2.5 times, hence a length exceeding 20 cm will result in some difficulty with intracorporal maneuvers.

Steps in Laparoscopic Suturing

Introduction of Needles

The cannula valve mechanism can trap the needle; therefore, it is recommended to use an introducer tube. An appropriate suture length (not more than 20 cm) is needed as too small or too long a length will be a problem. A length of 15—20 cm is recommended for a continuous suture. The essential steps start with the passage of the needle holder through the introducer to grasp the suture halfway from the needle tip, then withdrawing it completely (out of sight) into the introducer. The tube introducer is inserted into the port then extruding the needle and suture safely into the peritoneal cavity under visual supervision.

Needle Adjustment

Adjusting the intra-corporeal laparoscopic needle can be achieved in several ways. These include using the assisting hand instrument; touching the tip of the needle on a firm surface; compressing the middle of the needle on a safe surface using the needle holder; and putting some tension or traction on the suture with another instrument while the needle is being held with the needle holder.

Driving a Needle

Good technique in suturing involves approaching the tissue with the needle at a right angle while applying a perpendicular force to the cut tissue while maintaining a counter pressure. This avoids the deflection of the needle and facilitates the suturing process. A skillful choreography of needle positioning, entrance bite, needle extracting process, and exit bite is the desired routine followed by intra-corporeal knot tying. This is more challenging than an extra-corporeal knot application. A new disposable automated suturing device, the EndoStitch (Covidien) is reported to be significantly more cost-effective than traditional laparoscopic suturing techniques (Fig. 8.3) [6].

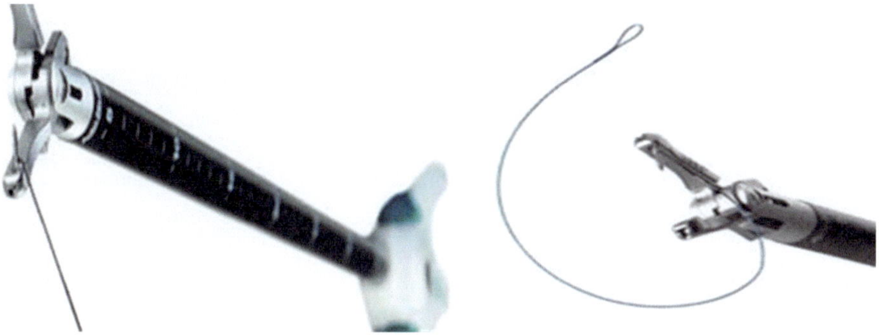

Fig. 8.3 Endo-stitch

It is important to watch out for the following errors in the laparoscopic suturing process: loosening of knots; unravelling of knots; short suture length; incorrect loop formation; crossing instruments; needle deflection; and complications of suturing (iatrogenic injury to tissue by the needle; lost needle.

Laparoscopic Staplers

Historically surgical stappling anastomosis was started in 1908 by a Hungarian surgeon, Humer Hultl [7]. However modern surgical staplers were developed in the Soviet Union in the 1950s [8]. Initial surgical staplers were developed for open surgery, however with the advancement in laparoscopic surgery, laparoscopic staplers were developed and this made it possible for complex gastrointestinal operations to be done laparoscopically. Laparoscopic staplers are mainly linear, however circular staplers used in open surgery can also be used to achieve laparoscopic gastrointestinal anastomosis like in esophagogastric surgery, or rectal surgery.

The laparoscopic linear stapler is a very useful device for tissue approximation. The stapler cartridges come in various sizes. Each of the different sizes is color-coded (Table 8.2 and Figs. 8.4 and 8.5) to allow for appropriate selection based on tissue thickness. This allows the surgeon to choose the appropriate homeostasis/ tissue apposition without significant ischemia or tissue destruction. The common staple cartridges used to accommodate different tissue thicknesses for appropriate tissue management are shown in Figs. 8.4 and 8.6. Based on the stapling height, the cartridges are in descending order: Black, Green, Gold, Blue, White, and Grey (Fig. 8.7). The black cartridge is used in thicker tissues such as the antrum of the stomach and Rectal transection while white and Grey are used in thin tissues such as small bowels and blood vessels.

If the closed staple height is too high, it may inadequately appose the tissues resulting in leakage, bleeding, and/or dehiscence. Conversely, if the staple height selected is too low, ischemia, serosal shearing, or "cheese wiring" may result,

Table 8.2 Stapler color codes and tissues sealed

Stapler color code	Tissues used to seal	Tissue thickness
White	Small bowel, blood vessels	Thin
Blue	Body and fundus of the stomach, colon	Medium thickness
Gold	Body of stomach	Medium thickness
Green	The antral region of the stomach and Rectum	Thick tissues
Black	Antral region of the stomach, Rectum	Thick tissues

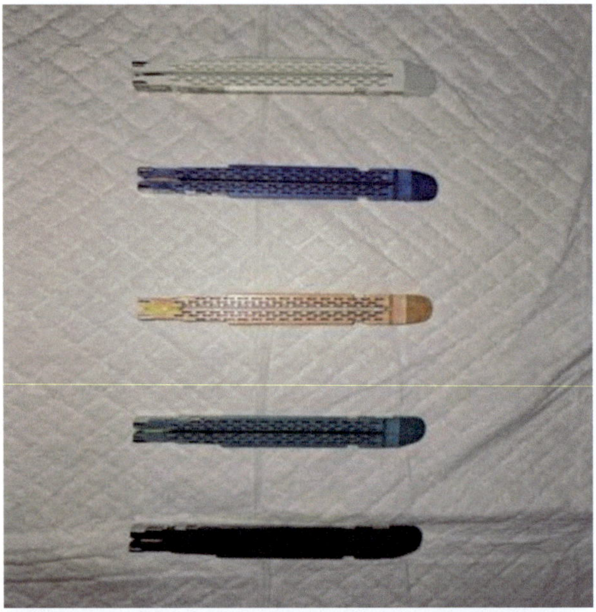

Fig. 8.4 Laparoscopic stapler reloads from above downward Viz; White, Blue, Gold, Green, and Black colors

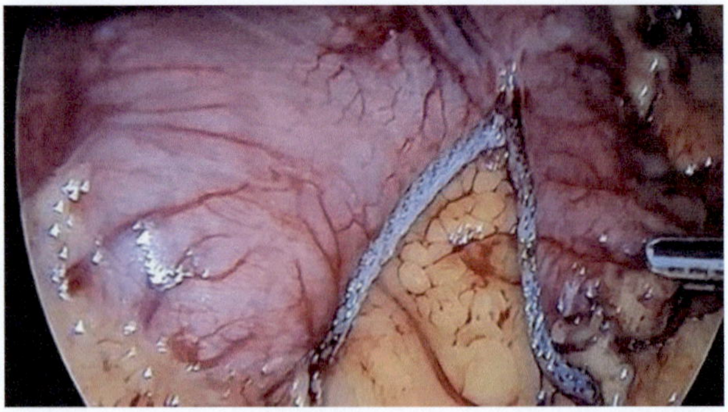

Fig. 8.5 Stapling gastric antrum during laparoscopic sleeve gastrectomy

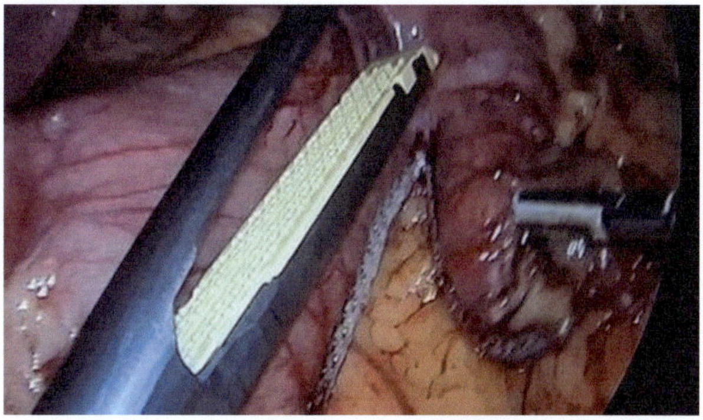

Fig. 8.6 Gold color reload used for second stapling greater curvature of the stomach adjacent to the incisura angularis during laparoscopic sleeve gastrectomy

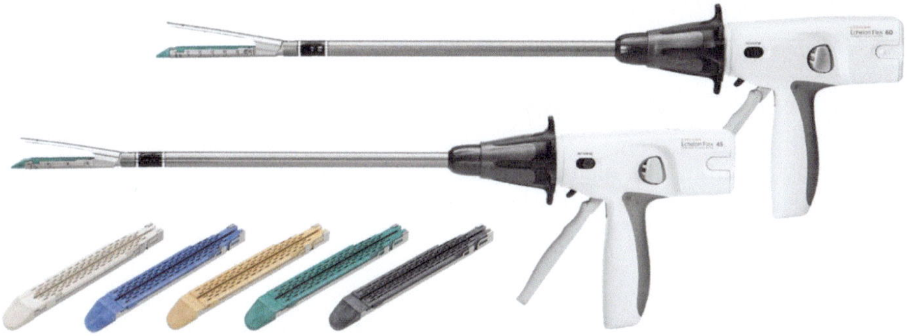

Fig. 8.7 Laparoscopic staplers handle with reloads

potentially leading to leakage or frank necrosis. Modern laparoscopic staplers are arranged in three rows with varying stapling heights. When fired, each staple is shaped into a B-shape staple form, which helps secure the tissue. However, staple malfunction can occur because staple leg bending depends on several tissue/stapler characteristics including tissue thickness, tissue viscosity, staple height, and other staple properties (thickness, bending characteristics, type of metal, etc). Staples are designed to form consistently, and staples that are not forming as intended should be investigated.

Other Tissue Approximation Devices

Though in use, other useful tools for tissue approximation do not necessarily diminish the importance of suturing. These include clips and clip appliers (Fig. 8.8), ligating instruments, fibrin glue, and a bio-fragmentable anastomosis ring [9–11].

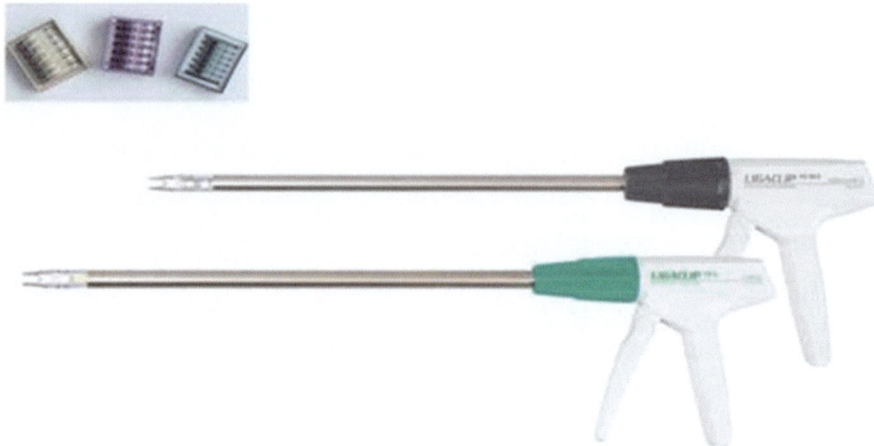

Fig. 8.8 Laparoscopic clips and clip Appliers

Ligating Instruments include diathermy, Harmonic scalpel, LigaSure, and Thunderbeat. These instruments also perform some form of tissue approximation [12, 13] (See in Chap. 3).

Recent Advances in Laparoscopic Suturing and Tissue Approximation

Virtual Reality Simulators Laparoscopic box trainers have been used to enhance skill acquisition in laparoscopic suturing and Tissue approximation, however, an innovative training tool—the Virtual Reality Simulators has recently proven to be more useful in making a seemingly complex process to be simple with better engagement of surgical trainees [14].

Suturing Techniques Laparoscopic suturing, extracorporeal, and intracorporeal knotting are used. In recent randomized controlled studies comparing intracorporeal and extracorporeal open and closed knotting techniques, students were found to have achieved significantly better results using extracorporeal knot tying as it was found to be faster, more precise, and associated with reduced knot-spread ability [15, 16]. Other tissue approximation innovations include barbed sutures, advances in hydrogel adhesives, and the "flip-flap" technique for laparoscopic port-site closure [17–19].

Novel Devices Novel methods of achieving tissue approximation by tissue fusion using infrared devices have been developed [20].

Prospects

Tissue Approximation Devices Although not yet used in humans, the Su2ura Approximation Device has been used in laboratory animals and found to have no safety concerns [21].

References

1. Mishra RK. Textbook of practical laparoscopic surgery. 3rd ed. New Delhi: Jaypee Brothers Medical Publishers; 2013. p. 120–39.
2. Mishra RK. Mastering the techniques of laparoscopic suturing and knotting. 1st ed. New Delhi: Jaypee Brothers Medical Publishers; 2009.
3. Bhatia P, John SJ, Deed JP. Step by step art of endo-suturing. 1st ed. New Delhi: Jaypee Brothers Medical Publishers; 2005. p. 10–24.
4. Croce E, Olmi S. Intra-corporeal knot-tying and suturing techniques in laparoscopic surgery: technical details. JSLS. 2000;4(1):17–22.
5. Kothari R, Somashekar U, Sharma D, Thakur DS, Kumar V. A simple and safe extracorporeal knotting technique. JSLS. 2012;16(2):280–2.
6. Hart S, Hashemi L, Sobolewski CJ. Effect of a disposable automated suturing device on cost and operating room time in benign Total laparoscopic hysterectomy procedures. JSLS. 2013;17:508–16.
7. Hültl H. II Kongress der Ungarischen Gesellschaft für Chirurgie. Budapest, Mai 1908. Pester Med Chir Presse. 1909;45:108–10, 121–122
8. Akopov A. Surgical staplers: the history of conception and adoption. Ann Thorac Surg. 2021;112(5):1716–21.
9. Freire DF, Taha MO, Soares JH, Simoes M, Fagundes AL, Fagundes DJ. The laparoscopy splenic injury repair. The use of fibrin glue in a heparinized porcine model. Acta Cir Bras. 2011;26(3):235–41.
10. Masoomi H, Luo R, Mills S, Carmichael JC, Senagore AJ, Stamos MJ. Compression anastomosis ring device in colorectal anastomosis: a review of 1,180 patients. Am J Surg. 2013;205(4):447–51.
11. Forde KA, Goodell KH, DellaBadia M. A 10-year single-institutional study of the biofragmentable anastomosis ring. Am J Surg. 2006;191(4):483–7.
12. Smith AV, Kondo MT, Kondo W, Cabrera R. Laparoscopic surgical devices: a review of the newest energies and instruments. Int J Med Sci Health Res. 2018;2:40–60.
13. Gyn PA. Principles of electrosurgery in laparoscopy. Pan. 2019;2(1):22–9.
14. Akritidou E, Lykoudis PM, Nastos C, Dellaportas D, Pararas N, Papaconstantinou D, Theofilogiannakou E, Davoutis E, Giannou AD, Pikoulis E. Virtual reality simulation training in laparoscopic suturing and knot-tying: a narrative review. Ann Laparosc Endosc Surg. 2024.
15. Labrosse KB, Marinho C, Fellmann-Fischer B, Geissler F, Schötzau A, HeinzelmannSchwarz V, Zwimpfer TA. Intracorporeal vs. extracorporeal open and closed knot tying techniques in laparoscopy: a randomized, controlled study. Heliyon. 2024;10(3)
16. Förster CE, Calabretti I, Gubser L, Schötzau A, Fellmann-Fischer B, HeinzelmannSchwarz V, Zwimpfer TA. Comparison of different suture techniques for laparoscopic vaginal cuff closure. Sci Rep. 2024;14(1):4860.
17. Vázquez FJ, Argüelles D, Muñoz JA, Genton M, Méndez Angulo JL, Climent F, Roquet I, Iglesias M, Velloso Álvarez A, Vitoria A, Bulnes F. Use of knotless barbed sutures in laparoscopic inguinal Hernioplasty in horses: 40 cases. Animals. 2024;14(12):1826.

18. Hu X, Grinstaff MW. Advances in hydrogel adhesives for gastrointestinal wound closure and repair. Gels. 2023;9(4):282.
19. Wani AA, Khuroo S, Jain SK, Heer VK, Rajput D, Maqsood S. The "Flip-Flap" technique for laparoscopic port-site closure—description of a novel, cost-effective technique with review of literature. Surg J. 2021;7(03):e168–71.
20. Cipolato O, Leuthold T, Zäch M, Männel G, Aegerter S, Sciascia C, Jessernig A, von Salis M, Sarcevic S, Rosendorf J, Liska V. Robotic laser tissue soldering for atraumatic soft tissue fusion guided by fluorescent nanothermometry. Adv Sci. 2024:2406671.
21. Ramot Y, Rousselle S, Steiner M, Lavie Y, Ezov N, Nyska A. Safety and performance evaluation of Su2ura approximation, a new suturing device, in pigs. Toxicol Pathol. 2022;50(2):211–7.

Chapter 9
Tissue/Organ Retrieval and Port Closure

Olanrewaju Samuel Balogun

Introduction

Laparoscopic surgery allows the execution of minimally invasive procedures using small "keyhole" incisions to assess the abdomen for diagnostic and therapeutic purposes. It is widely employed in several scenarios from tissue biopsy to removal of intact tissues and organs like in open surgical procedures. However, it requires minimal effort to remove tissue specimens in open surgery through a large incision created for access. Retrieval of larger tissues and organ specimens can be technically challenging for beginners in laparoscopy. Most times such specimens are larger than the access route used to gain entry into the abdomen. The extension of a surgical incision to accommodate a large specimen violates the basic principle and cosmetic aim of minimally invasive surgery [1]. It is also important to realize that infected and potentially malignant specimens should be prevented from direct contact with the anterior abdominal wall to avoid sepsis and port site implantation of mitotic cells. The choice of technique of tissue retrieval in laparoscopy is largely dependent on the size and nature of the tissue as well as the procedure type [2].

O. S. Balogun (✉)
Lagos University Teaching Hospital (LUTH), Lagos, Nigeria
e-mail: osbalogun@unilag.edu.ng

E. Ray-Offor, R. J. Rosenthal (eds.), *Principles and Practice of Laparoscopic Surgery*, https://doi.org/10.1007/978-3-031-96321-6_9

Tissue Retrieval Techniques

Laparoscopic Aspiration Needle

As an alternative to percutaneous needle biopsy, specimens may be obtained under direct visualization with the confirmation of hemostasis at laparoscopy using the laparoscopy aspiration needle (Fig. 9.1). An intraoperative ultrasound probe may be used to identify discrete liver lesions, confirm appropriate biopsy methods, and avoid venous structures. In the presence of ascitic fluid, this is aspirated and sent for cytology. Yet in the absence of ascites, 200 cc of normal saline can be instilled into the peritoneal cavity and aspirated from the pelvis and bilateral subdiaphragmatic spaces for cytologic examination [3].

Laparoscopy Biopsy Forceps

An effective method for small tissue biopsy involves using laparoscopic biopsy forceps (Fig. 9.2). This instrument comprises a spiked cup at the insertion tip and a terminal at the handle for connection to the electrosurgery unit. A wedge biopsy with cupped forceps is followed by coagulation.

Tissue Retrieval Bags

Several tissue-retrieval techniques using bags have been developed to facilitate the extraction of larger tissue specimens and organs from the abdomen. Tissue retrieval bags are of different types [4]. Some commercial retrieval bags in disposable pouches of various sizes are pre-loaded into 5 mm or 10 mm cylindrical introducers. A flat metal beam and purse-string sutures are swaged at the rim of the pouch to facilitate the opening and closing. Structurally, commercial retrieval bags are made from ripstop (reinforced)Nylon configured into a pouch system lined by polyurethane inner coating. Endo-pouches are available as simple bags or bags with opening and closing mechanisms. They include Endopouch® (Ethicon) and Endocatch® (Medtronic) (Fig. 9.3).

Endopouches are invaluable in the following settings:

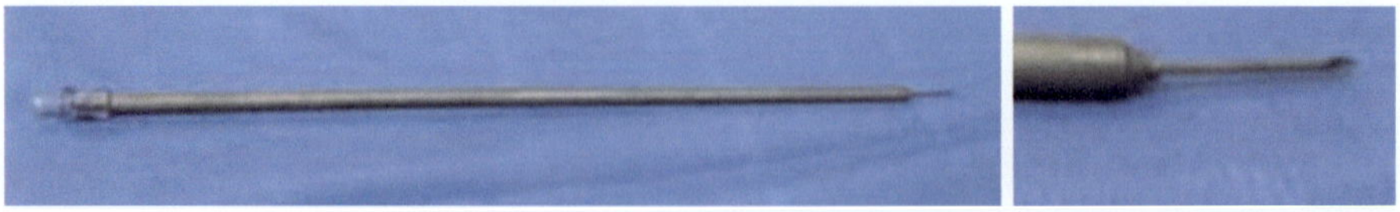

Fig. 9.1 Laparoscopic aspiration needle

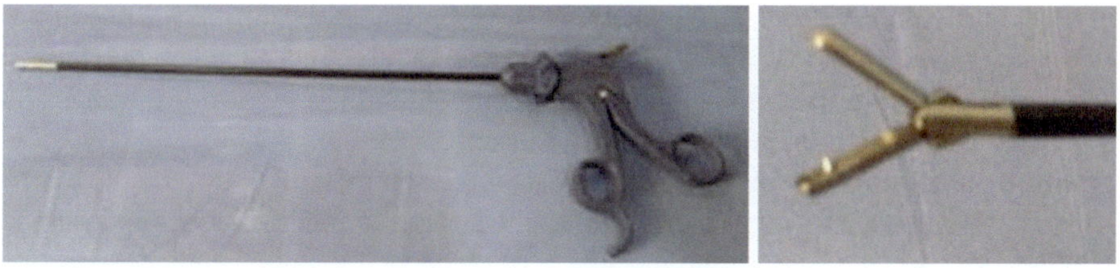

Fig. 9.2 Laparoscopic biopsy forceps

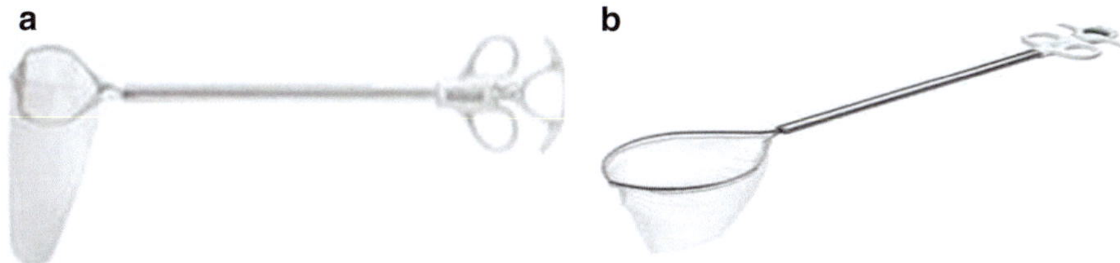

Fig. 9.3 Tissue retrieval bags (**a**) Endopouch (**b**) Endocatch

- When there is a need to extract infected tissue specimens such as the inflamed appendix
- Extraction of malignant tissues and organs to prevent port site implantation
- To contain spillage of gallstones during gallbladder extraction.
- To contain specimen that requires further fragmentation before removal. This method is employed during the extraction of splenic tissue or a large hydronephrotic kidney

The desirable properties in choosing an Endo bag include the size, opening and closing mechanisms, tenacity, ability to withstand considerable stretch without tearing or ripping, impermeability to fluids and microbial organisms, and ease of handling [5, 6].

Technique

The method of specimen extraction from the abdomen during laparoscopic surgery depends largely on the size and nature of the tissue or organ to be removed and the type of retrieval sac available.

The technique of using the retrieval bag entails:

1. Introduction of the bag through the trocar or the port site with the trocar removed
2. Once the introducer is inside the abdomen, the neck of the bag is opened by pushing forward on the plunger on the tail of the introducer. This deploys the bag in an open configuration inside the abdomen.
3. Placement of specimen inside the bag with the aid of a traumatic (Allis) grasper

4. Specimen entrapment inside the bag is accomplished by pulling on the suture string on the tail of the introducer. This closes the aperture of the bag and causes separation of the sac from the flexible metal beam at the mouth of the sac. The metal beam is then pulled back into the introducer.
5. Bag extraction containing specimen is accomplished by pulling it through the trocar and both withdrawn as a unit through the port site incision under endoscopic guidance. An extension of the incision is often needed to create enough space for the delivery of the bag and the specimen. In some instances, a reduction in the volume of the specimen in the bag may be required before extraction. In laparoscopic cholecystectomy, for example, a partially extracted bag may be secured and opened above the skin level. The gallbladder is then opened and containing stones are fragmented and extracted with sponge-holding forceps. In addition, bile in the gallbladder may be suctioned to reduce its bulk for extraction through the port site.

Morcellation

Tissue morcellation is used for large benign solid tissue specimens that do not have to be removed in whole for pathologic examination [2]. A partially extracted sac can be opened, and the content fragmented by ring forceps, clamps suction, or commercial mechanical morcellators while keeping the sac under direct laparoscopic vision. Retrieval bags used for morcellation are large and tough. The commercial morcellator consists of a power-driven cutting tube with selectable speed. Tissue extraction can be accomplished with this device within a short period. The device enables precise cutting of tissues without alteration of the internal architecture of the tissue [7]. Morcellation is used to retrieve large solid benign renal and splenic masses. Many morcellators have been withdrawn from the market due to vascular or solid organ injury associated with their use. While morcellation may appear as a laudable option for the removal of large specimens, evidence shows that it may facilitate the dissemination of infection and malignant cells [8, 9].

Mini Laparotomy

A mini-laparotomy is used when there is a need to remove intact tissue specimens with the preservation of their anatomy. The mini-laparotomy is performed by extending one of the port site incisions or by making a fresh incision elsewhere on the anterior abdominal wall. Examples of such sites include the left lower midline incision for removing the spleen after laparoscopic splenectomy and, the Pfannenstiel incision for removing the sigmoid colon during sigmoid colectomy. A major drawback of mini-laparotomy is the high risk of wound contamination by infected specimens and the risk of malignant tumor implantation during specimen extraction [10]. A wound protector system such as Alexis(Applied Medical) helps to minimize this risk. Wound protector systems have wide applications in colorectal and bariatric surgeries.

Natural Orifice Specimen Extraction Surgery (NOSES)

This surgical approach refers to the use of traditional laparoscopic instruments, transanal endoscopic microsurgery (TEM), or soft endoscopy to obtain specimens through a natural orifice (oral cavity, vagina, or anus) without the aid of an abdominal auxiliary incision after abdominal operation [11]. The trans-anal route is commonly used for colon extraction during low anterior and abdominoperineal resections. The transvaginal route is popular with Gynecologists and is employed for the removal of the ovary and uterus during laparoscopic-assisted procedures.

Untoward Events During Specimen Extraction

- Misplaced or loss of tissue specimen. After excision, tissue specimens should be kept in areas where they can easily be retrieved and may unlikely get lost within tissues. Some surgeons during laparoscopic cholecystectomy routinely drop gallbladder specimens on the right lobe of the liver for easy access during the extraction phase.
- Rupture of retrieval bags may occur with the use of excessive traction force in an attempt to extract the bag from the port site.
- Tissue specimen rupture and spillage of content with peritoneal and port site contamination.
- Injury to adjacent viscus may result from impalement or entrapment of organs during specimen extraction.
- Wound infection from spillage of infected contents and direct wound contamination
- Seedling of port sites with malignant cells leading to port site metastasis
- Port site hernias may follow if there is a failure to close 10–12 mm ports in adults or 5 mm ports in children or due to poor technique.

Improvisations in Low- Middle-Income Countries

Home-Made Retrieval Sacs

The use of washed sterilized condoms, sterilized polyethylene bags, surgical latex hand gloves, or finger of latex hand gloves have been applied as alternatives to commercial endo bags in low-resource settings or in circumstances where endo bags are not available [1, 5]. These homemade devices are safe to use and effective for trapping and retrieving tissue specimens during laparoscopic cholecystectomy and appendectomy. Surgical latex gloves can be made into sacs by tying the base of the digits together with 2 concentric sutures and cutting off the glove digits distal to the sutures. Some authors also run a continuous concentric monofilament suture at the open end of the gloves to facilitate bag closure at specimen extraction.

Through the Cannula Method

Small specimens can be delivered through most available port sites. Intact tissue specimens such as the appendix may be extracted through 10-12 mm trocars with the cannula acting as a barrier to prevent contact of an infected appendix with the anterior abdominal wall [12]. In the cannula method, no bag is used, and is suitable for benign and preferably collapsible tissue specimens or organs with considerable wall resilience such as gallbladder and grossly hydronephrotic kidney. There are concerns that this method may increase the incidence of port site infection but is valuable in low/middle-income countries where commercial endo bags are not available or affordable.

Port Closure

The closure of trocar wounds is performed at the end of laparoscopic surgery. A good technique is required for closing wounds created during trocar insertion to prevent or minimize complications such as post-operative port-site hernia and intestinal obstruction. It is estimated that the incidence of port site complications after laparoscopic surgery is 21 per 100,000 cases [13, 14]. Port site complications are highly dependent on the nature of the procedure, the size of the port, and the duration of surgery [15]. Port site complications include infection, hernia formation, tumor, and parasite implantation [14, 15]. As a rule, trocar wound size equal to or greater than 10-12 mm in adults and 5 mm or greater in children should be closed to prevent port site hernia [16, 17]. An ideal closure should include fascia and peritoneum approximation. However, fascia approximation can be difficult especially in obese patients due to the thick layer of fat on the anterior abdominal wall restricting access to deeper layers of fascia and peritoneum.

Port Closure Instruments

Techniques of trocar wound approximation range from direct closure with sutures to the use of purpose-built devices to assist the port closure, especially with fascia approximation. A variety of port closure devices have been designed for use in laparoscopic surgery. The selection of closure technique depends on the site and length of the incision, the patient's body build, and the surgeon's experience.

Port Closure Techniques

The common port closure techniques include:

A. *Direct fascia suturing*

   This is an open surgical procedure. The trocar wound is examined during desufflation, and fascial edges are grasped with traumatic clamps and sutured with simple sutures. The use of conventional open-surgery needles in fascia closure can be challenging in patients with thick anterior abdominal wall fat. This is due to the relatively high fascia depth to wound length ratio which restricts easy access to the fascia. The needle trajectory may miss anterior abdominal wall fascia incorporation during closure, this predisposes the patient to the development of port site hernia. Specialized J-type needles (Ethicon) were designed to facilitate fascia closure in this situation.

B. *Purpose-built port closure devices*

   These devices ensure the accuracy of trans-fascial suture placement when compared to direct needle closure. Port closure devices are of different types but are used in two different ways.

   (a) Port closure under direct laparoscopic guidance and visualization: the fascial defect is approximated using a device that is specifically designed for this purpose. These include suture passers (Fig. 9.4) [Carter-Thomason needle-point suture passer and the Endo-Close (Autosuture) suture carrier]. These devices are used to pass sutures across fascial and peritoneal defects for approximation under laparoscopic monitoring.
   (b) Port closure under the direct vision of the operating surgeon. This method requires good insufflation of the abdomen. Several techniques have been described under this approach. These include the suture carrier method, dual hemostat techniques, and Lowsley retractor with skin closure.

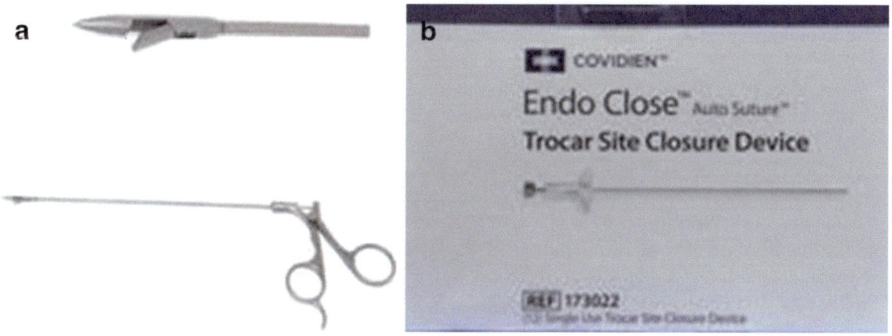

Fig. 9.4 (**a**) Laparoscopic Suture passer (**b**) EndoClose

C. *Skin closure*

Skin closure is the last step in tissue approximation during laparoscopic surgery. The quality of skin closure determines the eventual cosmetic appearance of the surgical scar. Subcuticular sutures have long been used for skin closure in laparoscopic surgery but other methods like skin staples, surgical tapes (Steri-strips), and tissue adhesives have shown good results. Skin approximation using Octyl cyanoacrylate after laparoscopic cholecystectomy is effective and economical. This method also leads to shorter operating times and greater efficiency when compared to monofilament sutures [18].

References

1. Schellpfeffer MA. A novel laparoscopic tissue retrieval device. J Soc Laparoendosc Surg. 2011;15:527–32.
2. Amer N, Amer M, Mishra K, R. Different techniques of tissue retrieval from abdominal cavity during minimal access surgery. World J Laparosc Surg with DVD. 2013;6:63–8.
3. Society of America Gastrointestinal and Endoscopic Surgeons (SAGES). Guidelines for diagnostic laparoscopy. SAGES guidelines [Internet]. 2022 [cited 2024 Nov 7]; Available from: sages.org/publications/guidelines/guidelines-for-diagnosticlaparoscopy.
4. Hye-Chun STH. Laparoscopic specimen retrieval bag in gyn surgery. Expert guidance on selection Surgical Technique. 2020;10:36–44.
5. Kao CC, Cha TL, Sun GH, Yu DS, Chen HI, Chang SY, et al. Cost-effective homemade specimen retrieval bag for use in laparoscopic surgery: experience at a single center. Asian J Surg. 2012;35:140–3.
6. Islam S, Bheem V, Maughn A, Harnarayan P, Dan D, Naraynsingh V. Surgical glove use for specimen removal in laparoscopy, the cheapest available: a prospective study. Trop Dr. 2020;50:94–9.
7. Stavroulis A, Memtsa M, Yoong W. Methods for specimen removal from the peritoneal cavity after laparoscopic excision. Obstetr Gynaecol. 2013;15:26–30.
8. Hall T, Lee SI, Boruta DM, Goodman A. Medical device safety and surgical dissemination of unrecognized uterine malignancy: morcellation in minimally invasive gynecologic surgery. Oncologist. 2015;20:1274–82.
9. Sizzi O, Manganaro L, Rossetti A, Saldari M, Florio G, Loddo A, et al. Assessing the risk of laparoscopic morcellation of occult uterine sarcomas during hysterectomy and myomectomy: literature review and the ISGE recommendations. Eur J Obstetr Gynecol Reprod Biol. 2018;220:30–8.
10. Binsaleh S. Specimen processing during laparoscopic renal surgery: a review of techniques and technologies. Clinics. 2014;69:862–6.
11. Tang Q, Zhu Y, Xiong H, et al. Natural orifice specimen extraction surgery versus conventional laparoscopic-assisted resection in the treatment of colorectal cancer: a propensity-score matching study. Cancer Manag Res. 2021;13:2247–57. Published 2021 Mar 9. https://doi.org/10.2147/CMAR.S291085.
12. Deziel DJCS-C. 8. Principles of specimen removal A. General considerations; 1999.
13. Aziz R. In: Ricardo A, Alvarez MA, editors. Practical manual of operative laparoscopy. 2nd ed. New York: Springer; 1992.
14. Karthik S, Augustine AJ, Shibumon MM, Pai MV. Analysis of laparoscopic port site complications: a descriptive study. J Minim Access Surg. 2013;9:59–64.
15. Chandra JN, Manivasagam SS, Choudhary S, Manocha P, Reddy BH. Insights into laparoscopic port site complications: a comprehensive review. Cureus. 2024;16:e63431.

16. Hamood MA, Mishra RK. Different port closure techniques in laparoscopy surgery. World J Laparosc Surg. 2009;2(3):29–38.
17. Krittiyanitsakun S, Nampoolsuksan C, Tawantanakorn T, Suwatthanarak T, Srisuworanan N, Taweerutchana V, et al. Is fascial closure required for a 12-mm trocar? A comparative study on trocar site hernia with long-term follow-up. World J Clin Cases. 2023;11:357–65.
18. Ben Safta Y, Maatouk M, Bouzidi MT, Sakly N, Mabrouk A, Bouafif M, et al. A randomized clinical trial to compare octyl cyanoacrylate with absorbable monofilament sutures for the closure of laparoscopic cholecystectomy port incisions. Int Wound J. 2020;17:449–54.

Chapter 10
Complications of Laparoscopic Surgery

Christopher N. Ekwunife

Introduction

The science and art of laparoscopic surgery have progressed rapidly over a relatively short period, transforming the surgical landscape. The surgeon adept at laparoscopic techniques must have invested a significant commitment and practice, perseverance, and patience to overcome the enormous challenges of the learning curve. This progress has been supported by advancements in technology, such as improved optical systems, enhanced energy devices, and the development of safer access tools, all of which have significantly mitigated some of the earlier challenges associated with this approach. The public recognizes the clear benefits of laparoscopic surgeries, such as reduced postoperative pain, shorter hospital stays, and faster recovery times. However, these perceived advantages may lead to unrealistic expectations. Complications, though less frequent than in open surgery, can temper these expectations and present significant challenges, particularly in otherwise healthy patient populations.

The risks associated with laparoscopic surgery are less than those from open surgery. However, the huge volume of laparoscopic surgeries being carried out now may magnify these risks. This becomes even more glaring when it happens in an otherwise healthy population of patients. Extensive research on complications of laparoscopic surgery can be derived from gynecologic literature. From the studies by Jansen et al., the mortality from laparoscopic surgery has been estimated at 8 per 100,000, which is significantly lower than the risk of death from abdominal operations [1]. Even during the early phase of adoption of minimal access surgery, laparoscopic cholecystectomy was reported to be associated with a 33% reduction in operative mortality compared to open cholecystectomy in Maryland, USA [1].

C. N. Ekwunife (✉)
Department of Surgery, Federal Medical Centre, Owerri, Imo State, Nigeria
e-mail: chrisekwunife@fthowerri.gov.ng

E. Ray-Offor, R. J. Rosenthal (eds.), *Principles and Practice of Laparoscopic Surgery*, https://doi.org/10.1007/978-3-031-96321-6_10

Currently, mortality appears to be more influenced by patient factors than by the surgical procedure itself [2].

The complexities of laparoscopic surgery are multifaceted and encompass anesthetic challenges, position-related risks, pneumoperitoneum management, safe access to the peritoneal cavity, and the potential for intraoperative and postoperative complications. This chapter aims to explore these complications comprehensively, offering strategies for prevention, early detection, and effective management to optimize patient outcomes.

Anaesthetic Complications

The majority of laparoscopic procedures are performed under general anesthesia. The pneumoperitoneum of laparoscopy can splint the diaphragm, leading to decreased pulmonary compliance and increased airway pressures. An in-depth discussion of the challenges related to anesthesia is discussed in Chap. 6. Regional Anaesthesia has become increasingly used.

Position-Related Complications

Optimal patient positioning is crucial in laparoscopic surgery to provide the surgeon with adequate access to the operative site. However, prolonged or extreme positions, such as the Trendelenburg or reverse Trendelenburg, can predispose patients to significant complications. The Trendelenburg position, often used in pelvic and colorectal surgeries, involves tilting the patient head-down to improve visualization of the operative field. However, this position increases venous return to the brain and head while reducing venous outflow, potentially leading to cerebral and upper airway edema. Over time, the elevated intracranial pressure may exacerbate pre-existing conditions such as intracranial hypertension or obstructive sleep apnea. Careful monitoring of the duration of Trendelenburg positioning is essential, and regular reassessment of the patient's hemodynamic status can help mitigate these risks. In procedures lasting more than 4 h in this position, compartment syndrome rarely may occur due to impaired arterial perfusion, compression of veins by the limb supports, and reduced venous drainage from the pneumoperitoneum. While periodic repositioning to the horizontal position every 2 h can help, additional preventive measures include the use of pneumatic compression devices to maintain lower limb circulation and ensuring that limb supports are padded and correctly positioned to minimize pressure on vascular structures. The reverse Trendelenburg position, commonly employed during upper gastrointestinal surgeries, also reduces venous return and may worsen hypotension in hypovolemic patients. This carries risks of myocardial or cerebral ischemia, necessitating close monitoring of blood pressure and volume status.

The increased risk of deep vein thrombosis from prolonged immobility and venous stasis in these positions further highlights the need for preventive strategies. Pharmacologic prophylaxis, such as lowmolecular-weight heparin, and mechanical prophylaxis, such as intermittent pneumatic compression devices, are recommended for high-risk patients.

Access Related Complications

Accessing the peritoneal cavity is a critical step in laparoscopic surgery. In a review of 25,764 laparoscopic gynecologic operations, Jansen et al. discovered that 57% of complications arose from access [3]. However, it is noteworthy that access-related injuries are reassuringly low, ranging from 5 per 10,000 to 3 per 1000 in large databases from France. However, they could be uncommonly fatal [4]. The placement of secondary trocars accounts for less than 5% of these injuries because they are inserted under direct vision. Nonetheless, there is no entry technique or device that is safe. The open technique of peritoneal access presents two major advantages over the Veress needle technique: injuries to major abdominal vessels are virtually eliminated, and visceral injuries are not only reduced but can be recognized and repaired immediately. The small bowel is the most commonly injured viscera in the access period, followed by the colon and the liver. Up to 50% of these bowel injuries may be unrecognized for more than 24 h postoperatively, leading to high morbidity and possible mortality. Immediate recognition and repair will ameliorate this condition. This can be done laparoscopically if visualization is adequate, and the surgeon is proficient. Otherwise, conversion to open surgery should be done. Vascular injuries tend to be more terrifying, in part due to the magnification inherent in laparoscopic surgery. Major vascular injuries during laparoscopic surgery are rare but potentially life-threatening, with an incidence of 0.09–0.14% and associated morbidity and mortality rates of 6–13% [5]. The most commonly affected vessels are the inferior epigastric vessels, followed by major vessels such as the right iliac vessels, inferior vena cava, and, less commonly, the abdominal aorta [6]. These injuries frequently occur during entry, particularly with the use of a Veress needle or trocar insertion. In the event of major vascular injury, conversion is the rule. However, attempts should be made initially to control the bleeding by direct pressure at the bleeding point with a sponge as preparation for conversion is being made. Several measures are necessary to prevent these complications. The surgeon should be aware of the patient's vascular anatomy. The patient should be adequately relaxed during the entry to reduce the axial force exerted by the surgeon. In patients who have had prior abdominal operations, first trocar entry should be away from previous incisions. The conically tipped and bladeless trocars are becoming more prevalent as they cause less trauma to the tissue. The choice of optical trocar permits the passage of the cannula through the abdominal wall under vision.

Pneumoperitoneum Related Complications

Important circulatory and respiratory changes occur during laparoscopic surgery. Pneumoperitoneum can decrease cardiac output and also cause hypercapnia and respiratory acidosis. When capnoperitoneum is maintained at 12–14 mmHg in ASA 1/11 patients, these changes are rarely clinically relevant. The monitoring of end-tidal CO_2 should be mandatory. In patients with limited pulmonary reserves, arterial blood gas monitoring is recommended, although laparoscopic surgery preserves post-operative pulmonary function better than open surgery. Gasless laparoscopy could be an alternative. The incidence of carbon dioxide embolism is very rare but potentially catastrophic. It can follow vessel injury during Veress needle insufflation, trocar placement, or intraoperatively. A sudden hypotension or drop in end-tidal CO_2 should alert the surgical team about this possibility; the 'millwheel' murmur is elicited on auscultation of the heart. Heart failure supervenes within minutes if appropriate measures are not taken. The remedial measures include stopping insufflation and deflating the abdomen, placing the patient head-down in the left decubitus position, giving 100% $O_{2,}$ and central venous catheterization with aspiration of carbon dioxide. Also, pneumomediastinum or pneumothorax can result from iatrogenic diaphragmatic injury or gas diffusion through a pre-existing diaphragmatic defect. More commonly, subcutaneous emphysema usually results from multiple attempts at initial abdominal entry, loose fitting cannulas, improper cannula placement, increased intra-abdominal pressures, and using the laparoscope as a lever [7].

Procedure-Related Intraoperative Complications

The gravity of intraoperative complications affects the complexity of laparoscopic procedures. Although about half of the complications that may occur may be unrelated to entry approaches, a quarter of these may be unrecognized at the time of surgery [3].

Bowel Injury

The small intestine is comparably the most injured bowel segment [8]. An injury can result when secondary ports are not placed under direct vision. Iatrogenic injury can also result during adhesiolysis. More commonly, they occur from electrosurgical current. Electrosurgical devices can cause thermal tissue damage through several mechanisms: unintended direct contact with tissue, current transmission through other conductive instruments (coupling), discharge due to insulation failure, and capacitive coupling, where accumulated charge from a monopolar electrode transfers energy to nearby tissue. Another established mechanism, antenna coupling, occurs when an active electrode emits energy that is passively captured by a nearby inactive wire [9].

Early recognition of bowel injury during laparoscopic surgery is crucial. Bowel contents may soil the peritoneal cavity if the injury site is visible, but this is not always the case. Management depends on the type of injury and the surgeon's expertise. Monopolar injuries, which tend to be extensive, typically require resection and anastomosis, while smaller bipolar injuries (involving less than half of the bowel's circumference) may allow for simple excision and closure. Experienced laparoscopic surgeons can often manage these laparoscopically; otherwise, conversion to open surgery is advised. If unrecognized intraoperatively, signs of injury may develop within 24 h post-surgery, including nausea, vomiting, increasing abdominal pain, distension, and reduced urine output, though fever may not yet be present. A lack of expected rapid recovery should prompt suspicion of a major abdominal complication. An urgent abdominal CT scan is recommended, and in many cases, immediate laparoscopy may be the most critical lifesaving intervention.

Vascular Injury

Vascular injuries can result from inadequate exposure to vascular structures or a lack of understanding of vascular abnormalities. The right hepatic artery may be mistaken for the cystic artery, during laparoscopic cholecystectomy. The iliac vessels may be injured during laparoscopic inguinal hernia repair, anterior resection, or pelvic lymphadenectomy. A transection of the inferior vena cava may result from urologic surgeries.

Bile Duct Injury (BDI)

The most important complication of laparoscopic cholecystectomy is biliary injury. Its incidence in laparoscopic cholecystectomy is 0.3–0.5% compared to 0.1–0.2% in open cholecystectomy [10]. However, there has been a trend towards a reduction in BDI over time [11]. It occurs more commonly when an operation is done in the presence of unclear biliary anatomy or acute cholecystitis. This complication can be suspected when there is bile in the operative field. In the postoperative period, peritonitis, jaundice, and sepsis may supervene. The appropriate intervention will depend on the type of injury, using the Strasberg classification as a guide. This will range from biliary stenting to bilio-enteric anastomosis. An immediate life-saving measure is the insertion of a drain intraoperatively. The surgeon should not ideally attempt a repair if he/she is not conversant with these repair procedures, the patient may benefit more from referral to specialist hepatobiliary surgeons. It is, however, more efficacious to prevent biliary injuries. Intraoperatively, adequate skeletonization of the structures in Calot's triangle to demonstrate the critical view of safety should be done before ligation of the cystic duct and artery. An intraoperative cholangiogram may come in handy where there is unclear anatomy of the biliary system.

Urinary Bladder Injury

Gynaecologic operations account for the bulk of these complications. It is also a rare complication of laparoscopic groin hernia repair. A good number of them are recognizable intraoperatively by the leakage of urine or the passage of blood and/or gas in the urethral catheter. In high-risk operations like laparoscopic hysterectomy, routine intravesical dye tests before the conclusion of the operation can help to detect inadvertent bladder injuries. Most laparoscopic surgeons should be able to close the bladder lacerations with a running absorbable suture.

Ureteric Injury

Ureteric injury can complicate colorectal, gynecology, and urology procedures. These injuries could result from transection, devitalization of blood supply, and electrothermal damage. With immediate recognition, repair should be done where expertise is readily available. A useful guide to preventing this injury is for the surgeon to identify the ureter before conducting dissection close to it. The insertion of preoperative ureteric stents in anticipated difficult procedures makes it easier for ureteric injuries to be detected early.

Splenic Injuries

The incidence of splenic iatrogenic injuries is a rare complication of radical gastrectomy, distal pancreatectomy as well as retroperitoneal urologic procedures. The more common minor capsular tears can easily be managed laparoscopically with pressure, argon plasma coagulation, and the application of hemostatic agents. More extensive injuries may warrant a splenectomy.

Postoperative Complications

Port-Site Infections

Surgical site infection is a recurring problem for all surgical wounds. Its incidence has been reduced by minimal access surgery. However, it still detracts from the obvious advantages of laparoscopic surgeries. It is reported that about 8% of laparoscopic cholecystectomies are complicated by umbilical port site infection. Thus, the umbilicus must be thoroughly scrubbed during skin preparation. The extraction of potentially infected tissues in retrieval bags should ensure the protection of the port sites. Adequate sterilization of ports and hand instruments or the use of disposable trocars/cannulas cannot be overemphasized.

Port Site Hernias

Port site hernias (PSHs) are an under-recognized complication of laparoscopic surgery, with reported incidence ranging from 0.57% to 1.47% [12]. However, high-quality studies suggest the true incidence may be as high as 40% [13]. These hernias carry a high risk of strangulation due to the small size of the defect. While most hernias occur at sites larger than 10 mm, cases have been reported at 5 mm port sites [14]. Preventing port-site hernias (PSHs) involves closing fascial defects of 10 mm or larger, ensuring the inclusion of both the peritoneum and fascia. Recommended strategies also include evaluating predisposing factors, applying precise surgical techniques, and utilizing fascial closure devices [15].

Port Site Metastasis

This complication is rarer than originally thought despite the increased volume of laparoscopic cancer operations being done. While the exact mechanism of port site metastasis (PSM) remains unclear, tumor aggressiveness is considered a leading factor [16]. Proposed theories for PSM include direct implantation, gas turbulence, tumor manipulation, and hematogenous spread [17]. The low incidence could be due to adherence to surgical oncologic principles, including utilization of wound protective devices. The presence of port site metastasis warrants a search for evidence of peritoneal tumor dissemination.

Postoperative Air Embolism

This complication is extremely rare. This can be explained by the sudden deflation of pneumoperitoneum, and thereafter the CO_2 trapped in the tissues forms bubbles that could be absorbed in the circulation. Patients may show hemodynamic changes in the postoperative period. This complication can be prevented by not using a high-pressure pneumoperitoneum during operation. It is also important to ensure initial gas injection at low flow.

References

1. Steiner CA, Bass EB, Talamini MA, Pitt HA, Steinberg EP. Surgical rates and operative mortality for open and laparoscopic cholecystectomy in Maryland. N Engl J Med. 1994;330(6):403–8.
2. Fakhoury HMA, Yousef Z, Tamim H, Daher S, Attasi AA, Al Ajlan A, et al. The combined effect of age and body mass index on postoperative mortality and morbidity in laparoscopic cholecystectomy patients. Front Surg. 2023;10:1243915.
3. Jansen FW, Kapiteyn K, Trimbos-Kemper T, Hermans J, Trimbos JB. Complications of laparoscopy: a prospective multicentre observational study. BJOG. 1997;104(5):595–600.
4. Champault G, Cazacu F, Taffinder N. Serious trocar accidents in laparoscopic surgery a French survey of 103,852 operations. Surg Laparosc Endosc. 1996;6(5):367–70.
5. King NR, Lin E, Yeh C, Wong JMK, Friedman J, Traylor J, et al. Laparoscopic major vascular injuries in gynecologic surgery for benign indications: a systematic review. Obstetr Gynecol (New York 1953). 2021;137(3):434–42.
6. Asfour V, Smythe E, Attia R. Vascular injury at laparoscopy: a guide to management. J Obstet Gynaecol. 2018;38(5):598–606.
7. Ott DE. Subcutaneous emphysema—beyond the pneumoperitoneum. JSLS. 2014;8(1):17.
8. Muntener M, Romero FR, Kavoussi LR. Complications in laparoscopic surgery. Berlin/Heidelberg: Springer; 2007. p. 349–63.
9. Cassaro S. Delayed manifestations of laparoscopic bowel injury. Am Surg. 2015;81(5):478–82.
10. MacFadyen BV, Vecchio R, Ricardo AE, Mathis CR. Bile duct injury after laparoscopic cholecystectomy: the United States experience. Surg Endosc. 1998;12:315–21.
11. Pucher PH, Brunt LM, Davies N, Linsk A, Munshi A, Rodriguez HA, Fingerhut A, Fanelli RD, Asbun H, Aggarwal R, SAGES Safe Cholecystectomy Task Force. Outcome trends and safety measures after 30 years of laparoscopic cholecystectomy: a systematic review and pooled data analysis. Surg Endosc. 2018;32:2175–83.
12. Owens M, Barry M, Janjua AZ, Winter DC. A systematic review of laparoscopic port site hernias in gastrointestinal surgery. Surgeon (Edinburgh). 2011;9(4):218–24.
13. Holihan JL, Chen JS, Greenberg J, Hehir D, Johnston SM, Marcus D, Ryan H, Tsuda S, Liang MK. Incidence of port-site hernias: a survey and literature review. Surg Laparosc Endosc Percutan Tech. 2016;26(6):425–30.
14. de Jager E, Wing G, Ho Y-H. Incarcerated 5-mm port site hernia: a systematic literature review and case report. Int Surg. 2019;104(11–12):550–5.
15. De Alwis D, Ades A, Nanayakkara P. Laparoscopic port-site hernia: an Underrecognized iatrogenic complication of laparoscopic surgery. Obstet Gynecol Surv. 2021;76(12):751–9.
16. Sooriakumaran P, Kommu SS, Anderson C, Rane A. Port-site metastasis after laparoscopic surgery: what causes them and what can be done to reduce their incidence? BJU Int. 2009;103(9):1150–3.
17. Ramirez PT, Wolf JK, Levenback C. Laparoscopic port-site metastases: etiology and prevention. Gynecol Oncol. 2003;91(1):179–89.

Chapter 11
Simulation and Training in Laparoscopic Surgery

Elad Boaz, Noam Kahana, Ana Pena, Samuel Szomstein, Emanuele Lo Menzo, and Raul J. Rosenthal

Introduction

Laparoscopic surgery, or minimally invasive surgery, has revolutionized the field of surgical procedures. The advent of laparoscopic cholecystectomy in the late 1980s resulted in a rapid demand to introduce the procedure into clinical practice due to

E. Boaz · N. Kahana
Department of General Surgery, The Bariatric and Metabolic Institute, Ellen Leifer Shulman and Steven Shulman Digestive Disease Center, Cleveland Clinic Florida, Weston, FL, USA

Department of General Surgery, Shaare Zedek Medical Center, Faculty of Medicine, Hebrew University of Jerusalem, Jerusalem, Israel

A. Pena
Department of General Surgery, The Bariatric and Metabolic Institute, Ellen Leifer Shulman and Steven Shulman Digestive Disease Center, Cleveland Clinic Florida, Weston, FL, USA

S. Szomstein
Department of General Surgery, The Bariatric and Metabolic Institute, Ellen Leifer Shulman and Steven Shulman Digestive Disease Center, Cleveland Clinic Florida, Weston, FL, USA

Herbert Wertheim College of Medicine, Florida International University, Miami, FL, USA

E. Lo Menzo
Minimally Invasive and Bariatric Surgery, The Bariatric and Metabolic Institute, Ellen Leifer Shulman and Steven Shulman Digestive Disease Center, Weston, FL, USA

Department of General Surgery, General Surgery Residency Program, Cleveland Clinic Florida, Weston, FL, USA

Florida Atlantic University College of Medicine, Boca Raton, FL, USA

Florida International University College of Medicine, Miami, FL, USA

R. J. Rosenthal (✉)
Division of General Surgery, Ronald Reagan UCLA Medical Center, David Geffen School of Medicine, Los Angeles, CA, USA
e-mail: rosentr@ccf.org

E. Ray-Offor, R. J. Rosenthal (eds.), *Principles and Practice of Laparoscopic Surgery*, https://doi.org/10.1007/978-3-031-96321-6_11

numerous advantages over traditional open surgery, including smaller incisions, reduced pain, shorter hospital stays, and quicker recovery times. Consequently, laparoscopic surgery is a current requirement in the basic skill set that a surgeon must acquire during training. While traditional surgical education followed the "see one, do one, teach one" Halstead's principle, laparoscopic surgery demands a unique skill set distinct from open surgery. It involves working with real-time images on a monitor using endoscopic instruments, navigating and manipulating outside the line of vision, camera handling, depth perception, and tissue manipulation [1].

The implementation of worktime regulations worldwide has restricted the duration a trainee can dedicate to gaining skills in the hospital [2]. Various factors such as economic, social, cultural, and legal constraints further contribute to limiting opportunities for trainees to develop essential skills in the operating room (OR). Consequently, simulation and training have become integral components in preparing surgeons for the challenges of laparoscopy. Proficiency in laparoscopy surgery involves stepwise deliberate practice due to the distinct skill set required. The learning curve is prolonged, necessitating structured training. Simulations offer a non-threatening environment for trainees to repeatedly practice skills without compromising patient safety. Teaching laparoscopy skills during actual operations is challenging due to safety concerns, varying case complexity, and additional time requirements [3]. Several studies demonstrate the transferability of technical skills learned in simulation environments to the OR [4, 5].

Various training and assessment modalities exist, including laparoscopic surgery courses, fellowships, on-site mentoring programs, and accredited residency programs. Current surgical trainees routinely gain experience in basic laparoscopic procedures like appendectomy and cholecystectomy. This chapter explores the significance of simulation in laparoscopic surgery training, diverse simulation methods and technologies, and the future of simulation-based training.

Importance and Benefits of Simulation Training

The aviation industry has an extensive history of researching and utilizing simulation, aiming to transfer skills in real scenarios while minimizing costs and risks to lives and aircraft. This successful approach was embraced by the surgical field in the late twentieth century, particularly for teaching minimally invasive procedures. Training simulations create a structured and effective learning environment without compromising patient safety [6]. The application of simulation techniques relies on breaking down complex activities into simple parts and encouraging deliberate and repeated practice, along with standardized and monitored assessments. Additionally, simulation facilitates effective feedback from educators. Surgical skill training, when conducted through simulation prior to actual procedures, has demonstrated more effective learning in the OR. Simulation holds the potential to enhance experiential learning, improve patient safety, replicate infrequently encountered scenarios, and assess trainees' skills and competence in diverse situations [7]. Mental training in laparoscopic surgery has become increasingly recognized as a valuable component of surgical education and skill development. This approach is defined as the “cognitive rehearsal of a task in the absence of overt physical movement.” [8]. The combination of motor and mental training sessions has been validated as a tool to enhance surgical performance [9, 10]. Key benefits of simulation in surgery include the following:

- **Risk Reduction**: Surgeons can make and learn from mistakes without endangering patients and minimizing errors during real procedures.
- **Skill Development**: Trainees can practice specific techniques, such as suturing or knot tying, repeatedly until mastery is achieved.
- **Procedure Familiarization**: Simulators help surgeons become familiar with laparoscopic instruments, camera systems, different procedures, and the associated OR setup.
- **Team Training**: Simulation is a valuable tool for training entire surgical teams, fostering effective communication and teamwork.
- **Assessment and Feedback:** Instructors can objectively assess trainees’ performance, providing constructive feedback for continuous improvement.

Types of Laparoscopic Simulators

A wide range of simulation methods and technologies are available for laparoscopic surgery training, each with its advantages and limitations.

Physical Box Trainers

Physical box simulators are containers designed for the placement and manipulation of objects or organs using surgical instruments (Fig. 11.1). These cost-effective devices provide a simple yet effective replication of the laparoscopic environment. Typically, these simulators incorporate traditional laparoscopic instruments and are particularly valuable for novice surgeons in the early stages of learning laparoscopic skills. The simulation model utilizes synthetic materials, animal organs, and tissues to create a realistic training scenario. Basic skills, including instrument handling, camera

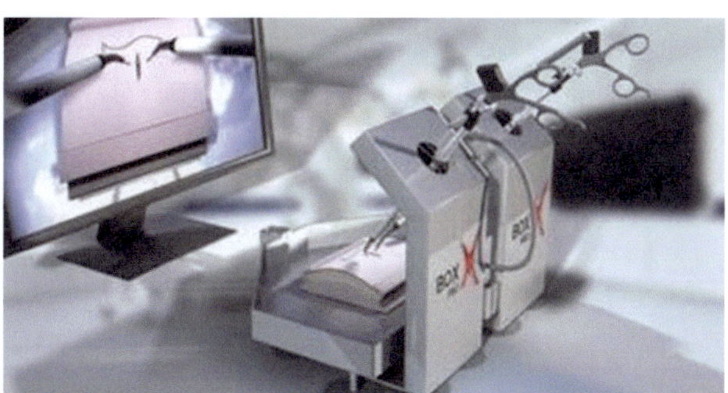

Fig. 11.1 Lap-X Box®- a traditional box trainer

manipulation, and hand-eye coordination, are developed using these trainers. While the tactile feedback quality is perceived to be akin to that experienced in the OR, a notable drawback is the absence of robust assessment metrics and objective feedback.

Virtual Reality Simulators

Virtual reality simulators (VRS) immerse trainees in a computer-generated laparoscopic environment, offering a realistic 3D experience for practicing various procedures. These simulators, like the well-validated Minimally Invasive Surgical Trainer-Virtual Reality (MIST-VR; Mentice Inc., San Diego, CA) and the newer LapSim Basic Skills and Dissection (Surgical Science, Gothenburg, Sweden) (Fig. 11.2) utilize abstract graphics to create high-fidelity simulations suitable for both training and assessment purposes [11]. Present laparoscopic VRS software replicates essential psychomotor skills, including cutting, grasping, and suturing, enabling trainees to acquire the skills necessary for real-time procedures. Reports generated by these simulators often include metrics such as error rates, time taken, and economy of instrument motion. They track individual performance and present results through graphs and tables promptly. VRS systems may lack realistic haptic feedback and vary in fidelity, cost, tasks, and metrics, influencing their availability and utilization.

Augmented Reality (AR) Simulators

AR simulators superimpose digital information onto the actual laparoscopic view, enriching training by offering guidance, highlighting structures, and providing step-by-step instructions during procedures. These laparoscopic simulators utilizing AR not only deliver realistic haptic feedback but also offer objective assessments after each performance.

Hybrid Simulators

Hybrid simulation combines physical box trainers with VR or AR elements (Fig. 11.3). This approach provides the benefits of both physical and virtual training, allowing trainees to interact with physical objects while benefiting from the advantages of digital simulation.

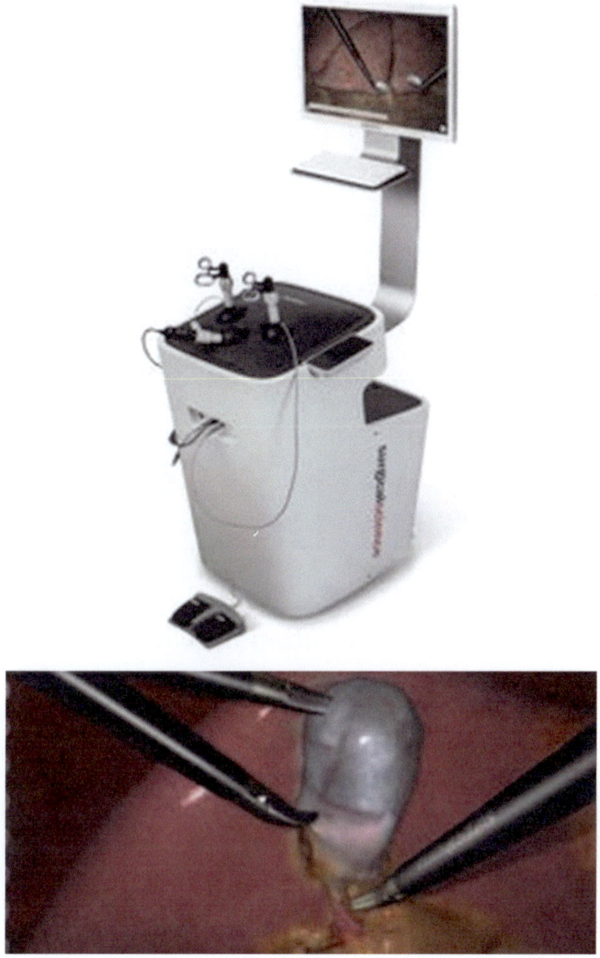

Fig. 11.2 Virtual laparoscopic cholecystectomy on the LapSim® virtual reality (VR) simulator

Animal and Cadaver Models

While not true simulations, animal and cadaver models are used for advanced laparoscopic training. These models offer the closest approximation to real surgical conditions, allowing trainees to practice on living tissue. Animal models play a significant role in surgical training and education. Live animal surgery remains the most realistic training model, offering a realistic anatomy and tissue haptics (high fidelity) unmatched by other kinds of simulation models, but are limited by costs and ethical concerns. Simulations in animal labs are unique portals in surgical training that allow learners to work on live tissues in real OR-simulated situations.

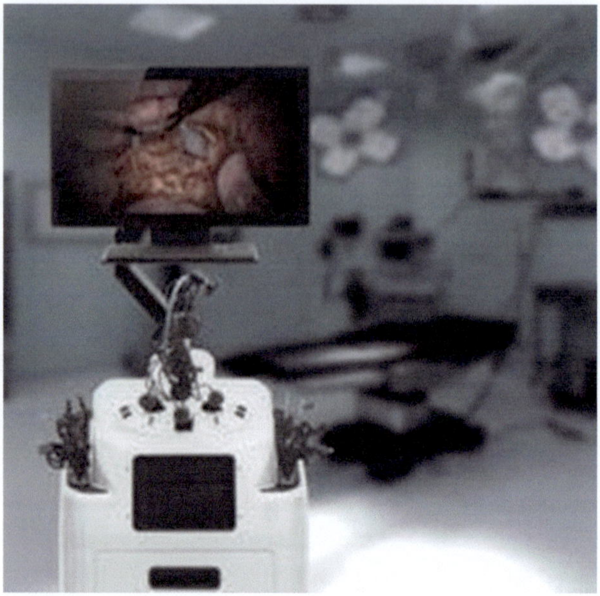

Fig. 11.3 Laparo Apex PRO® hybrid simulator

Integration of Simulation into Surgical Education

The advancements in laparoscopic surgery have prompted the emergence of a new paradigm, acknowledging the vital necessity for skills acquisition beyond the confines of the OR. The primary objective of any simulation program is to effectively transfer acquired skills to real-life scenarios. Several validation studies consistently report the efficacy of simulation in surgical education, showcasing the successful transfer of skills to the OR, enhanced performance, and reduced errors. For example, in randomized controlled trials (RCTs) focusing on inguinal hernia repair, simulation-based education was associated with decreased operative time, improved surgical performance, reduced complications, and shorter hospital stays compared to the control group [12, 13]. Similar positive results were reported in RCTs evaluating simulation training for laparoscopic cholecystectomy [14], bariatric surgery [15], and laparoscopic colectomy [16]. A systematic review, which included RCTs assessing various simulation methods in real operating theaters, suggested that simulation-based training contributes to improved operating performance among novice surgeons [4].

Fundamentals of Laparoscopic Surgery Course

Introduced at the Society of American Gastrointestinal and Endoscopic Surgeons (SAGES) Conference in 2004, the Fundamentals of Laparoscopic Surgery (FLS) course was designed to impart essential skills for laparoscopic surgery. Since

2009, this program has been established as a prerequisite for the American Board of General Surgery Qualifying Examination. Comprising both theoretical and practical components, the FLS course includes standardized exercises on a bench model (Fig. 11.4), involving tasks like moving objects between positions and performing intra- and extra-corporeal suturing. A study by Hafford et al. revealed that only 30% of active surgeons who had not received training in simulation were able to pass the FLS course, highlighting a distinct deficiency in laparoscopic technical skills compared to trained surgeons [17]. The FLS program has been widely validated, demonstrating its correlation with basic technical skills in the OR. FLS certification serves as a potential patient safety measure for surgeons engaged in minimally invasive surgery. Consequently, there is growing interest among medical insurance carriers to encourage surgeons to obtain FLS certification.

Despite these positive findings, notable variability exists across training programs in the adoption and integration of simulation for technical skills acquisition and proficiency assessment. One significant reason for this variability lies in the absence of strict methodologies aimed at ensuring the reliability and validity of assessment tools. In the realm of simulation, it is essential to establish the cost-effectiveness of a surgical simulation program for the institution. Studies have shown that simulation programs, especially those utilizing bench models and virtual simulators with more than 10 residents, prove to be more profitable than exclusive conventional training [18].

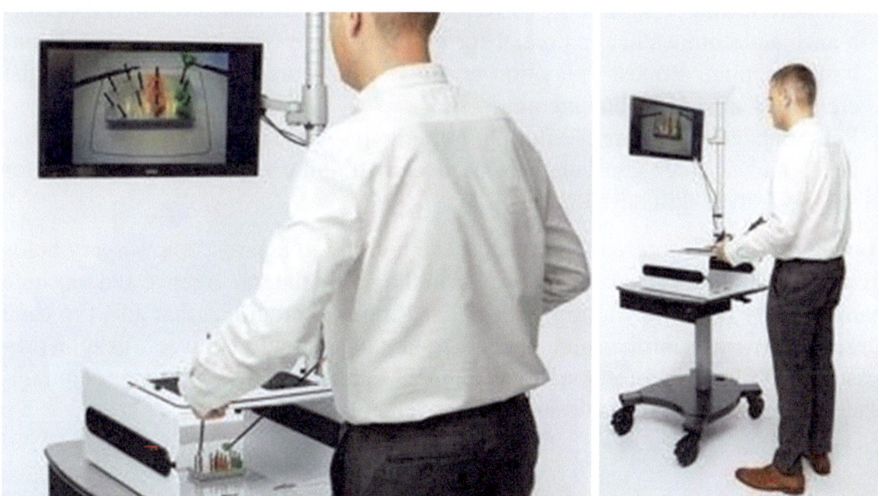

Fig. 11.4 Fundamentals of Laparoscopic Surgery (FLS) trainer system

Challenges and Future Directions

Surgical education is undergoing a transformative shift, with most residency programs focusing on increasing surgical practice within constrained schedules while upholding patient safety standards and integrating minimally invasive surgery into traditional training. Simulation emerges as a promising solution to this challenging task, offering the opportunity to shorten learning curves in a safe and controlled environment by transferring skills acquired during training to the OR.

The scope of surgical simulation should extend beyond residency programs. Instead, it should be integrated into medical undergraduate programs for basic procedures and utilized by practicing surgeons seeking continuous training and learning. Despite the numerous advantages of simulation-based training in laparoscopic surgery, there are challenges to overcome, including the following:

- **Cost**: High-quality simulators can be costly to acquire and maintain, necessitating efforts to address cost barriers and ensure broader access to simulation training.
- **Realism**: Simulators should strive for greater realism to provide trainees with a more authentic experience. This includes improvements in haptic feedback and realistic tissue behavior.
- **Integration into Curriculum**: Successfully incorporating simulation into surgical training programs requires careful planning and curriculum development to ensure seamless integration with existing educational frameworks.
- **Validation and Assessment**: Developing objective measures of trainee performance and competence is crucial for ensuring the effectiveness of simulation-based training. Robust validation and assessment processes contribute to the credibility of simulation outcomes.
- **Personalized Training**: Tailoring training programs to individual learners' needs and abilities can enhance the overall training experience, allowing for more effective skill development.

Looking ahead, the future of simulation and training in laparoscopic surgery holds promise. Technological advancements, including artificial intelligence and machine learning, may pave the way for personalized training programs that adapt to each surgeon's progress. Furthermore, the integration of simulation into certification processes and ongoing professional development is likely to become more commonplace, contributing to the continuous improvement of surgical skills.

References

1. Hasson HM. Core competency in laparoscopic surgery. JSLS. 2006;10(1):16–20.
2. Collins JP 2nd. International conference on surgical education and training. International consensus statement on surgical education and training in an era of reduced working hours. Surgeon. 2011;9(Suppl 1):S3–5.

3. Scott DJ, Cendan JC, Pugh CM, Minter RM, Dunnington GL, Kozar RA. The changing face of surgical education: simulation as the new paradigm. J Surg Res. 2008;147(2):189–93. https://doi.org/10.1016/j.jss.2008.02.014.
4. Spiliotis AE, Spiliotis PM, Palios IM. Transferability of simulation-based training in laparoscopic surgeries: a systematic review. Minim Invasive Surg. 2020;2020:5879485. https://doi.org/10.1155/2020/5879485.
5. Palter VN, Orzech N, Reznick RK, Grantcharov TP. Validation of a structured training and assessment curriculum for technical skill acquisition in minimally invasive surgery: a randomized controlled trial. Ann Surg. 2013;257(2):224–30. https://doi.org/10.1097/SLA.0b013e31827051cd.
6. Scott DJ. Patient safety, competency, and the future of surgical simulation. Simul Healthc. 2006;1(3):164–70. https://doi.org/10.1097/01.sih.0000244453.20671.f2.
7. Zendejas B, Brydges R, Hamstra SJ, Cook DA. State of the evidence on simulation-based training for laparoscopic surgery: a systematic review. Ann Surg. 2013;257(4):586–93. https://doi.org/10.1097/SLA.0b013e318288c40b.
8. Arora S, Aggarwal R, Sirimanna P, Moran A, Grantcharov T, Kneebone R, Sevdalis N, Darzi A. Mental practice enhances surgical technical skills: a randomized controlled study. Ann Surg. 2011;253(2):265–70.
9. Immenroth M, Bürger T, Brenner J, Nagelschmidt M, Eberspächer H, Troidl H. Mental training in surgical education: a randomized controlled trial. Ann Surg. 2007;245(3):385–91. https://doi.org/10.1097/01.sla.0000251575.95171.b3.
10. Rosenthal R, Rosales A, Menzo E, Dip F. Mental conditioning to perform common operations in general surgery training. New York: Springer; 2020.
11. Van Dongen KW, Tournoij E, Van der Zee DC, et al. Construct validity of the LapSim: can the LapSim virtual reality simulator distinguish between novices and experts? Surg Endosc. 2007;21:1413–7.
12. Zendejas B, Cook DA, Bingener J, et al. Simulation-based mastery learning improves patient outcomes in laparoscopic inguinal hernia repair: a randomized controlled trial. Ann Surg. 2011;254(3):502–11. https://doi.org/10.1097/SLA.0b013e31822c6994.
13. Kurashima Y, Feldman LS, Kaneva PA, et al. Simulation-based training improves the operative performance of totally extraperitoneal (TEP) laparoscopic inguinal hernia repair: a prospective randomized controlled trial. Surg Endosc. 2014;28(3):783–8. https://doi.org/10.1007/s00464-013-3241-8.
14. Seymour NE, Gallagher AG, Roman SA, et al. Virtual reality training improves operating room performance: results of a randomized, double-blinded study. Ann Surg. 2002;236(4):458–64. https://doi.org/10.1097/00000658-200210000-00008.
15. Duran Espinoza V, Belmar Riveros F, Jarry Trujillo C, et al. Five-year experience training surgeons with a laparoscopic simulation training program for bariatric surgery: a quasi-experimental design. Obes Surg. 2023;33(6):1831–7. https://doi.org/10.1007/s11695-023-06616-0.
16. Palter VN, Grantcharov TP. Development and validation of a comprehensive curriculum to teach an advanced minimally invasive procedure: a randomized controlled trial. Ann Surg. 2012;256(1):25–32. https://doi.org/10.1097/SLA.0b013e318258f5aa.
17. Hafford ML, Van Sickle KR, Willis RE, et al. Ensuring competency: are fundamentals of laparoscopic surgery training and certification necessary for practicing surgeons and operating room personnel? Surg Endosc. 2013;27(1):118–26. https://doi.org/10.1007/s00464-012-2437-7.
18. Orzech N, Palter V, Reznick R, Aggarwal R, Grantcharov T. A comparison of 2 ex vivo training curricula for advanced laparoscopic skills: a randomized controlled trial. Ann Surg. 2012;255:833–9.

Part II
Applications of Laparoscopic Techniques

Chapter 12
Diagnostic Laparoscopy

Ademola Adeyeye and Ogbu E. Ngim

Introduction

Diagnostic laparoscopy (DL) represents a major milestone in the evolution of surgery. Combining the principles of minimally invasive surgery (MIS) with the diagnostic capabilities of direct visual inspection has transformed the management of a wide spectrum of abdominal and pelvic conditions. Historically, the first recorded laparoscopic procedure in humans was performed by Hans Christian Jacobaeus in the early twentieth century (almost a hundred years ago) [1, 2]. Over time, advancements in optics, instrumentation, and anesthetic techniques have greatly enhanced the safety and utilization of laparoscopy.

Today, diagnostic laparoscopy bridges the gap between non-invasive imaging techniques (such as abdominal ultrasound and CT scans) and exploratory laparotomy, thus, offering a higher diagnostic accuracy with reduced patient morbidity [3]. Diagnostic Laparoscopy is a safe and well-tolerated procedure that can be performed in an inpatient or outpatient setting under general or occasionally local anesthesia with intravenous sedation in carefully selected patients with a reported diagnostic accuracy of 90–100% [4, 5]. The main limitation of the procedure is in

A. Adeyeye (✉)
Department of Colorectal Surgery, King's College Hospital, London, UK

Faculty of Life Sciences and Medicine, King's College, London, UK

Afe Babalola University, Ado-Ekiti, Ekiti State, Nigeria
e-mail: ademola.adeyeye1@nhs.net

O. E. Ngim
Department of Surgery, University of Calabar, Calabar, Cross River State, Nigeria

Department of Surgery, University of Calabar Teaching Hospital (UCTH), Calabar, Cross River State, Nigeria

E. Ray-Offor, R. J. Rosenthal (eds.), *Principles and Practice of Laparoscopic Surgery*, https://doi.org/10.1007/978-3-031-96321-6_12

the evaluation of retroperitoneal structures such as the pancreas, where additional dissection and tissue manipulation are needed, increasing the surgical risk and implications for patients.

The role of diagnostic laparoscopy has expanded with the integration of cytology, biopsy techniques, and imaging adjuncts such as fluorescence-guided visualization [4, 5].

Indications

Diagnostic laparoscopy is particularly suited for cases where clinical and imaging findings are lacking and inconclusive. These commonly include the following conditions:

Acute Conditions

Acute Abdomen

The panoramic view of the abdomen offered by the laparoscope aids accurate diagnosis of suspected acute abdominal conditions such as acute appendicitis (Fig. 12.1), acute cholecystitis, acute diverticulitis (for Hinchey I and IIa), perforated peptic ulcer disease, ruptured amoebic liver abscess, pelvic inflammatory disease (PID), endometriosis and adnexal pathologies [4–6].

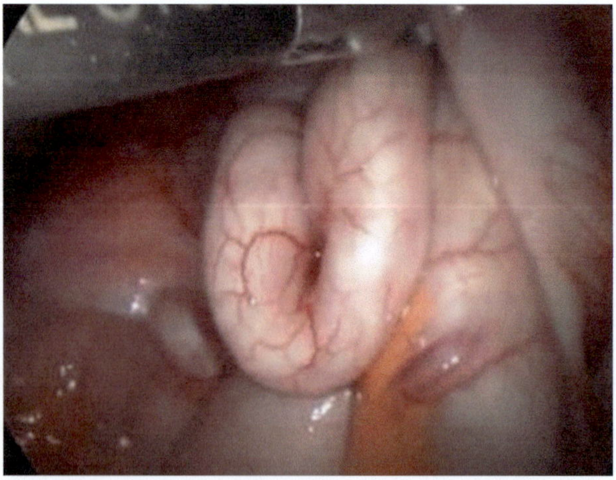

Fig. 12.1 Inflamed appendix kinked from adhesions

Vascular Disorders

Diagnostic laparoscopy has proven to be a reliable means in diagnosing mesenteric vascular ischemia where adjunctive tools for assessing blood flow, including computed tomography angiography, are not readily available. Clinical assessment in this condition is often non-specific and a prompt diagnostic laparoscopy can settle the diagnosis thereby guiding appropriate treatment and avoiding unnecessary exploratory laparotomy with its attendant morbidity, especially in the elderly who often have other comorbidities [7].

Abdominal Trauma

Diagnostic laparoscopy is indicated in suspected but unproven intra-abdominal injury after blunt or penetrating abdominal trauma. The use of diagnostic laparoscopy in trauma has remained a topical issue though it is generally accepted that such patients should be hemodynamically stable before undergoing the procedure. Injuries to the flank, epigastric regions, and retroperitoneum are often missed by diagnostic laparoscopy compared to laparotomy. However, there are certain situations in which laparoscopy is valuable, including diaphragmatic and small bowel injuries, which don't typically present clearly on traditional imaging. In the case of diaphragmatic injuries, laparoscopic access is often easier and faster compared to the open approach. The sensitivity, specificity, and diagnostic accuracy of diagnostic laparoscopy when used to predict the need for laparotomy is reported to be as high as 75–100% [4]. Patients with penetrating abdominal trauma who are stable can be discharged within 24–48 h of diagnostic laparoscopy in contrast to open laparotomy for which they will spend several days in the hospital [3, 4].

Intensive Care Unit (ICU)

The main indications for diagnostic laparoscopy in ICU patients are unexplained sepsis, systemic inflammatory response syndrome, and multisystem organ failure. However, laparotomy should be considered in cases of pneumoperitoneum, massive gastrointestinal bleeding, and small bowel obstruction [8].

Cancer Staging (Staging Laparoscopy)

Staging laparoscopy is useful in the evaluation of intra-abdominal malignancies such as peritoneal carcinomatosis from gastric, pancreatic, and ovarian cancer (Fig. 12.2) [9–11]. Its deployment also helps in determining operability by evaluating resectability, thus avoiding unnecessary laparotomy if the tumor is unresectable. A Cochrane review found that diagnostic laparoscopy before laparotomy with

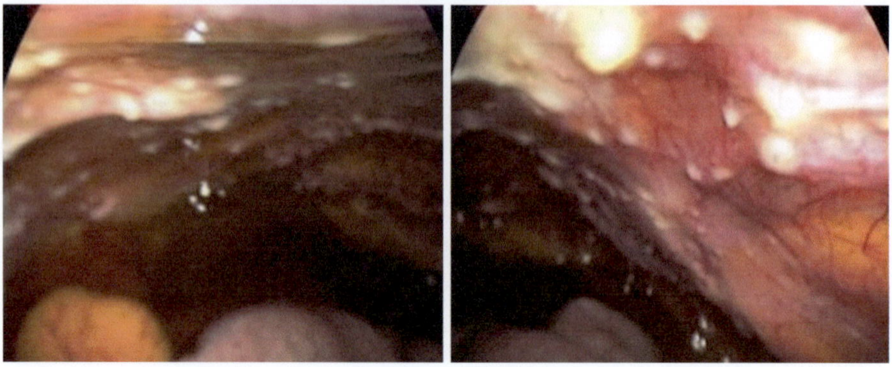

Fig. 12.2 Carcinomatosis peritonei from a rectal cancer

laparoscopic ultrasound scan as an adjunct can decrease the rate of unnecessary laparotomy from 17% to 40% in patients with pancreatic and periampullary cancer diagnosed as a resectable disease from abdominal CT scan [12]. This procedure also enables guided visual biopsies to be taken as well as diagnose occult intraabdominal metastasis.

Chronic Abdominal Conditions

Chronic Pelvic Pain

Chronic pelvic pain can be associated with multiple etiologies and is defined as pelvic pain lasting more than 6 months. It is a complex disorder caused by a myriad of causes ranging from endometriosis, PID, and fallopian tube pathologies such as inflammation, adhesions as well as tubal blockade. Benign gynecologic disorders offer an array of applications for DL. Studies have shown greater than 90% sensitivity and specificity in determining the cause of chronic pelvic pain. The commonest findings on laparoscopy were adhesions in 40%, endometriosis in 18%, and pelvic congestion syndrome in 20% of cases while 10% of the patients had a normal pelvis [13–15].

Adhesions/Adhesive Bowel Obstruction

Accurate diagnosis of recurrent bowel obstructions from post-operative adhesions or other reasons can be facilitated by DL (Fig. 12.3). This approach offers a minimized risk of postoperative recurrence compared to laparotomy.

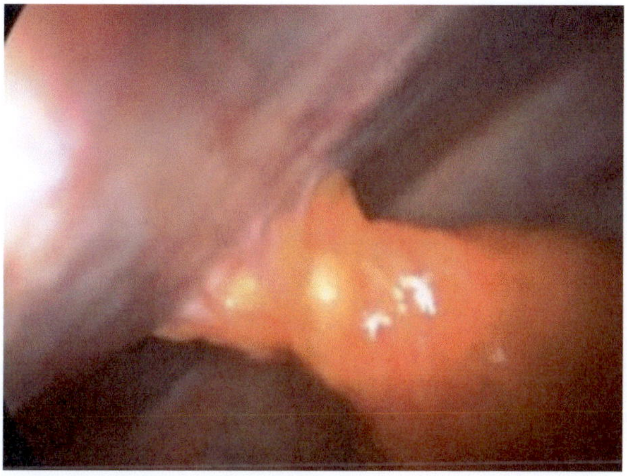

Fig. 12.3 Adhesion to Lanz incision site

Liver Disease

Diagnostic laparoscopy with the aid of intraoperative ultrasound scan has been used in the diagnosis of a wide range of liver pathologies such as liver cirrhosis, and discrete liver masses (metastatic cancer, hepatoma, benign masses, etc) with the added advantage of ultrasound-guided biopsy of these lesions [14] (Fig. 12.4).

Infertility

Diagnostic laparoscopy is a useful adjunct in the investigation of infertility. Its role in the laparoscopic dye test cannot be overemphasized as tubal patency is well demonstrated by the spillage of dye into the peritoneal cavity under direct vision. Diagnostic laparoscopy is also important in evaluating other causes of female infertility such as endometriosis and adhesions involving the fallopian tubes.

Cryptorchidism

Laparoscopy has a sensitivity of 99–100% for the diagnosis of undescended testes [16].

Patent Processus Vaginalis

The evaluation of a contralateral patent processus vaginalis is feasible.

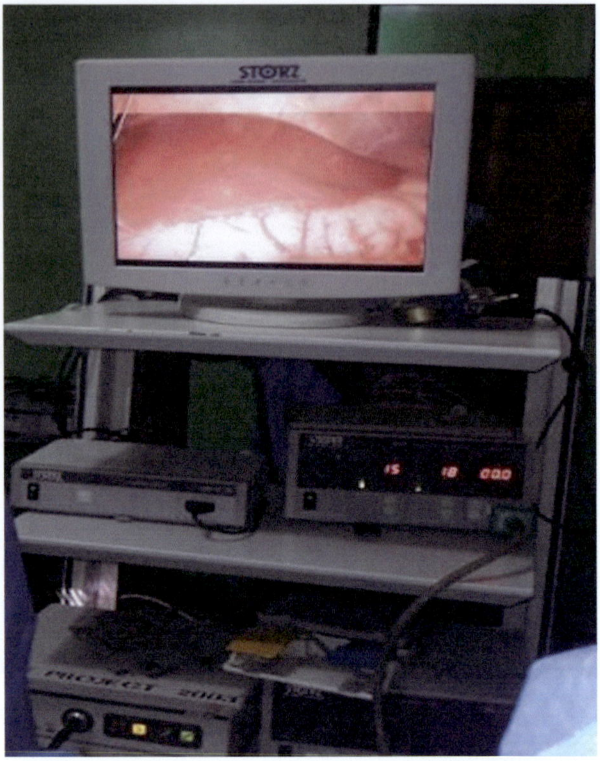

Fig. 12.4 Diagnostic laparoscopy—liver surface

Others

Second Look (Re-Look)

A re-look diagnostic laparoscopy can be performed within 24–48 h of an abdominal surgery (open or laparoscopic) if the patient's condition demands. Following laparoscopic surgery, DL can be used to determine the presence of anastomotic leaks or collections when imaging is equivocal [17]. Relook DL is also used extensively post-treatment with chemotherapy or radiotherapy where residual disease may be detected which ultimately influences treatment options in these patients.

Palpable Intra-Abdominal Mass

DL is useful in this scenario where other imaging techniques fail to establish a diagnosis in addition to the possibility of taking a biopsy of the mass.

Contraindications [4]

These may be relative or absolute depending on some limiting factors.

Absolute Contraindications

- Uncorrected coagulopathy: Increased risk of bleeding.
- Uncorrectable hypercapnia >50 torr
- Severe cardiopulmonary instability: Intolerance to pneumoperitoneum, shock
- Peritonitis requiring immediate laparotomy: DL diagnostic delays or may worsen outcomes.
- Hemodynamically unstable trauma patients: They require immediate laparotomy
- Abdominal wall dehiscence
- Abdominal compartment syndrome

Relative Contraindications

- Dense intra-abdominal adhesions: Higher risk of visceral or vascular injury.
- Morbid obesity: Technical challenges in port placement and visualization.
- Advanced pregnancy: Altered anatomy increases procedural complexity.
- ICU patients who are too ill to withstand the procedure and anesthesia
- Presence of anterior abdominal wall infection (cellulitis or soft-tissue infection)
- Multiple anterior abdominal wall surgeries with marked scarring
- Aortoiliac aneurysmal disease (may be associated with increased risk of vascular rupture)
- Pregnancy (2nd or 3rd trimester)
- Cardiopulmonary compromise

Pre-procedure Preparation

Adequate pre-operative preparation includes:

- Detailed history and examination
- Relevant baseline and specific investigations, based on the patient's medical history and comorbidities, including complete blood count and chemistry ECG, Chest X-ray, urinalysis, and coagulation profile among others.

- An Informed consent must be obtained on admission and specific complications peculiar to laparoscopic surgery (e.g. fatal gas embolism, hypercarbia, postoperative crepitus, and pneumothorax, etc) should be explained to patients in addition to other possible complications of the surgical intervention and anesthesia.
- Mandatory fasting for at least 6 h for solid food, and 2 h for clear liquids, to minimize the risk of aspiration except in hemodynamically stable trauma patients where appropriate anesthetic technique is deployed.
- Thromboprophylaxis and antibiotic prophylaxis should be administered as indicated
- The possibility of conversion to open surgery due to unforeseen conditions such as uncontrollable hemorrhage or visceral injury should also be made known to the patient
- The World Health Organisation surgery safety checklist should be adhered to [18]
- Availability and functionality of all relevant instruments/equipment required for the procedure should be ascertained before the commencement of DL

Technique

Anesthesia

General anesthesia is usually employed although local anesthesia (with sedation) can be used in some circumstances including very ill patients in ICU and selected trauma patients. Placing a nasogastric tube and/or urethral catheter is optional but generally recommended. A close monitoring of blood pressure, pulse, respiratory rate, oxygen saturation, ECG, and level of sedation is necessary.

Positioning

The patient is usually placed supine with the ability to tilt the position of the operating table. For example, a pelvic examination is best done with the patient in a Lithotomy position and a manipulator can be introduced into the cervix or a rectal probe, if necessary, for further retraction (Fig. 12.5). These instruments are usually not used during conscious sedation.

Access and Port Placement

Primary peritoneal access by the Veress needle technique is rapid and less invasive in a virgin abdomen. Usually through Palmer's point (located approximately 3 cm distal to the left costal margin in the mid-clavicular line) or a periumbilical incision.

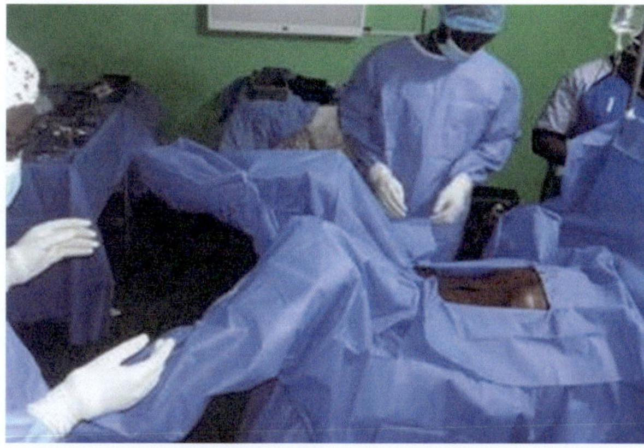

Fig. 12.5 Modified Lithotomy (Lloyd-Davies) with Trendelenburg position under general anesthesia

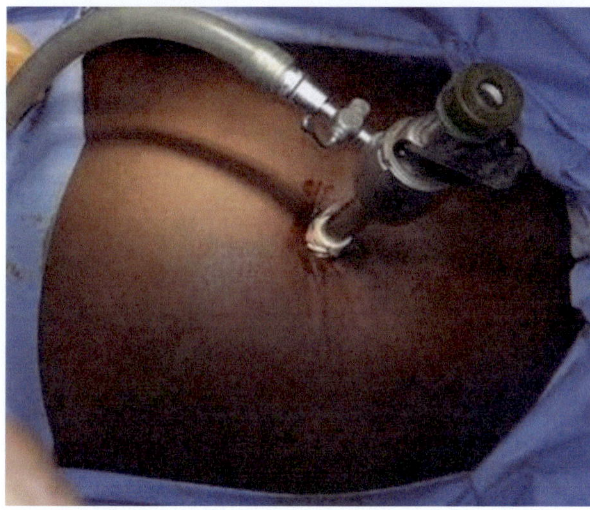

Fig. 12.6 Umbilical port for pneumoperitoneum inserted via Hasson technique

The Hasson's open technique is usually at the umbilicus and is preferred in patients with prior abdominal surgeries (Fig. 12.6). Alternatively, the optical trocar option allows clear dissection of the anterior abdominal wall under vision during access. This primary trocar position could be either a 10 or 5 mm port depending on the size of the telescope. A 30^0 telescope is preferred to a 0^0 telescope for DL because of the wider field of vision it offers.

Pneumoperitoneum is created usually with carbon dioxide (CO_2) at a flow rate of 1-3 L/min and a pressure of 12–15 mmHg. Lower pressure settings (<8 mmHg) are used if the procedure is being done under local anesthesia with sedation. Working ports are placed under direct vision. A key consideration in port placement is the number of ports needed. Generally, one camera port is required and at least one 5 mm working port is used. A typical configuration is an umbilical camera port, and a secondary port in the left lower quadrant. Other ports are inserted as required

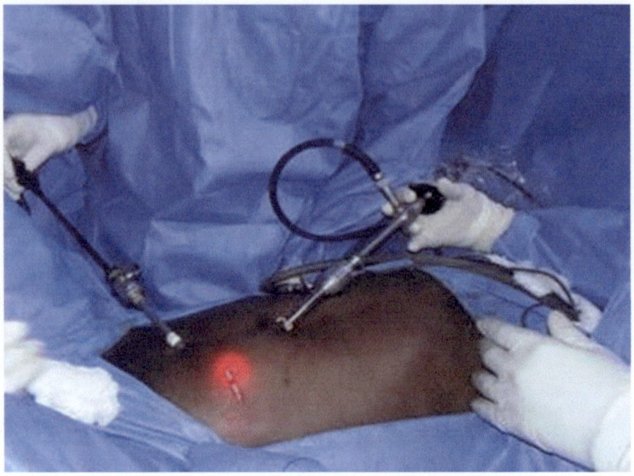

Fig. 12.7 Placement of additional ports

(Fig. 12.7). To enhance operative dexterity, the ports should be placed to form an equilateral triangle or a diamond, with the camera and the distance to the operative target considered. Sometimes in penetrating abdominal trauma, the injury site could be used as an entry port before the positions of other ports are determined.

Systematic Inspection

A systematic inspection is done once access to the peritoneal cavity is obtained. Begin with the diaphragm and liver, progressing systematically to evaluate all quadrants as well as the peritoneal surface of the anterior abdominal wall. Peritoneal washings should be collected before instrument manipulation. The use of an atraumatic grasper to manipulate organs and assess mobility. For malignant conditions, the primary site is sought, metastasis to the liver and other intra-abdominal organs. Biopsies of suspected lesions can be done at this stage and hemostasis secured. Targeted biopsies are performed on suspicious lesions using laparoscopic forceps. It is important to note that biopsies should not be attempted if appropriate hemostatic equipment is not available to avoid uncontrollable hemorrhage, which may turn out to be fatal. On completion of the procedure, the capnoperitoneum is released and any port more than 7 mm should be closed. Local infiltration of the port site with local anesthetic is practiced by some surgeons before proper dressing of these sites.

Post-operative Care

Urinary catheters and nasogastric tubes are removed soon after surgery before the patient is fully conscious except otherwise indicated. Suppository non-steroidal anti-inflammatory drugs (NSAIDs) and paracetamol are effective with the addition of opioids if pain is severe. Bowel sounds usually return hours after surgery; however, oral sips can be commenced 4–6 h after surgery. Patients are usually discharged on the same day after surgery after satisfactorily tolerating oral fluids and light feeds but are instructed to return to the hospital if they have any symptoms of concern such as severe abdominal pain. Port site sutures are handled as appropriate during the post-op visit and any biopsy results and other findings should be discussed with the patient.

Useful Tips for Beginners

- Instrument Familiarity: Practice on simulators to develop dexterity
- Ensure all the instruments you require are available and working before you scrub for the surgery
- Access for primary trocar must be done with care, especially in patients with previous abdominal scars. Palmer's position may be a safe option
- Patient positioning: Adjust table angles to optimize organ visibility.
- Avoiding Injury: Use blunt dissection and avoid over-retraction.
- Position your ports to allow for adequate triangulation
- Use atraumatic graspers
- Hold (gently) the mesentery rather than the bowel
- Follow a rule of "2" in assessing (or running!) the bowel: 2 sides (mesenteric and antimesenteric), 2 junctions (duodenojejunal junction and ileocecal junction), 2 passes (checking at least twice), 2 independent observers (ideally).
- Recognizing limitations: Do not hesitate to convert if there is a grave danger to the patient e.g. from uncontrollable hemorrhage and there is no experienced laparoscopic surgeon around
- Remember "conversion *(preferably proactive rather than reactive)* is not a failure" and "First do no harm"

References

1. Hatzinger M, Kwon ST, Langbein S, Kamp S, Häcker A, Alken P. Hans Christian Jacobaeus: inventor of human laparoscopy and thoracoscopy. J Endourol. 2006;20(11):848–50. https://doi.org/10.1089/end.2006.20.848.
2. Alkatout I, Mechler U, Mettler L, Pape J, Maass N, Biebl M, Gitas G, Laganà AS. Damaris Freytag the development of laparoscopy—a historical overview. Front Surg. 2021:799442. https://doi.org/10.3389/fsurg.2021.799442.
3. Agresta F, Ansaloni L, Baiocchi GL, et al. Laparoscopic approach to acute abdomen from the Consensus Development Conference of the Società Italiana di Chirurgia Endoscopica e nuove tecnologie (SICE), Associazione Chirurghi Ospedalieri Italiani (ACOI), Società Italiana di Chirurgia (SIC), Società Italiana di Chirurgia d'Urgenza e del Trauma (SICUT), Società Italiana di Chirurgia nell'Ospedalità Privata (SICOP), and the European Association

for Endoscopic Surgery (EAES). Surg Endosc. 2012;26:2134–64. https://doi.org/10.1007/s00464-012-2331-3.
4. Society of American Gastrointestinal Endoscopic Surgeons guidelines for diagnostic Laparoscopy. https://www.sages.org/. Accessed online 6 Jan 2025.
5. Stefanidis D, Richardson WS, Chang L, Earle DB, Fanelli RD. The role of diagnostic laparoscopy for acute abdominal conditions: an evidence-based review. Surg Endosc. 2009;23:16–23.
6. Simko S, Wright KN. The future of diagnostic laparoscopy—cons. Reprod Fertil. 2022;3(2):R91–5. https://doi.org/10.1530/RAF-22-0007. PMID: 35706581; PMCID: PMC9175578
7. Gonenc M, Dural CA, Kocatas A, Buyukasik S, Karabulut M, Alis H. The impact of early diagnostic laparoscopy on the prognosis of patients with suspected acute mesenteric ischemia. Eur J Trauma Emerg Surg. 2013;39(2):185–9.
8. Alemanno G, Prosperi P, Di Bella A, et al. Bedside diagnostic laparoscopy for critically ill patients in the intensive care unit: retrospective study and review of literature. J Minim Access Surg. 2019;15(1):56–62.
9. Van Hootegem SJM, Chmelo J, van der Sluis PC, Lagarde SM, Phillips AW, Wijnhoven BPL. The yield of diagnostic laparoscopy with peritoneal lavage in gastric adenocarcinoma: a retrospective cohort study. Eur J Surg Oncol. 2024;50(4):108233.
10. Morris S, Gurusamy KS, Sheringham J, Davidson BR. Cost-effectiveness of diagnostic laparoscopy for assessing resectability in pancreatic and periampullary cancer. BMC Gastroenterol. 2015;15:44.
11. Tse KY, Ngan HY. The role of laparoscopy in the staging of different gynecological cancers. Best Pract Res Clin Obstet Gynaecol. 2015;29(6):884–95.
12. Allen VB, Gurusamy K, Takwoingi Y, Kalia A, Davidson BR. Diagnostic accuracy of laparoscopy following computed tomography (CT) scanning for assessing the resectability with curative intent in pancreatic and periampullary cancer. Cochrane Database Syst Rev. 2016;(7):Art. No.: CD009323.
13. Levy L, Tsaltas J. Recent advances in benign gynecological laparoscopic surgery. Fac Rev. 2021;10:60. https://doi.org/10.12703/r/10-60. PMID: 34409423; PMCID: PMC8361750
14. Richardson WS, Stefanidis D, Chang L, Earle DB, Fanelli RD. The role of diagnostic laparoscopy for chronic abdominal conditions: an evidence-based review. Surg Endosc. 2009;23(9):2073–7.
15. Sharma D, Dahiya K, Duhan N, Bansal R. Diagnostic laparoscopy in chronic pelvic pain. Arch Gynecol Obstet. 2011;283(2):295–7. https://doi.org/10.1007/s00404-010-1354-z. Epub 2010 Jan 14
16. Tasian GE, Copp HL, Baskin LS. Diagnostic imaging in cryptorchidism: utility, indications, and effectiveness. J Pediatr Surg. 2011;46(12):2406–13.
17. Hussain A, El-Hasani S. Diagnostic laparoscopy or CT scan to diagnose the leak following bariatric surgery. Obes Surg. 2016;26:617–8.
18. World Health Organization WHO Surgical Checklist. https://www.who.int/teams/integratedhealth-services/patient-safety/research/safe-surgery/tool-and-resources. Accessed online 6 Jan 2025.

Chapter 13
Laparoscopic Appendicectomy

Emeka Ray-Offor, Sameh H. Emile, Zoe Garoufalia, and Nir Horesh

Introduction

Dating from the first report on the management of acute appendicitis by Reginald Fitz in 1886, appendicectomy remains the gold standard treatment for acute appendicitis [1]. This common surgical emergency has been traditionally treated by open appendicectomy. In 1983, Kurt Semm, a German gynecologist, performed the first laparoscopic appendicectomy [2]. Over the next two decades, there was a paradigm shift towards the closed cavity approach of laparoscopic appendicectomy (LA) in

E. Ray-Offor (✉)
College of Health Sciences, University of Port Harcourt, Choba, Rivers State, Nigeria

Minimal Access Surgery Program, University of Port Harcourt Teaching Hospital (UPTH), Port Harcourt, Rivers State, Nigeria

Department of Surgery, UPTH, Port Harcourt, Rivers State, Nigeria

Oak Endoscopy Centre and Radiodiagnostics, Port Harcourt, Rivers State, Nigeria
e-mail: emeka.ray-offor@uniport.edu.ng

S. H. Emile
Cleveland Clinic Florida, Weston, FL, USA

Schmidt College of Medicine, Florida Atlantic University, Boca Raton, FL, USA

Faculty of Medicine, Mansoura University, Mansoura, Egypt

Z. Garoufalia
Ellen Leifer Shulman and Steven Shulman Digestive Disease Center, Cleveland Clinic Florida, Weston, FL, USA

N. Horesh
Ellen Leifer Shulman and Steven Shulman Digestive Disease Center, Cleveland Clinic Florida, Weston, FL, USA

Faculty of Medicine, Tel Aviv University, Tel Aviv, Israel

E. Ray-Offor, R. J. Rosenthal (eds.), *Principles and Practice of Laparoscopic Surgery*, https://doi.org/10.1007/978-3-031-96321-6_13

developed countries. Evidence-based studies demonstrated that LA has a high diagnostic value and is associated with less pain, shorter hospital stays, an earlier resumption of oral intake, an earlier return to work, and better cosmesis [3, 4]. In addition, LA is associated with a reduced incidence of superficial wound infection, incisional hernia, and adhesive bowel obstruction. However, there were concerns about longer operating times, increased costs, and higher rates of intrabdominal abscess in complicated acute appendicitis [5].

The classification of appendicitis is essential for an effective treatment strategy. Based on pre-operative, intra-operative, and histopathological findings, patients with appendicitis are categorized as uncomplicated or complicated appendicitis. Complicated appendicitis refers to patients with appendiceal perforation, intraabdominal abscess or purulent peritonitis, a gangrenous inflamed appendix, or periappendicular contained phlegmon [6]. Several studies show the feasibility and safety of non-operative antibiotic treatment for uncomplicated appendicitis in the general population, [7]. Although more frequently performed, the current state of the evidence does not justify a change of the standard therapy from surgery to conservative treatment. There is a risk of recurrence in a third of patients treated with antibiotics requiring subsequent appendicectomy [8]. LA is the preferred approach in appendicectomy for uncomplicated and complicated acute appendicitis when laparoscopic equipment and expertise are available.

Anatomic Considerations

The vestigial appendix is identified at the confluence of the three taenia coli in the caecum, about 2-3 cm below and posterior to the ileocaecal junction (Fig. 13.1). Its arterial supply is from the appendiceal artery, typically located in the free margin of the mesentery of the appendix. Securing this artery in the mesoappendix is a key step in appendicectomy. The retrocecal position is the most common

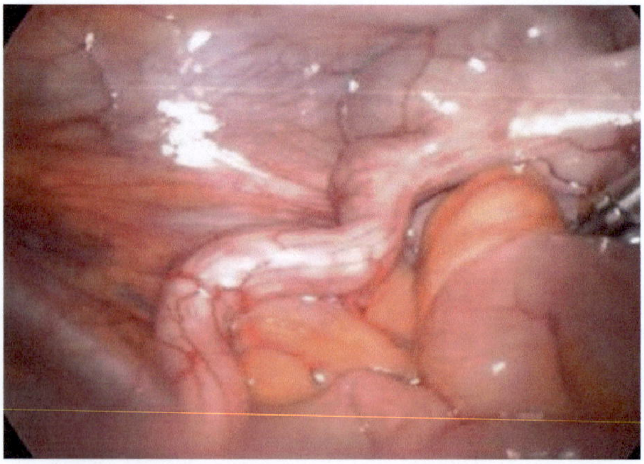

Fig. 13.1 Inflamed appendix

location when the appendix is within the peritoneal space. Dense adhesions in the setting of a retrocecal appendix may necessitate a retrograde technique of removal involving the transection of the appendix stump before securing the mesoappendix.

Intraoperative grading systems help guide post-operative treatment regarding antibiotic therapy which may affect outcomes [9]. However, the intraoperative diagnosis alone is insufficient for identifying unexpected diseases hence routine histopathology is necessary. Evidence from a meta-analysis showed an overall negative appendectomy rate of 13% after laparoscopic surgery [10].

Indications

The indications for LA are similar to those for open appendicectomy. Patients with uncomplicated acute appendicitis may benefit the most from LA including:

Females

Where the requisite expertise is available, the panoramic view of LA, in women of childbearing age with acute lower abdominal pain, non-specific lower abdominal pain, or suspected appendicitis, is helpful. This view offers a more accurate diagnosis based on the likelihood of pelvic pathologies and a lower rate of negative appendicectomy [11].

Obesity

Obesity poses a unique set of surgical challenges that affect intraoperative and postoperative outcomes. The laparoscopic technique in obese adult patients is associated with reduced mortality (RR 0.19), reduced overall morbidity (RR 0.49), reduced superficial SSI (RR 0.27), and shorter operating times and postoperative length of hospital stay, compared to OA [6].

Elderly

The reduced physiological reserves and impaired inflammatory response in the elderly favor the minimally invasive approach of appendicectomy [12].

Patients with Comorbidities

Surgical outcomes can be adversely affected by significant co-morbidities. For high-risk ASA-3 and ASA-4 patients, LA has proven to be safe, feasible, and associated with lower rates of postoperative mortality and morbidity, and shorter hospitalization [6].

Contraindications

Appendicectomy for acute appendicitis may be associated with fetal loss in early pregnancy. However, LA is feasible in pregnancy with acceptable outcomes, especially in early and mid-trimester pregnancies, with sophisticated hands and experienced centers [13, 14].

Preoperative Preparation

A diagnosis of acute appendicitis is based on clinical, biochemical, and radiology studies. The biochemical parameters include elevated, white blood cell count and C-reactive protein. Given varied clinical presentations and multiple differential diagnoses, predictive scoring systems have been advocated and used to reduce the rate of negative appendicectomy. This consists of clinical and biochemical parameters and include ALVARADO, Adult Appendicitis Score, and Appendicitis Inflammatory Response systems. The suspected cases of appendicitis are categorized into either low, moderate, or high-risk status. Ultrasound (US), abdominal computed tomography (CT) scans, and magnetic resonance imaging (MRI) are useful additional investigations in patients at moderate risk for appendicitis. A low-dose unenhanced CT scan is equivalent to standard-dose CT with intravenous contrast agents yet has a higher sensitivity than the US. This may be required in patients with an equivocal US or if perforation is suspected. The five cardinal findings of perforated appendicitis from a CT scan with IV contrast are extraluminal appendicolith, abscess, extraluminal air, appendiceal wall enhancement defect, and periappendiceal fat stranding [15].

Although the feasibility and safety of non-operative management for uncomplicated appendicitis has been demonstrated in the general population using antibiotic therapy, however, with nearly 3 out of 10 reported patients undergoing appendectomy within 90 days [16]. This is critical information to share with the patient for informed consent. The optimal timing of surgery is as soon as possible within 24 h after diagnosis [17]. Data from the American College of Surgeons National Surgical Quality Improvement Program demonstrate that appendectomies performed after 48 h of admission had increased 30-day mortality and all major postoperative complications, in comparison with operations done within 24–48 h of admission [18]. However, emergency operations for appendicular abscess and phlegmon can lead to a higher rate of morbidity when compared with interval appendicectomy [19]. Patients with previous abdominal operations, obesity, and complicated appendicitis should be counseled about the higher risk of conversion [20]. Prophylactic antibiotics, comprising third-generation cephalosporin and metronidazole, are typically administered 30 minutes before the induction of anesthesia. The urinary bladder should be emptied before surgery to avoid bladder injury during port placement.

Technique for Conventional LA

The operating room is set up with the patient positioned supine and having the left upper limb adducted to the side for the ease of the surgeon positioned on this left side. A monitor is set to face the surgeon in coaxial alignment with the target site (Fig. 13.2). The assistant surgeon is positioned opposite at start of surgery but relocates to the right side of the surgeon after peritoneal access is achieved. General anesthesia is then administered with good abdominal muscle relaxation. Intraperitoneal local anesthetics can be used in LA as it is associated with less postoperative pain and a reduction in postoperative adverse events [21].

Access is created by closed or open technique via an 11-mm infra-umbilical incision. A 30^0 10-mm laparoscope is inserted. Capnoperitoneum is slowly established and maintained at 12–15 mmHg. This step is followed by inserting 5-mm working ports in the suprapubic and left lower abdomen. This sectoral position is not observed to affect the learning curve compared to the umbilical centralization of the optical port with the working ports in the right lumbar quadrant and left lower abdomen [22]. A diagnostic laparoscopy is then performed to confirm the diagnosis and

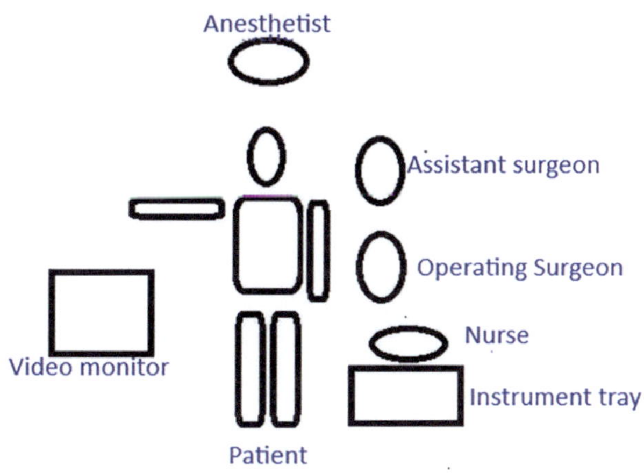

Fig. 13.2 Operating room set up for laparoscopic appendicectomy

exclude double pathology (Table 13.1). In the event a plastron appendix is encountered, an interval appendectomy is a wise decision to avoid post-operative fistula complications.

The patient is repositioned in a Trendelenburg position with a left lateral tilt. The appendix is identified at the confluence of the taeniae in the caecum and grasped with Babcock forceps and any adhesions are released. Monopolar electrocoagulation and bipolar energy are effective techniques to mobilize the appendix and secure the mesoappendix. The mesoappendix is safely divided using bipolar energy device shears from its free margin up to the base of the appendix (Fig. 13.3).

In low-budget settings, a window can be created in the mesoappendix close to the base of the appendix with the diathermy-activated tip of a Maryland forceps (Fig. 13.4). Two close intra-corporeal or extra-corporeal hand knots are made with polyglactin 2/0 to secure the appendiceal artery in the mesoappendix through the window. The vessel is then cut in between knots. Two close pretied endo-loops are secured around the base of the appendix which is now severed 5–10 mm distal to the lowest (Fig. 13.5). Careful attention is made to ligate the base of the appendix using the confluence of the taenia as a landmark. The appendix is then severed in between the pretied knots. The stump should be no longer than 0.5 cm and cecal taenia should be followed onto the appendix at removal to ensure complete resection preventing stump appendicitis. Fluid is instilled into the surgical field with the amputated stump buried within testing for leak evidenced by a bubble sign.

An Endo GIA stapler, when available, is a quick method to secure the mesoappendix, appendix base resection, and simultaneous stump closure. Using single or double polymeric clips (Hem-o-Lok) is also another effective method that can save time. The rate of postoperative complications of all methods of appendiceal stump closure is similar [23]. Intracorporeal and extracorporeal knotting are cheap and effective but less time-efficient than the above-mentioned methods.

The 10-mm laparoscope is withdrawn and replaced with a 5-mm laparoscope through one of the working ports. This facilitates the introduction of a tissue retrieval bag through the umbilical port to extract the severed appendix. The cannula technique is a viable alternative where the switch of the laparoscope is not needed, as the

Table 13.1 Laparoscopic grading system of acute appendicitis

Non-complicated appendicitis
Grade 0 Normal looking appendix (Endoappendicitis/periappendicitis)
Grade 1 Inflamed Appendix (Hyperemia, edema ± fibrin without or little pericolic fluid).
Complicated appendicitis
Grade 2 Necrosis A—Segmental necrosis ((without or little pericolic fluid)) B—Base necrosis ((without or little pericolic fluid))
Grade 3 Inflammatory/A—Phlegmons
Tumor B Abscess < 5 cm without intraperitoneal free air
C Abscess > 5 cm without intraperitoneal free air
Grade 4 Perforated—Diffuse Peritonitis with or without intraperitoneal free air

Gomes et al. 2015 [9]

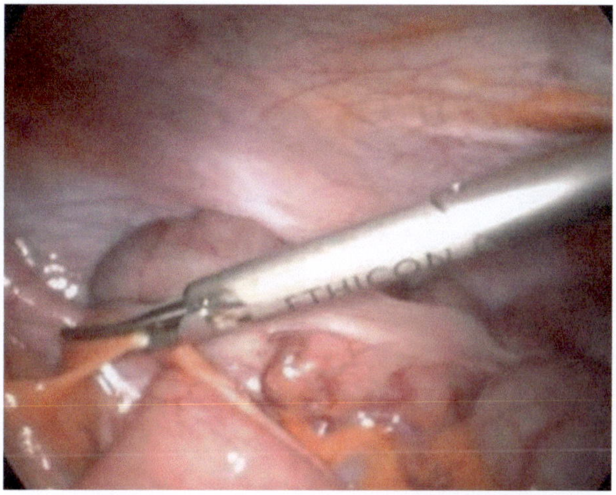

Fig. 13.3 Securing the mesoappendix

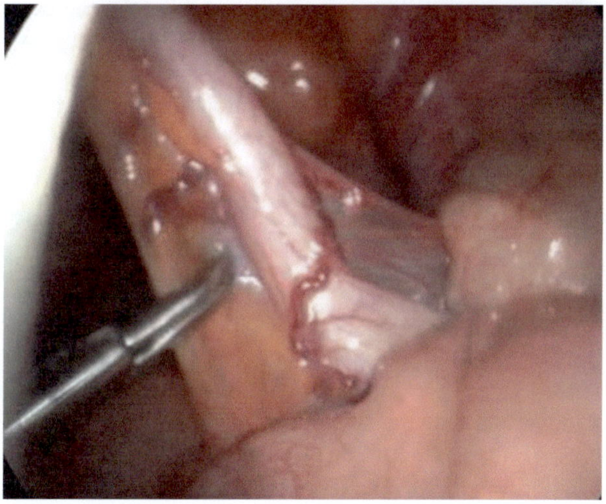

Fig. 13.4 Creating a window in the mesoappendix

resected appendix is grasped at its proximal end through the suprapubic port and railroaded into the 11-mm umbilical port while withdrawing the laparoscope. The specimen is kept under the protective cover of the cannula during the process of extraction.

When there is perforation and abscess, aspiration and appendicectomy are satisfactory treatments. However, peritoneal irrigation with 4–6 L of isosmotic fluid and suction is recommended to reduce bacterial peritoneal contamination. Ensuring the instilled amount of irrigating fluid tallies with the volume of fluid evacuated mitigates retention of collections. Peritoneal drainage following LA for complicated appendicitis is not recommended. Drainage not only increases the incidence of wound infection and aggravates patients' postoperative pain, but also prolongs the

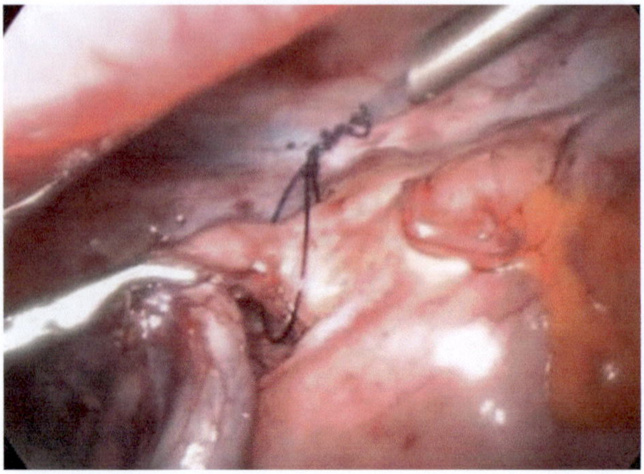

Fig. 13.5 Correct positioning of Endo loop at the base of the appendix

operative and recovery times, and hospitalization [24]. Conversion to open surgery rates are generally low in experienced hands; the common reasons for conversion include appendicular base perforation, adherences, inability to find the appendicular base, appendicular plastron, and profuse bleeding.

Finally, an inspection is made for hemostasis and iatrogenic injury. The capnoperitoneum is released, and the fascia at the 11-mm port is closed with PDS 1 (preferable); then, subcutaneous skin closure and dressings are applied.

Post-operative Care

Bowel function is expected to return within 12 h, then oral sips are started. Postoperative pain management should follow the protocols for pain management after abdominal surgery. The risk of complications is higher in complicated appendicitis with an incidence ranging from 3.0% to 28.7% [6]. Complications include adhesive small bowel obstruction, wound infection, intra-abdominal abscess, stump leakage, and stump appendicitis.

Initial conservative management of post-operative complications is advised before surgical intervention. However, in case of lack of improvement or deterioration, a more invasive strategy should be applied, including percutaneous drainage or surgical (laparoscopic) drainage. Postoperative administration of antibiotics significantly reduces the rate of SSI in complicated appendicitis. However, the appropriate duration of postoperative antibiotics for complex appendicitis is unclear. The increasing global threat of antimicrobial resistance warrants restrictive antibiotic use. High-level evidence shows that 2 days of postoperative intravenous antibiotics for complex appendicitis is non-inferior to 5 days in terms of infectious complications and 90-day mortality [25]. There is a paucity of evidence in support of routine postoperative administration of antibiotics in uncomplicated appendicitis after one preoperative dose.

Patients are usually sent home on POD 1–2 after surgery. However, in some centers day-case appendectomy is practiced. A definitive histologic diagnosis is needed at the follow-up visit as unexpected findings in pathology include carcinoids, diverticulitis, tuberculosis appendix, endometriosis, adenocarcinoma, and mucinous cystadenoma [26]. Treatment of the uncommon findings in resected pathological specimens may include right hemicolectomy and hyperthermic intraperitoneal chemotherapy (HIPEC) [27].

Newer Techniques

The scar-less technique of Single Port Laparoscopic Appendicectomy (SPLA) is a more recent innovation. The conventional 3-port laparoscopy is reduced to one umbilical incision with a single multi-port device. SPLA or single-incision laparoscopic appendicectomy can also be performed with multiple fascial incisions and port insertion through a single skin incision. Optimal cosmetic results are obtained through intra-umbilical incision as the scar will be concealed within the umbilicus, but a major concern may be injury to the epigastric vessels. The challenge of triangulation is overcome with roticulating or curved instruments. Percutaneous sutures or wires can be used to 'assist' the operation. Despite conclusive evidence that SPLA efficacy and safety are comparable to conventional LA in the management of uncomplicated appendicitis, it is associated with a slightly longer operative time and learning curve [28, 29]. The claims of enhanced recovery and reduced pain, blood loss, and complication compared to conventional LA and open procedures have yet to be objectively substantiated [30].

The quest for scarless surgery has led to Natural Orifice Transluminal Endoscopic Surgery (NOTES) which involves the removal of the appendix through the natural orifice of the vagina, rectum, or stomach by multidisciplinary teams in research centers [31]. The anticipated advantages of this method include shorter convalescence, reduction in postoperative pain, wound infection, abdominal wall hernias, and the absence of scars. Much work remains to determine if NOTES provides any additional advantages over the laparoscopic approach to appendicectomy.

Robotic platforms are increasingly applied to various procedures across surgical specialties without an exception to appendicectomy. This stable platform which offers 3D visualization, optimal ergonomic positioning, and precise instrument manipulation is mostly used in elective settings. However, there is a growing interest in applying this minimally invasive technique to acute care general surgery [32]. Robot-assisted laparoscopic appendicectomy compared to LA has double direct and total costs but similar postoperative outcomes are reported [33].

Laparoscopic Appendicectomy in Low and Middle-Income Countries LMICs

Globally, acute appendicitis is the most common surgical emergency with no exception to LMICs that have a higher surgical mortality rate. Appendicectomy is routinely performed by the open technique in less developed countries, however, the practice of minimally invasive surgery is gaining ascendancy [21, 34, 35]. A ready pool of appendicectomy cases offers an effective therapeutic laparoscopic skill training procedure to junior and trainee surgeons who perform the bulk of appendicectomies [36].

In these climes, the diagnosis and decision to operate on suspected acute appendicitis is mostly clinically based though an abdominal ultrasound scan is often useful, being cheap and readily available. The routine practice of CT scans and MRIs in suspected cases of perforated/complicated appendicitis is marred by the cost of service and non-ready availability of equipment. It is estimated that CT imaging equipment costs 2500 times more and MRI costs 4500 times more than laparoscopy equipment. This makes laparoscopy clinically and economically effective as a diagnostic and therapeutic tool.

The cost of equipment, paucity of support staff, and lack of political will in government owned tertiary health facilities are some of the factors mitigating the widespread application of this evidence-based improvement in surgical care [37]. Beyond the startup cost of acquisition of laparoscopy set and infrastructure set-up, the shorter hospital stay, early return to work, patient satisfaction, and improved quality of surgery are benefits worth coveting. Local adaptations and the use of reusable instruments are realities of cost in low/middle-income countries [38, 39]. The use of an Endo GIA stapler to secure the appendix stump adds significantly to the cost of surgery. Alternatively, the application of extra/intracorporeal knots or pretied endoloop to secure the base of the appendix with the use of monopolar/bipolar electrosurgery to secure the mesoappendix is widely reported.

Overcoming the local challenges to minimally invasive surgery technology is necessary for the widespread application of this improved quality of surgical care offered by laparoscopic appendicectomy. These include reducing operating time with surgeon's experience, training of support staff, and local maintenance of equipment.

References

1. Loveland JE. Reginald Heber Fitz, the exponent of appendicitis. Yale J Biol Med. 1937;9(509):b1–520.
2. Semm K. Endoscopic appendectomy. Endoscopy. 1983;15:59–64.
3. Wei HB, Huang JL, Zheng ZH, Wei B, Zheng F, Qiu WS, et al. Laparoscopic versus open appendectomy: a prospective randomized comparison. Surg Endosc. 2010;24:266–9.
4. Jaschinski T, Mosch CG, Eikermann M, Neugebauer EA, Sauerland S. Laparoscopic versus open surgery for suspected appendicitis. Cochrane Database Syst Rev. 2018;11:CD001546.

5. Sauerland S, Jaschinski T, Neugebauer EA. Laparoscopic versus open surgery for suspected appendicitis. Cochrane Database Syst Rev. 2010;10:CD001546.
6. Di Saverio S, Podda M, De Simone B, et al. Diagnosis and treatment of acute appendicitis: 2020 update of the WSES Jerusalem guidelines. World J Emerg Surg. 2020;15(1):27. Published 2020 Apr 15. https://doi.org/10.1186/s13017-020-00306-3.
7. Poon SHT, Lee JWY, Ng KM, Chiu GWY, Wong BYK, Foo CC, Law WL. The current management of acute uncomplicated appendicitis: should there be a change in paradigm? A systematic review of the literature and analysis of treatment performance. World J Emerg Surg. 2017;12:46.
8. Doleman B, Fonnes S, Lund JN, Boyd-Carson H, Javanmard-Emamghissi H, Moug S, Hollyman M, Tierney G, Tou S, Williams JP. Appendectomy versus antibiotic treatment for acute appendicitis. Cochrane Database Syst Rev. 2024;4(4):CD015038.
9. Gomes CA, Sartelli M, Di Saverio S, Ansaloni L, Catena F, Coccolini F, Inaba K, Demetriades D, Gomes FC, Gomes CC. Acute appendicitis: proposal of a new comprehensive grading system based on clinical, imaging, and laparoscopic findings. World J Emerg Surg. 2015;10:60.
10. Henriksen SR, Christophersen C, Rosenberg J, Fonnes S. Varying negative appendectomy rates after laparoscopic appendectomy: a systematic review and metaanalysis. Langenbeck's Arch Surg. 2023;408(1):205.
11. Gaitán HG, Reveiz L, Farquhar C, Elias VM. Laparoscopy for the management of acute lower abdominal pain in women of childbearing age. Cochrane Database Syst Rev. 2014;2014(5):CD007683. 13.
12. Fugazzola P, Ceresoli M, Agnoletti V, Agresta F, Amato B, Carcoforo P, Catena F, Chiara O, Chiarugi M, Cobianchi L, Coccolini F, De Troia A, Di Saverio S, Fabbri A, Feo C, Gabrielli F, Gurrado A, Guttadauro A, Leone L, Marrelli D, Petruzzelli L, Portolani N, Prete FP, Puzziello A, Sartelli M, Soliani G, Testini M, Tolone S, Tomasoni M, Tugnoli G, Viale P, Zese M, Ishay OB, Kluger Y, Kirkpatrick A, Ansaloni L. The SIFIPAC/WSES/SICG/SIMEU guidelines for diagnosis and treatment of acute appendicitis in the elderly (2019 Edition). World J Emerg Surg. 2020;15(1):19.
13. Adamina M, Andreou A, Arezzo A, Christogiannis C, Di Lorenzo N, Gioumidou M, Glavind J, Iavazzo C, Mavridis D, Muysoms FE, Preda D, Smart NJ, Syropoulou A, Tzanis AA, Van de Velde M, Vermeulen J, Antoniou SA. EAES rapid guideline: systematic review, meta-analysis, GRADE assessment, and evidence-informed European recommendations on appendicitis in pregnancy. Surg Endosc. 2022;36(12):86998712.
14. Zeng Q, Aierken A, Gu SS, Yao G, Apaer S, Anweier N, Wu J, Zhao JM, Li T, Tuxun T. Laparoscopic versus open appendectomy for appendicitis in pregnancy: systematic review and meta-analysis. Surg Laparosc Endosc Percutan Tech. 2021;31(5):637644.
15. Kim HY, Park JH, Lee YJ, Lee SS, Jeon JJ, Lee KH. Systematic review and metaanalysis of CT features for differentiating complicated and uncomplicated appendicitis. Radiology. 2018;287(1):104–15.
16. Collaborative CODA, Flum DR, Davidson GH, Monsell SE, Shapiro NI, Odom SR, Sanchez SE, Drake FT, Fischkoff K, Johnson J, Patton JH, Evans H, Cuschieri J, Sabbatini AK, Faine BA, Skeete DA, Liang MK, Sohn V, McGrane K, Kutcher ME, Chung B, Carter DW, Ayoung-Chee P, Chiang W, Rushing A, Steinberg S, Foster CS, Schaetzel SM, Price TP, Mandell KA, Ferrigno L, Salzberg M, DeUgarte DA, Kaji AH, Moran GJ, Saltzman D, Alam HB, Park PK, Kao LS, Thompson CM, Self WH, Yu JT, Wiebusch A, Winchell RJ, Clark S, Krishnadasan A, Fannon E, Lavallee DC, Comstock BA, Bizzell B, Heagerty PJ, Kessler LG, Talan DA. A randomized trial comparing antibiotics with appendectomy for appendicitis. N Engl J Med. 2020;383(20):1907–19. https://doi.org/10.1056/NEJMoa2014320. Epub 2020 Oct 5
17. Calpin GG, Hembrecht S, Giblin K, Hehir C, Dowling GP, Hill ADK. The impact of timing on outcomes in appendicectomy: a systematic review and network metaanalysis. World J Emerg Surg. 2024;19(1):24.
18. Alore EA, Ward JL, Todd SR, Wilson CT, Gordy SD, Hoffman MK, Suliburk JW. Population-level outcomes of early versus delayed appendectomy for acute appendicitis using the

American College of Surgeons National Surgical Quality Improvement Program. J Surg Res. 2018;229:234–42. https://doi.org/10.1016/j.jss.2018.04.011.
19. Akingboye AA, Mahmood F, Zaman S, Wright J, Mannan F, Mohamedahmed AYY. Early versus delayed (interval) appendicectomy for the management of appendicular abscess and phlegmon: a systematic review and meta-analysis. Langenbeck's Arch Surg. 2021;406(5):1341–51.
20. Wilasrusmee C, Sukrat B, McEvoy M, Attia J, Thakkinstian A. Systematic review and meta-analysis of safety of laparoscopic versus open appendicectomy for suspected appendicitis in pregnancy. Br J Surg. 2012;99:1470–9.
21. Abdelhakim AM, Elghazaly SM, Lotfy A. Efficacy and safety of intraperitoneal local anesthetics in laparoscopic appendectomy: a systematic review and meta-analysis. J Pain Palliat Care Pharmacother. 2020;34(1):32–42.
22. Ray-Offor E, Okoro PE, Gbobo I, Allison AB. Pilot study on laparoscopic surgery in Port-Harcourt. Nigeria Niger J Surg. 2014;20(1):23–5.
23. Ihnát P, Tesař M, Tulinský L, Vávra P. Technical modifications of appendiceal transection during laparoscopic appendectomy. Rozhl Chir. 2020;99(12):534–8.
24. Wu H, Liao B, Cao T, Ji T, Luo Y, Huang J, Ma K. Advantages comparison of peritoneal drainage versus no drainage after laparoscopic appendectomy for complicated appendicitis: a meta-analysis. BMC Gastroenterol. 2024;24(1):411.
25. de Wijkerslooth EML, Boerma EG, van Rossem CC, van Rosmalen J, Baeten CIM, Beverdam FH, Bosmans JWAM, Consten ECJ, Dekker JWT, Emous M, van Geloven AAW, Gijsen AF, Heijnen LA, Jairam AP, Melles DC, van der Ploeg APT, Steenvoorde P, Toorenvliet BR, Vermaas M, Wiering B, Wijnhoven BPL, van den Boom AL, APPIC Study Group. 2 days versus 5 days of postoperative antibiotics for complex appendicitis: a pragmatic, open-label, multicentre, non-inferiority randomised trial. Lancet. 2023;401(10374):366–76.
26. Chandrasegaram MD, Rothwell LA, An EI, Miller RJ. Pathologies of the appendix: a 10-year review of 4670 appendicectomy specimens. ANZ J Surg. 2012;82:844–7.
27. Gorter RR, Eker HH, Gorter-Stam MA, et al. Diagnosis and management of acute appendicitis. EAES consensus development conference 2015. Surg Endosc. 2016;30(11):4668–90.
28. Zaman S, Mohamedahmed AYY, Srinivasan A, Stonelake S, Sillah AK, Hajibandeh S, Hajibandeh S. Single-port laparoscopic appendicectomy versus conventional threeport approach for acute appendicitis: a systematic review, meta-analysis and trial sequential analysis of randomised controlled trials. Surgeon. 2021;19(6):365–79.
29. Cirocchi R, Cianci MC, Amato L, Properzi L, Buononato M, Di Rienzo VM, Tebala GD, Avenia S, Iandoli R, Santoro A, Vettoretto N, Coletta R, Morabito A. Laparoscopic appendectomy with single port vs conventional access: systematic review and metaanalysis of randomized clinical trials. Surg Endosc. 2024;38(4):1667–84. https://doi.org/10.1007/s00464-023-10659-w. Epub 2024 Feb 8. Erratum in: Surg Endosc. 2024 Apr;38(4):2305
30. Aly OE, Black DH, Rehman H, Ahmed I. Single incision laparoscopic appendicectomy versus conventional three-port laparoscopic appendicectomy: a systematic review and meta-analysis. Int J Surg. 2016;35:120–8.
31. Tabutsadze T, Kipshidze N. New trend in endoscopic surgery: transvaginal appendectomy NOTES (natural orifice transluminal endoscopic surgery). Georgian Med News. 2009;168:7–10.
32. Myla K, Bou-Ayash N, Kim WC, Bugaev N, Bawazeer M. Is implementation of roboticassisted procedures in acute care general surgery cost-effective? J Robot Surg. 2024;18(1):223.
33. Quilici PJ, Wolberg H, McConnell N. Operating costs, fiscal impact, value analysis and guidance for the routine use of robotic technology in abdominal surgical procedures. Surg Endosc. 2022;36(2):1433–43.
34. Ali R, Khan MR, Pishori T, Tayeb M. Laparoscopic appendectomy for acute appendicitis: is this a feasible option for developing countries? Saudi J Gastroenterol. 2010;16:25–9.
35. Adisa AO, Alatise OI, Arowolo OA, Lawal OO. Laparoscopic appendectomy in a Nigerian teaching hospital. J Soc Laparoendosc Surg. 2012;16:576–80.

36. Ray-Offor E, Jebbin NJ. Appendicectomy for appendicitis and laparoscopy training. J Gastrointest Dig Syst. 2017;7:1–3.
37. Ray-Offor E, Fiebai PO. Routine laparoscopic surgery: why not? Abstracts from the 61st Meeting of the Nigerian Surgical Research Society Calabar Nigeria, July 2012. Niger J Surg. 2012;18(2):110–1.
38. Carrillo Montenegro AF, Aristizabal Rojas S, Pulido Segura JA, Pedraza M, Padilla L, Lozada-Martinez ID, Rafael Narvaez-Rojas A, Cabrera-Vargas LF. Single incision laparoscopic appendectomy with surgical-glove port is cost-effective and reliable in complicated acute appendicitis: a case-control multicenter study in Colombia. Heliyon. 2023;9(1):e12972.
39. Domene CE, Volpe P, Santana AV. Laparoscopic appendicectomy without the use of disposable materials—a low-cost alternative—1,552 cases operated in 20 years. Rev Col Bras Cir. 2022;49:e20222446.

Chapter 14
Laparoscopic Cholecystectomy

Adewale O. Adisa

Introduction

Laparoscopic cholecystectomy represents a pivotal development in the evolution of minimally invasive surgical techniques within general surgery. Its introduction and global adoption catalyzed a significant transformation in surgical practice, leading to the widespread expansion of minimally invasive methods across various surgical subspecialties. Although open cholecystectomy has been a reliable procedure for over a century, the laparoscopic approach introduced distinct advantages that have profoundly altered the management of gallbladder diseases [1].

Compared to the traditional open approach, laparoscopic cholecystectomy involves less extensive tissue dissection and minimizes disruption to anatomical planes. These attributes contribute to reduced postoperative pain, shorter hospitalizations, and expedited return to normal daily activities. Additional benefits of minimally invasive surgery include reduced rates of wound complications and superior cosmetic outcomes, further enhancing patient satisfaction and recovery [1, 2].

Empirical data suggest that the advent of laparoscopy has led to an increased volume of cholecystectomy procedures performed at healthcare institutions. Furthermore, laparoscopic cholecystectomy has become a foundational procedure for developing laparoscopic skills among surgeons and surgical trainees, underscoring its educational value [3, 4].

However, the initial implementation of laparoscopic cholecystectomy was met with skepticism. Concerns were raised regarding the steep learning curve associated with mastering laparoscopic techniques and the incidence of bile duct injuries during the early adoption phase [2, 5]. Over time, these apprehensions were mitigated as rigorous studies demonstrated significantly low rates of bile duct injuries globally, supporting the safety and efficacy of the procedure.

A. O. Adisa (✉)
Department of Surgery, Obafemi Awolowo University, Ile Ife, Nigeria
e-mail: ao.adisa@oauife.edu.ng

E. Ray-Offor, R. J. Rosenthal (eds.), *Principles and Practice of Laparoscopic Surgery*, https://doi.org/10.1007/978-3-031-96321-6_14

Currently, laparoscopic cholecystectomy is universally recognized as the gold standard for treating gallbladder pathologies. The practice has further evolved, with many cases now being performed on a day-surgery basis, reflecting advancements in surgical protocols and perioperative care.

Anatomical Variations

The extrahepatic biliary tree has one of the most documented anatomic variations in the body, posing great challenges to the surgeon. Awareness of the normal and suspicion of the possibility of variation will aid in safe cholecystectomy while avoiding injury to the bile ducts and arterial supply. The normal anatomy is as shown in Fig. 14.1a. The gallbladder, comprising its fundus, body, and neck drains through the cystic duct which joins the common hepatic duct to form the common bile duct. A fusiform dilatation of the neck region, Hartman's pouch, is prominent in gallbladder pathologies, particularly with gallstones [6]. The Calot's triangle is a very important anatomical landmark for dissection [7]. It is bounded by the cystic duct laterally, the common hepatic duct medially, and the inferior surface of the liver superiorly. The cystic artery normally passes through the triangle. The hepatocystic triangle is the larger bed bounded medially by the common hepatic duct, laterally by the cystic duct and the gallbladder, and superiorly by the inferior surface of the liver, hence the Calot's triangle is the lower part of the hepatocystic triangle and occasionally both triangles are used interchangeably. Both the ductal and vascular structures in the area can present with variability in origin, course, length, and divisions as

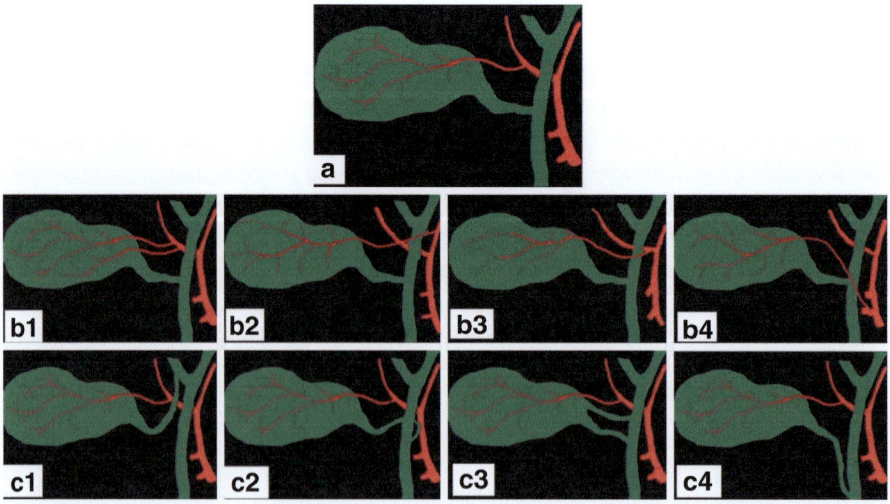

Fig. 14.1 Some anatomical variations in the extrahepatic biliary tree arrangement of the cystic artery (B1–B4) and the cystic duct (C1–C4)

depicted in Fig. 14.1. A high index of suspicion aided by precise dissection in a clear operating field can enhance recognition and avoidance of injuries. The selective use of intraoperative imaging in these cases is highly recommended.

Indications for Laparoscopic Cholecystectomy

The indications for laparoscopic cholecystectomy are largely the same as those of open surgery including congenital and acquired benign diseases of the gallbladder particularly gallstone diseases and its complications [8, 9]. These are listed in Table 14.1. It is also recognized as the optimal treatment for the incidentally detected and very early cancers of the gallbladder. While gallstones are prevalent, the majority are asymptomatic and will remain so for life. The ease and safety of laparoscopy made it possible to offer the procedure to asymptomatic patients. While some have justified this by the challenges, morbidity, and mortality associated with complicated gallstones, others have hinged the argument on the theoretical risk of developing gallbladder cancer over time. The necessity of cholecystectomy in patients with asymptomatic gallstones remains controversial except in peculiar patients including those with immune depression in whom acute cholecystitis should be prevented and sickle cell anemia patients who are at risk of more stone formation from hemolysis [10–13].

Table 14.1 Indications and contraindications of laparoscopic cholecystectomy

Indications for laparoscopic cholecystectomy
Calculous cholecystitis
Acalculous cholecystitis
Gallstone pancreatitis
Asymptomatic cholelithiasis in specific patient populations
Gallbladder empyema
Gallbladder polyps
Gallbladder mucocele
Cholesterosis
Gallbladder dyskinesia
Porcelain gallbladder
Incidentally detected gallbladder cancer
Typhoid carrier state
As part of other procedures e.g. Whipple's procedure
Contraindications
Severe cardio-respiratory compromise
Hemodynamic instability
Uncorrected coagulopathy
Previous upper abdominal surgery with very extensive adhesions
Late pregnancy

Poor surgical risk patients unfit for general anesthesia may also be unsuitable for laparoscopic cholecystectomy and of particular interest are those with a severe cardiorespiratory disease that may preclude the safety of pneumoperitoneum. Many other previously listed contraindications have become relative to the surgeon's experience.

Preoperative Preparations

The preoperative history and physical findings are very important. It is important to have clear radiological evidence of gallstones and detailed information about possible complications including empyema, pericholecystic collection, gallbladder wall thickness, common bile duct diameter, and presence of stones in the common bile duct using various investigation modalities including abdominal ultrasonography, Computerized Tomography scan, and Magnetic Resonance Cholangiopancreatography MRCP. The preoperative identification of choledocholithiasis or common bile duct dilatation is an indication for preoperative Endoscopic Retrograde Cholangiopancreatography (ERCP) and stone retrieval [14]. When a choledochoscope is available, laparoscopic cholecystectomy and common bile duct exploration are an options [15]. Routine pre-anesthetic requests including preoperative complete blood count, serum urea, creatinine and electrolytes, liver function test, and serology for viral hepatitis are important. Other routine investigations including chest x-ray, and electrocardiogram should be carried out.

Techniques

Cholecystectomy has been traditionally performed laparoscopically by the 4-port technique but different modifications including three-port, two-port, and single incision or single port laparoscopic techniques are commonly reported [16]. Robotic cholecystectomy and natural orifice transluminal endoscopic (NOTES) cholecystectomy which includes transgastric and transvaginal techniques have been described. The 4-port technique is the most practiced and will be described here.

The operating room set-up is equally variable. Many surgeons stand to the left of the patient, facing the gallbladder with the patient's left upper limb adducted for easy maneuverability of the surgeon and assistant. The monitor is placed on the upper right hand of the patient as depicted in Fig. 14.2a. A variation (French position) is for the surgeon to stand in between the legs of the patient as in many other upper abdominal surgeries (Fig. 14.2b). Intravenous prophylactic antibiotics should be administered at the induction of anesthesia. General anesthesia is the technique of choice and as for all laparoscopic operations, adequate muscle relaxation is important for patients to tolerate sustained pneumoperitoneum. Regional anesthesia has also been used for laparoscopic cholecystectomy with reports of good outcomes. A supine position is required at the start of the operation and nasogastric intubation

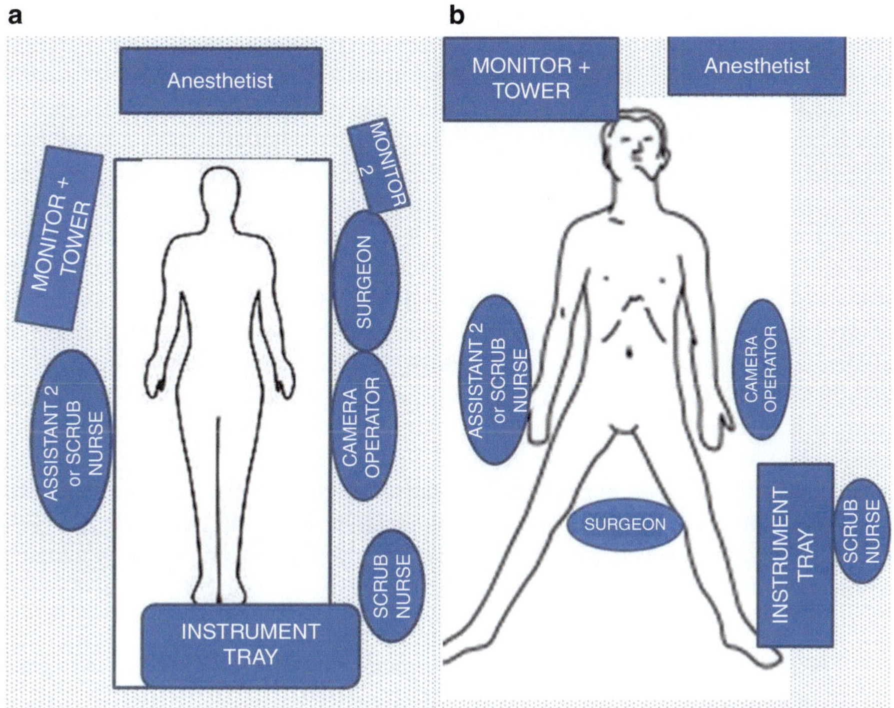

Fig. 14.2 Operating room set-ups for laparoscopic cholecystectomy. (**a**) Regular arrangement (**b**) French position

helps in decompressing the stomach and duodenum which is particularly useful when there are significant adhesions between the gallbladder, duodenum, greater omentum, and or the transverse colon. A urinary catheter is usually not required except when a possibility of conversion to open surgery is envisaged or other longer procedures are being performed concurrently.

A peritoneal access can be gained by the open dissection of Hasson's technique or by use of a Veress needle following which carbon dioxide insufflation and pneumoperitoneum up to the desired intraabdominal pressure. Hasson's technique is useful in patients who have had previous upper abdominal surgery and adhesions are envisaged, while using optical trocar is a good option. The primary port is typically 11 mm just below the umbilicus while the working ports are aligned along the right subcoastal line two inches below the ribs. Under vision, an 11 mm epigastric port is placed just to the left of the falciform ligament (which may be pierced). Two other 5 mm ports in the midclavicular and anterior axillary lines are usually adequate. These three working ports are best positioned after assessing the liver and the gallbladder as their location may need to be altered with hepatomegaly or grossly distended gallbladder. The epigastric port may also be 5 mm when a small cystic duct is envisaged and a 5 mm clip applicator is used. The choice of a straight-looking or angled telescope for the procedure is left to the discretion of the operating surgeon.

It is important to confirm the emptying of the stomach and duodenum and to position the patient supine in 30 degrees reverse Trendelenburg with a left lateral tilt facing the left. A quick inspection of the peritoneal cavity is generally advocated. The surgeon's attention is then turned towards the gallbladder which is grasped at the fundus and retracted upwards and laterally through the most lateral port (Fig. 14.3). Any adhesions of the omentum to the gallbladder are then dissected down until the infundibulum is exposed. Grasping on the infundibulum with gentle lateral retraction will aid further dissection. It is useful to open the peritoneal cover above and below the gallbladder at the level of the infundibulum. This exposes the structures in the Calot's triangle at the neck of the gallbladder and careful use of the hook electrode helps to separate the cystic duct and the cystic arteries ensuring that all dissection is carried out close to the gallbladder. The lymph node of Lund when identified in the Calot's triangle is a good guide to the inferior part of the cystic artery. Dissections are carried upwards along the peritoneal lining to expose the cystic plate and demonstrate the "Critical View of Safety" (CVS, Fig. 14.4). To achieve this, the surgeon must dissect the hepatocystic triangle, expose at least the lower one-third of the cystic plate, and demonstrate that only the cystic duct and cystic artery are attached to the gallbladder. By definition, the CVS is attained when [17]:

(a) **The hepatocystic triangle is cleared of fat and fibrous tissue**
(b) **The lower one-third of the gallbladder is separated from the liver to expose the cystic plate**
(c) **Two and only two structures (cystic duct and cystic artery) are seen entering the gallbladder.**

Proponents of the critical view of safety emphasize that no structure is clipped or ligated until these criteria are fulfilled [17–20]. When the view is attained, titanium clips are applied on the cystic duct, deploying one above and two below while carefully avoiding the common bile duct which may inadvertently be pulled upwards with the retraction on the infundibulum. An appropriate technique is reducing

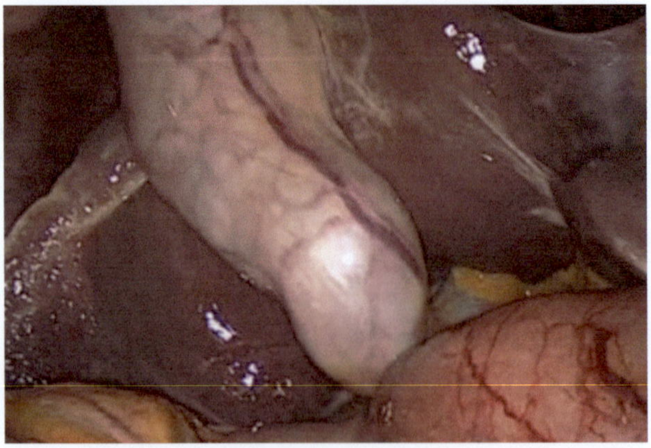

Fig. 14.3 Laparoscopic view of the gallbladder following initial traction on the fundus

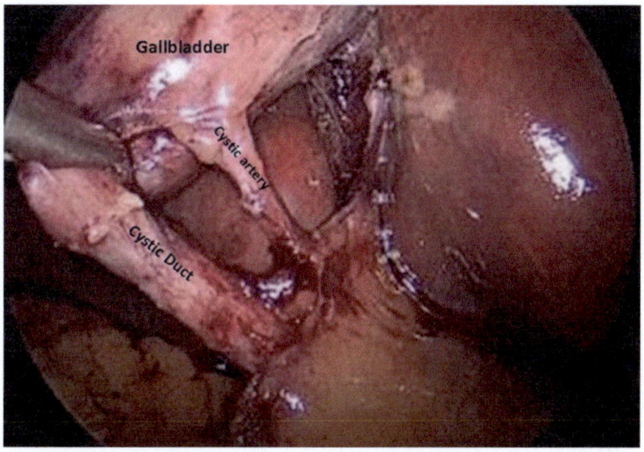

Fig. 14.4 The critical view of safety

traction on the gallbladder when deploying the clips and visually tracing the confluence of the cystic and common hepatic duct and staying at least 3–5 mm away from it. This may be challenging when the cystic duct is unusually short or there are dense adhesions in the Calot's triangle. It is safer to apply the clips as close to the infundibulum as possible or to consider a fundus-first approach. Clips are also applied in a similar pattern on the cystic artery before it is divided. The L-hook electrode or harmonic scalpel is then carefully used in excising the gallbladder from its bed on the liver. The dissection is carried out within the thin layer of fatty tissue overlying the bed to prevent damage to the capsule of the liver which usually provokes bleeding. In all instances, hemostasis should be ensured before the end of the surgery. The uninflamed gallbladder containing a few small stones can safely be aspirated with a laparoscopic needle aspirator and extracted through the 11 mm umbilical port. An inflamed or inadvertently perforated gallbladder and the presence of large or multiple stones mandate the compulsory use of a retrieval bag which is similarly extracted through the umbilical port site.

Special Considerations

There are occasions when a difficult gallbladder is encountered. Such includes one with severe adhesions or a markedly contracted gallbladder. Severe adhesions may require carefully controlled adhesiolysis with good judgment of where to use or avoid electrocautery particularly when bowel adhesions are present. A contracted gallbladder may be better handled with a claw grasper. Other challenging cases include empyema of the gallbladder in which care must be taken to avoid spillage. Both empyema and mucoceles can distend the gallbladder and make it very difficult to grasp in which case careful drainage with a needle aspirator may be useful. Occasionally a large and floppy left lobe of the liver obscures vision. This may require re-aligning the working ports or inserting the other for liver retraction.

An unclear anatomy of the Calot's triangle is one of the most common causes of injuries in laparoscopic surgery [9, 10, 21, 22]. Also, confusing findings such as very short or dilated cystic ducts may be encountered. This may be due to acute or chronic inflammation-inducing changes in the normal anatomy. Several strategies may be useful including adopting the "fundus first" (top-down) approach and ligating the structures just below the infundibulum of the gallbladder. An intraoperative laparoscopic ultrasound scan and the use of a cholangiogram where readily available will aid dissection of the structures. In some instances, subtotal cholecystectomy is an option, but if all else fails, conversion to an open procedure should be seen as good judgment and not a sign of failure.

Safety in Laparoscopic Cholecystectomy

A lot of concerns were raised following reports of bile duct injuries with the advent of laparoscopic cholecystectomy. Though rates of injuries have declined over time, the peculiarity of laparoscopic view and unexpected complications are still reported. The six major considerations for safety during laparoscopic cholecystectomy as recommended by the Society of American Gastrointestinal Endoscopic Surgeons (SAGES) include [17]:

- Use the Critical View of Safety (CVS) method of identification of the cystic duct and cystic artery during laparoscopic cholecystectomy
- Considering an Intra-operative Time-Out during laparoscopic cholecystectomy before clipping, cutting, or transecting any ductal structures
- Understand the potential for aberrant anatomy in all cases.
- Make liberal use of cholangiography or other methods to image the biliary tree intra-operatively
- Recognize when the dissection is approaching a zone of significant risk and halt the dissection before entering the zone. Finish the operation by a safe method other than laparoscopic cholecystectomy if conditions around the gallbladder are too dangerous.
- Get help from another surgeon when the dissection or conditions are difficult.

These recommendations have been widely used and found to improve outcomes and reduce complications of laparoscopic cholecystectomies.

Intraoperative Cholangiography

The indications for intraoperative cholangiography are listed in Table 14.2. These can include preoperative findings which allow for a planned cholangiography or intraoperative findings necessitating emergency cholangiography [23, 24].

Table 14.2 Indications for intraoperative cholangiography during laparoscopic cholecystectomy

Indications for intraoperative cholangiography	
Preoperative findings	History of jaundice Imaging findings of common bile duct stones Gallstones with a history of pancreatitis Deranged liver function tests Dilated common bile duct >7 mm
Intraoperative findings	Cystic duct larger than 3 mm diameter Short cystic duct Unclear anatomy Recognition of anatomical variations Inability to attain the critical view of safety Suspected or detected bile duct injury or leak

Laparoscopic Common Bile Duct Exploration

A preplanned exploration of the common bile duct can be performed laparoscopically but the decision can equally be taken intraoperatively. Preoperatively detected stones on imaging may be an indication, particularly in those whose ERCP and stone extraction have failed. The intraoperative decision is usually based on findings from cholangiography or laparoscopic ultrasonography. There are diverse opinions on the treatment of preoperatively detected choledocholithiasis. The use of preoperative ERCP followed by laparoscopic cholecystectomy has been compared with laparoscopic cholecystectomy and CBD exploration, or intraoperative ERCP in many studies with variable outcomes [17, 19, 25, 26].

Complications of Laparoscopic Cholecystectomy

Specific complications include challenges with access, creation, and maintenance of pneumoperitoneum, and technical issues with equipment failure. Trocar injuries have been reported and different solutions have been advocated including the adoption of open dissection and the use of optical trocars. Trocar insertion under vision is the most important way of avoiding bowel injury.

Intraoperative hemorrhage can occur from dissection of dense adhesions, damage to the cystic artery or right hepatic artery as well as from the gallbladder bed on the liver. Uncontrolled bleeding can be challenging as safe dissection in laparoscopy depends on maintaining a clear vision. The judicious use of electrocautery, rather than stripping, application of pressure, use of pledgets, hydro-dissection, and deployment of energy devices including bipolar cautery, ultrasonic energy, argon beam, and laser may be required. The best way to maintain hemostasis during dissection is through careful dissection to prevent bleeding proactively.

Bile leak and bile duct injury are perhaps the most feared complications of laparoscopic cholecystectomy [27, 28]. Despite recent advances in training and augmented intraoperative pattern recognition, bile duct injuries still occur in 0.5–3% of laparoscopic cholecystectomies in many series. Many of these injuries result from non-recognition of aberrant anatomy or adhesions from severe acute or chronic inflammation. Injuries may follow dissection in wrong planes, clipping, ligation, or transection of the wrong structures or from direct and indirect heat of electrocautery. Various classifications of these injuries and their management have been described [29]. These include Bismuth, Strasberg, McMahon, and Stewart-Way, etc. The best outcome is usually guaranteed when such injuries are detected intra-operatively and repaired simultaneously. Unrecognized injuries leading to biliary peritonitis or obstruction should be promptly recognized and treated. Imaging of the biliary tree to determine the type of injury, peritoneal drainage, and biliary stenting are options to be considered. With the prospect of biliary stricture, biliary cirrhosis, and hepatic failure attending these injuries in the long term, early recognition and surgical intervention in a recognized hepatobiliary center.

Other complications include gallbladder perforation leading to spillage and or dropped stones. This should be prevented to avoid peritonitis and possible subphrenic abscess. Wound complications are often negligible but wound contamination at the extraction site can produce significant surgical site infection. In our series in Nigeria, hypertrophic scars and keloids have also been documented particularly at the epigastric port site. Shoulder tip pain has been commonly reported in the past with many proposed interventions including intraperitoneal local anesthetic infiltration.

Artificial Intelligence and Laparoscopic Cholecystectomy

Since its introduction, continuous efforts have been directed towards enhancing the safety of laparoscopic cholecystectomy (LC). Recently, the integration of Artificial Intelligence (AI) and Machine Learning (ML) into LC has shown significant potential for improving safety and patient outcomes [30]. These technologies have been successfully applied to tasks such as anatomical recognition, surgical phase identification, and verification of the Critical View of Safety (CVS) during the procedure [31].

The accurate recognition of CVS is particularly critical, as it not only minimizes the risk of incorrect dissection but also provides robust documentation. This documentation serves as a valuable tool for training purposes, allowing phase recognition and the assessment of performance among surgical trainees.

Looking ahead, the utilization of AI in laparoscopic cholecystectomy is anticipated to expand further, particularly in the areas of surgical training and ensuring safe procedural practices [32]. These advancements hold promise for standardizing outcomes and enhancing both surgical precision and educational methodologies.

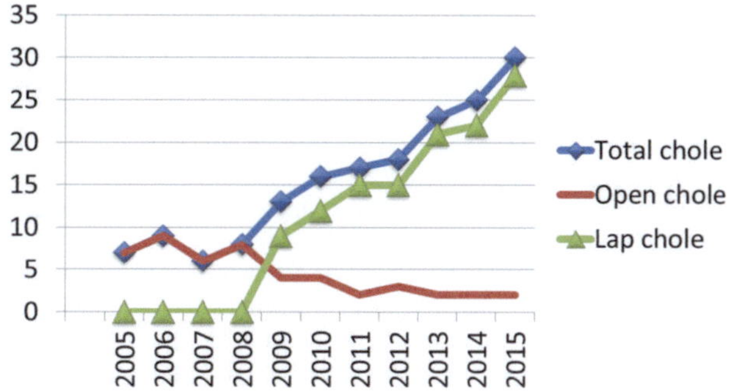

Fig. 14.5 Upward trend in cholecystectomy rates in a Nigerian tertiary hospital [37]

Challenges and Opportunities for Laparoscopy in Low- and Middle-Income Countries

Despite the global adoption of laparoscopic techniques for cholecystectomy and other abdominal procedures, laparoscopy remains underutilized in many low- and middle-income countries (LMICs) [33, 34]. In these settings, the preference for open cholecystectomy often stems from the limited availability of laparoscopic equipment and expertise. Nevertheless, our clinical experience highlights the substantial benefits of laparoscopic surgery for patients in low socio-economic groups, where the advantages of reduced morbidity, quicker recovery, and minimized post-operative costs are particularly impactful. This perspective is aptly summarized by the assertion, "It is more important for a poor person to have laparoscopy than a rich person," as evidenced in our patient outcomes [35].

The introduction of laparoscopic surgery in healthcare facilities within LMICs has demonstrated a notable increase in the volume of cholecystectomies performed (Fig. 14.5) [36, 37]. This rise not only enhances the opportunities for surgeons to refine their technical skills but also creates avenues for resident training in laparoscopic techniques. These advancements extend beyond cholecystectomy, contributing to the broader adoption and application of minimally invasive surgery (MIS) in various procedures.

References

1. Nam C, Lee JS, Kim JS, et al. Evolution of minimally invasive cholecystectomy: a narrative review. BMC Surg. 2024;24:378. https://doi.org/10.1186/s12893-024-02659-x.
2. Osborne DA, Alexander G, Boe B, Zervos EE. Laparoscopic cholecystectomy: past, present, and future. Surg Technol Int. 2006;15:81–5.
3. Singh BP, Pandey A, Sarda H, Hareesh SN, Regmi S. An institutional approach to thick wall gall bladder and our experience of 5450 gallstone disease. J Minim Access Surg. 2024; https://doi.org/10.4103/jmas.jmas_209_24.
4. Caskey RC, Owei L, Rao R, Riddle EW, Brooks AD, Dempsey DT, Morris JB, Neylan CJ, Williams NN, Dumon KR. Integration of hands-on team training into existing curriculum

improves both technical and nontechnical skills in laparoscopic cholecystectomy. J Surg Educ. 2017;74(6):915–20. https://doi.org/10.1016/j.jsurg.2017.05.007.
5. Udwadia TE. Laparoscopic cholecystectomy—the new surgery. Hepato-Gastroenterology. 1992;39(4):287–8.
6. Nagral S. Anatomy relevant to cholecystectomy. J Minim Access Surg. 2005;1(2):53–8. https://doi.org/10.4103/0972-9941.16527.
7. Abdalla S, Pierre S, Ellis H. Calot's triangle. Clin Anat. 2013;26(4):493–501. https://doi.org/10.1002/ca.22170.
8. Pisano M, Allievi N, Gurusamy K, Borzellino G, Cimbanassi S, Boerna D. 2020 World Society of Emergency Surgery updated guidelines for the diagnosis and treatment of acute calculus cholecystitis. World J Emerg Surg. 2020;15(1):61.
9. Overby DW, Apelgren KN, Richardson W, Fanelli R. Society of American gastrointestinal and endoscopic surgeons. SAGES guidelines for the clinical application of laparoscopic biliary tract surgery. Surg Endosc. 2010;24(10):2368–86. https://doi.org/10.1007/s00464-010-1268-7.
10. Alberton A, Peltz ED. Cholecystectomy. Surg Clin North Am. 2024;104(6):1203–15. https://doi.org/10.1016/j.suc.2024.04.011.
11. Sandler BJ, Davis KA, Schuster KM. Symptomatic human immunodeficiency virus-infected patients have poorer outcomes following emergency general surgery: a study of the nationwide inpatient sample. J Trauma Acute Care Surg. 2019;86(3):479–88. https://doi.org/10.1097/TA.0000000000002161.
12. Meshikhes AW. Asymptomatic gallstones in the laparoscopic era. J R Coll Surg Edinb. 2002;47(6):742–8.
13. Martins RA, Soares RS, Vito FBD, Barbosa VDF, Silva SS, Moraes-Souza H, Martins PRJ. Cholelithiasis and its complications in sickle cell disease in a university hospital. Rev Bras Hematol Hemoter. 2016;39(1):28–31. https://doi.org/10.1016/j.bjhh.2016.09.009.
14. Dasari BV, Tan CJ, Gurusamy KS, Martin DJ, Kirk G, McKie L, Diamond T, Taylor MA. Surgical versus endoscopic treatment of bile duct stones. Cochrane Database Syst Rev. 2013;2013(12):CD003327. https://doi.org/10.1002/14651858.CD003327.pub4.
15. Lei C, Lu T, Yang W, Yang M, Tian H, Song S, Gong S, Yang J, Jiang W, Yang K, Guo T. Comparison of intraoperative endoscopic retrograde cholangiopancreatography and laparoscopic common bile duct exploration combined with laparoscopic cholecystectomy for treating gallstones and common bile duct stones: a systematic review and meta-analysis. Surg Endosc. 2021;35(11):5918–35. https://doi.org/10.1007/s00464-021-08648-y.
16. Pallati P, Oleynikov D. Laparoscopic cholecystectomy. In: Soper NJ, Scott-Conner CEH, editors. The SAGES manual: Volume 1 basic laparoscopy and endoscopy. p. 255. https://doi.org/10.1007/978-1-4614-2344-7_20.
17. The SAGES cholecystectomy program: Strategies for Minimizing Bile Duct Injuries: Adopting a Universal Culture of Safety in Cholecystectomy.www.sages.org/safe-cholecystectomy-program/. Accessed 27 Feb 2018.
18. Tsalis K, Antoniou N, Koukouritaki Z, Patridas D, Christoforidis E, Lazaridis C. Open-access technique and "critical view of safety" as the safest way to perform laparoscopic cholecystectomy. Surg Laparosc Endosc Percutan Tech. 2015;25(2):119–24.
19. Soper NJ, Scott-Conner CEH, editors. The SAGES manual, volume 1, basic laparoscopy and endoscopy. 3rd ed. New York: Springer; 2012.
20. Pucher PH, Brunt LM, Fanelli RD, Asbun HJ, Aggarwal R. SAGES expert Delphi consensus: critical factors for safe surgical practice in laparoscopic cholecystectomy. Surg Endosc. 2015;9(11):3074–85.
21. Esposito F, Scoleri I, Cattan R, Cook MC, Sacrieru D, Meziani N, Del Prete M, Kabbej M. Systematic intraoperative cholangiography during elective laparoscopic cholecystectomy: is it a justifiable practice? Ann Hepatobiliary Pancreat Surg. 2023;27(2):166–71. https://doi.org/10.14701/ahbps.22-099.
22. Gurusamy KS, Davidson C, Gluud C, Davidson BR. Early versus delayed laparoscopic cholecystectomy for people with acute cholecystitis. Cochrane Database Syst Rev. 2013;6:CD005440.

23. Edebo A, Andersson J, Gustavsson J, Jivegård L, Ribokas D, Svanberg T, Wallerstedt SM. Benefits and risks of using laparoscopic ultrasonography versus intraoperative cholangiography during laparoscopic cholecystectomy for gallstone disease: a systematic review and meta-analysis. Surg Endosc. 2024;38(9):5096–107. https://doi.org/10.1007/s00464-024-10979-5.
24. Hall C, Amatya S, Shanmugasundaram R, Lau NS, Beenen E, Gananadha S. Intraoperative cholangiography in laparoscopic cholecystectomy: a systematic review and meta-analysis. JSLS. 2023;27(1):e2022.00093. https://doi.org/10.4293/JSLS.2022.00093.
25. Zhu J, Li G, Du P, Zhou X, Xiao W, Li Y. Laparoscopic common bile duct exploration versus intraoperative endoscopic retrograde cholangiopancreatography in patients with gallbladder and common bile duct stones: a meta-analysis. Surg Endosc. 2021;35(3):997–1005. https://doi.org/10.1007/s00464-020-08052-y.
26. Lyu Y, Cheng Y, Li T, Cheng B, Jin X. Laparoscopic common bile duct exploration plus cholecystectomy versus endoscopic retrograde cholangiopancreatography plus laparoscopic cholecystectomy for cholecystocholedocholithiasis: a meta-analysis. Surg Endosc. 2019;33(10):3275–86. https://doi.org/10.1007/s00464-018-06613-w.
27. Philip Rothman J, Burcharth J, Pommergaard HC, Viereck S, Rosenberg J. Preoperative risk factors for conversion of laparoscopic cholecystectomy to open surgery—A systematic review and meta-analysis of observational studies. Dig Surg. 2016;33(5):414–23.
28. Adisa AO, Olasehinde O, Alatise OI, Ibitoye BO, Faponle AF, Lawal OO. Conversions and complications of elective laparoscopic cholecystectomy in a West African population. Egypt J Surg. 2018;37(4):440–4.
29. St CK. Recent classifications of the common bile duct injury. Korean J Hepatobiliary Pancreat Surg. 2014;18(3):69–72. https://doi.org/10.14701/kjhbps.2014.18.3.69.
30. Fernicola A, Palomba G, De Capuano M, Palma GGD, Aprea G. Artificial intelligence applied to laparoscopic cholecystectomy: what is the next step? A narrative review. Updat Surg. 2024;76:1655–67.
31. Petracchi EJ, Olivieri SE, Varela J, Canullan CM, Zandalazini H, Ocampo C, Quesada BM. Use of artificial intelligence in the detection of the critical view of safety during laparoscopic cholecystectomy. J Gastrointest Surg. 2024;28(6):877–9. https://doi.org/10.1016/j.gassur.2024.03.018. Epub 2024 Mar 18
32. Protserov S, Hunter J, Zhang H, Mashouri P, Masino C, Brudno M, Madani A. Development, deployment and scaling of operating room-ready artificial intelligence for real-time surgical decision support. NPJ Digit Med. 2024;7(1):231. https://doi.org/10.1038/s41746-024-01225-2.
33. Gyedu A, Bingener J, Dally C, Oppong J, Price R, Reid-Lombardo K. Starting a laparoscopic surgery programme in the second largest teaching hospital in Ghana. East Afr Med J. 2014;91(4):133–7.
34. Falola AF, Fadairo RT, Dada OS, Adenikinju JS, Ogbodu E, Effiong-John B, Akande DG, Okere MO, Adelotan A, Ndong A. Current state of minimally invasive general surgical practice in Africa: a systematic review and meta-analysis of the laparoscopic procedures performed and outcomes. World J Surg. 2024;48(7):1634–50. https://doi.org/10.1002/wjs.12195.
35. Adisa AO, Lawal OO, Arowolo OA, Alatise OI. Local adaptations aid establishment of laparoscopic surgery in a semi-urban Nigerian Hospital. Surg Endosc. 2013;27:390–3.
36. Yankunze Y, Mwachiro MM, Lando JO, Bachheta N, Mangaoang D, Bekele A, Parker RK. Laparoscopy experience in East, Central, and Southern Africa: insights from operative case volume analysis. Surg Endosc. 2024;38(8):4415–21. https://doi.org/10.1007/s00464-024-10960-2.
37. Adisa AO, Lawal OO, Adejuyigbe O. Trend over time for cholecystectomy following the introduction of laparoscopy in a Nigerian tertiary hospital. Nig J Surg. 2017;23(2):102–5.

Chapter 15
Difficult Cholecystectomy

Adedapo Osinowo

Introduction

Laparoscopic cholecystectomy (LC) has become the gold standard treatment for symptomatic cholelithiasis. It is customarily a basic laparoscopic procedure but, in some situations, it becomes an advanced one. This is the situation in a difficult gall bladder as it incurs an increased surgical risk compared with basic or standard cholecystectomy [1]. LC can be more difficult in situations that obscure normal biliary anatomy (e.g., acute, or chronic cholecystitis) or operative exposure (e.g., obesity or prior upper abdominal surgery). Several conditions have been associated with difficult gallbladder and these include acute cholecystitis, severe chronic cholecystitis, Mirizzi syndrome, cirrhosis, and other non-gall bladder-related factors such as morbid obesity and extensive previous upper abdominal surgery. Other predictors of surgical difficulty are male gender, increased age, and increased number of 'attacks' that have been identified as risk factors for severe inflammation [2–4]. An appraisal of pre-operative data and diagnostic imaging using operating time or the open conversion rate as indicators of surgical difficulty in symptomatic cholelithiasis identified body mass index, non-visualized gallbladder on preoperative cholangiography, cyst duct length, temperature, and abnormal findings on computed tomography as five factors that significantly affected the time required for cholecystectomy [5]. Additionally, other studies identified gallbladder wall thickening (>4–5 mm on ultrasound), incarcerated stones in the GB neck, and duration of elevated C-reactive protein contributed to prolonged operating time [6]. These factors could be considered surrogate markers of the degree of inflammation. Similarly, another study found that the rates of open conversion and complications were significantly higher in Tokyo Guidelines 13 (TG13) Grade II and III cases compared with Grade I cases

A. Osinowo (✉)
Lagos University Teaching Hospital, Idi Araba, Lagos State, Nigeria
e-mail: aosinowo@unilag.edu.ng; adedapo.osinowo@npmcn.edu.ng

E. Ray-Offor, R. J. Rosenthal (eds.), *Principles and Practice of Laparoscopic Surgery*, https://doi.org/10.1007/978-3-031-96321-6_15

[7]. Based on the foregoing surgical difficulty can be predicted pre-operatively on the following factors: preoperative imaging and blood tests, and TG13 grade. Whilst arguably more technically challenging than basic LC, simple strategies can be employed to optimize patient outcomes. Preoperative recognition and awareness of these situations as well as modifications of technical strategies are important to a successful outcome and avoiding major complications in these patients. The underpinnings of these strategies are the following:

1. Cholelithiasis is a benign disease.
2. There are good and safe ways of completing an intended cholecystectomy without removing the gallbladder.
3. The harm of an iatrogenic biliary injury exceeds the benefit of completing a cholecystectomy many times over.

Accordingly, there must always be a "Culture of Safety in Cholecystectomy" [8] (COSIC) which includes the following:

(a) Putting safety first
(b) A reliable method of cyst duct identification such as the critical view of safety (CVS) must always be employed.
(c) The possibility of aberrant anatomy must always be considered
(d) Recognizing when dissection is approaching a zone of great danger and halting before entering the zone.
(e) It means getting help from another surgeon when things are difficult
(f) It means sometimes finishing the operation by a safe method other than cholecystectomy.

In the elective setting, the following conditions are associated with difficult gallbladder:

A. Morbid obesity
B. Acute cholecystitis
C. Severe chronic cholecystitis (contracted gall bladder)
D. Cirrhosis
E. Mirizzi's syndrome
F. Previous upper abdominal surgery

Task Analysis of Basic Laparoscopic Cholecystectomy

1. Preparation of the patient: The patient is positioned in either the American or French style. In the American style, with the patient supine the surgeon and camera operator position themselves to the patient's left while the assistant stands to the right. Conversely, the French setup involves the patient supine with the legs abducted, the surgeon positioned between the legs, the camera operator on the left, and the assistant on the right. The pneumoperitoneum is created by the Veress needle or the Hasson technique.

   (a) Standard 4 port technique: Optical (primary) port with a 30^0 laparoscope, epigastric port (10 mm), and two 5 mm ports, one subcostal trocar in the right upper quadrant and another 5 mm trocar lower at the right anterior axillary line.
   (b) Reverse Trendelenburg position and rotation to the left is instituted to give maximal exposure to the right upper quadrant.

2. Initial diagnostic laparoscopy
3. Retraction of the gallbladder fundus to expose the entire gallbladder using a grasper through the lateral 5 mm trocar in the anterior axillary is used for the retraction over the liver towards the right shoulder. Adhesions to the gall bladder should be taken down by blunt and sharp dissections (up to down to avoid duodenal injuries) to expose the entire gall bladder.
4. Another grasper in the medial 5 mm port is used to retract the infundibulum caudolaterally. This maneuver straightens the cyst duct (i.e., retracts it at 90^0 from the common bile duct (CBD) and helps protect the CBD from inadvertent injury.
5. Exposure and delicate dissection of the Calot's triangle to achieve the critical view of safety. It needs to identify clearly the common bile duct, the cystic duct, and the cystic artery.

   (a) Dissection of the cystic pedicle should be started with anteromedial traction by the lefthand grasper placed on the anterior edge of Hartmann's pouch. The peritoneum of the posterior leaf of the cystic pedicle is divided superficially as far back as the liver. The posterior leaf is dissected first because it is relatively less vascular and the bleeding if any, will not soil the anterior peritoneum, whereas if the anterior peritoneum is tackled first, it will make the dissection area of the posterior peritoneum filled with blood difficult. Once the visceral peritoneum is dissected an Endo Peanut or Maryland dissector is used for blunt dissection.
   (b) Cystic duct and cystic artery should be skeletonized, and a window created between them. The window should be near the gall bladder-cystic duct junction to avoid injury to the CBD. The lower third of the gallbladder must be freed from the cystic plate. This is the only way a dangerous anomaly in which the cystic duct drains directly into a variant right hepatic duct (or sectional or segmental duct) is identified.
   (c) A secure anatomy identification of the cystic duct and cystic artery through the establishment of the critical view of safety (CVS) before clipping any biliary structures must be achieved.

6. Clipping and division of the cyst duct and cystic artery. The medial clips should be placed first, before the lateral clips, to avoid lateral pinching of the common bile duct or the right branch of the hepatic artery.
7. Dissection of gall bladder from the liver bed
8. Extraction of the gall bladder and any spilled stone in a bag
9. Irrigation and suction of the operating field
10. Final diagnostic laparoscopy

Morbid Obesity

One of the risk factors for cholelithiasis is obesity, the incidence of which is increasing worldwide [9]. Therefore, surgeons are increasingly likely to encounter a growing number of obese patients who require cholecystectomy for symptomatic cholelithiasis. Hitherto, obesity was a relative contraindication because the technical difficulties were thought to be associated with higher morbidity and mortality as well as increased open conversion rates [10, 11]. The abdominal wall thickness increases the difficulty of access and torque on trocars, and the umbilicus is often displaced caudad which increases the distance of the laparoscopic camera from the gallbladder.

Furthermore, for patients with central obesity, an abundance of visceral fat may obscure the lower part of the gall bladder, and the liver may be bulky and fatty hence less flexible and harder to elevate to expose the gall bladder. The gall bladder is also often intrahepatic, which makes it more difficult to dissect from the liver bed. Nevertheless, with increasing experience in laparoscopic surgery and better instruments, several contemporary studies have demonstrated that LC can be safely performed [12–14].

Simple Strategies for Overcoming the Challenges of Morbid Obesity

(a) The camera port is not inserted at the umbilicus but rather roughly halfway between the umbilicus and xiphisternum or 15 cm below the xiphoid process
(b) A standard 4-trocar technique should be used but an additional trocar should be prepared for. In addition, there may be a need to ligate the fat-laden falciform ligament if it is obstructing the view.
(c) The patient may be positioned in steep reverse Trendelenburg to help displace the omentum and bowel loops caudally and improve operative vision.
(d) Extra equipment may be required such as an optical trocar, long Veress needle, liver retractor (to retract the omentum, transverse colon, and stomach), and extra 5 mm port.

Acute Cholecystitis (AC)

Acute cholecystitis is the most common cause of a difficult gallbladder [15]. The difficulties of LC in acute cholecystitis are related to the acute inflammatory process that can obscure the hepatocystic triangle and lead to difficulty in manipulating and retracting the gallbladder due to edema, large stones, or necrosis (Fig. 15.1). Accordingly, laparoscopic cholecystectomy in AC is not a basic laparoscopic surgery but rather an advanced laparoscopic procedure as severe inflammation of the gallbladder and its surroundings increases both the difficulty of LC and the frequency of postoperative complications. During the early inflammatory phase, the

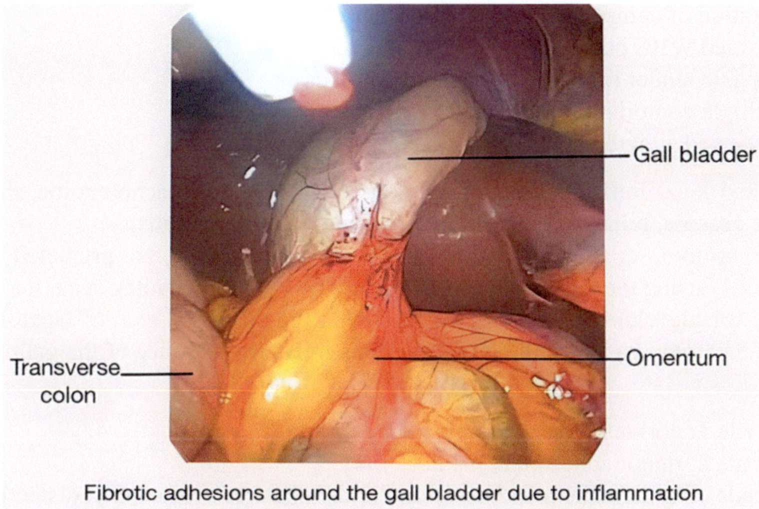

Fig. 15.1 Parkland Grade 3 acute cholecystitis

gallbladder is edematous, which makes dissection easier, whereas later in the process it becomes more vascular and fibrotic hence several societies have proposed early laparoscopic cholecystectomy. The timing of cholecystectomy in patients presenting with acute cholecystitis has been under intense investigation, with "early" cholecystectomy variably defined in the literature as gallbladder surgery performed within 3, 7, or 10 days of symptom onset and "delayed" cholecystectomy as that performed 7 or 45 days, or 6 weeks, after initial diagnosis [16]. However, the updated 2018 Tokyo Guidelines concluded that in patients for whom more than 72 h have passed since symptom onset, there are still benefits to performing cholecystectomy early, and recommended early cholecystectomy in low-risk patients with acute calculous cholecystitis regardless of how much time has passed since symptom onset [17].

The results of several randomized trials and subsequent meta-analyses have shown that LC performed for AC within 7 days from presentation appears as safe and effective as delayed LC for acute cholecystitis and may shorten total hospital stay [16, 18–22]. However, when acute local inflammation prevents the safe identification of the cyst duct and artery, surgeons should consider bail-out options. A bail-out procedure should also be undertaken when the Calot's triangle is appropriately defined but the critical view of safety (CVS) cannot be achieved because of the presence of severe fibrosis or non-dissectable scarring (chronic cholecystitis with biliary inflammatory fusion (BIF). The surgical difficulty of AC varies greatly depending on the severity of inflammation and fibrosis. Correspondingly, the risk of biliary duct injury (BDI) has been shown to increase with the severity of AC [23].

Surgeons must intuitively recognize the risk factors for increased difficulty of cholecystectomy for acute cholecystitis:

1. Duration of complaints greater than 72 h
2. Elevated WBC count (>18,000/mm^3)
3. Palpable tender mass in the right upper quadrant*
4. Multiple comorbidities,
5. Suspected gangrenous cholecystitis [24].

* Marked local inflammation (gangrenous cholecystitis, pericholecystic abscess, hepatic abscess, biliary peritonitis, emphysematous cholecystitis).

Furthermore, crucially the degree of difficulty could be predicted intra-operatively using the Parkland grading scale. The Parkland grading scale for cholecystitis was developed and validated to predict the difficulty level of laparoscopic cholecystectomy based on the initial (intraoperative) appearance of the gallbladder [25, 26]:

(a) Grade 1: normal
(b) Grade 2: minor adhesion at the neck only
(c) Grade 3: hyperemia, pericholecystic fluid, adhesions to the body, distention
(d) Grade 4: adhesion obscuring the majority of the gallbladder, or Grade I-III with abnormal liver anatomy, intrahepatic gallbladder, or impacted stone (Mirizzi)
(e) Grade 5: perforation, necrosis, or inability to visualize gallbladder [27]

Technical difficulties associated with LC for AC include the following:

(a) Dense adhesions
(b) Increased vascularity of tissues
(c) Difficulty in grasping the gallbladder
(d) Impacted stone in the gallbladder neck or cystic duct
(e) Shortening and thickening of the cystic duct
(f) Approximation of the CBD to the gallbladder

Important points that will prevent biliary injury in AC

1. *Early LC before fibrosis:* LC for AC should be performed at an early stage before florid inflammation and fibrosis develop to avoid biliary duct injury (BDI). Frequently, the adhesions to the gallbladder that occur as a reaction to inflammatory attacks are usually avascular. Dissection of these adhesions should begin at the fundus of the gallbladder and should then proceed down toward the neck of the gallbladder. The best way to take them down is to grasp the gallbladder with grasping forceps at the site where the adhesions attach and gradually place traction on the adhesions with the other hand.
2. *Decompression of the gallbladder should be done early if it is distended***.** This could be done by needle aspiration using a Veress needle or Spinal needle gauge 14 or puncture of the fundus with a 5 mm trocar. This allows better grasping and retraction of the gallbladder and thus good exposure of the Calot's triangle.
3. *Dissection of the Calot's triangle should be done carefully with a suction-irrigation device*. This is particularly useful in defining anatomy around a grossly inflamed duct. This may be the safest technique. A laparoscopic peanut or laparoscopic Kittner dissector can also be used for blunt dissection.

4. *Dissection along the GB surface with the following landmarks*: The plane of dissection should be on the gallbladder. If the GB surface is difficult to identify in the Calot's triangle, an attempt should first be made to identify the GB surface from the dorsal side of the neck of the GB. If the GB surface is still difficult to identify, bail-out procedures should be considered.
5. *Creation of the CVS* must be achieved (Fig. 15.2).
6. *Troubleshooting:* Control of short or wide cyst duct. Edema and acute inflammation may lead to thickening and foreshortening of the cyst duct, with subsequent difficulties in dissection and ligation. If the duct is edematous or wide, clips may

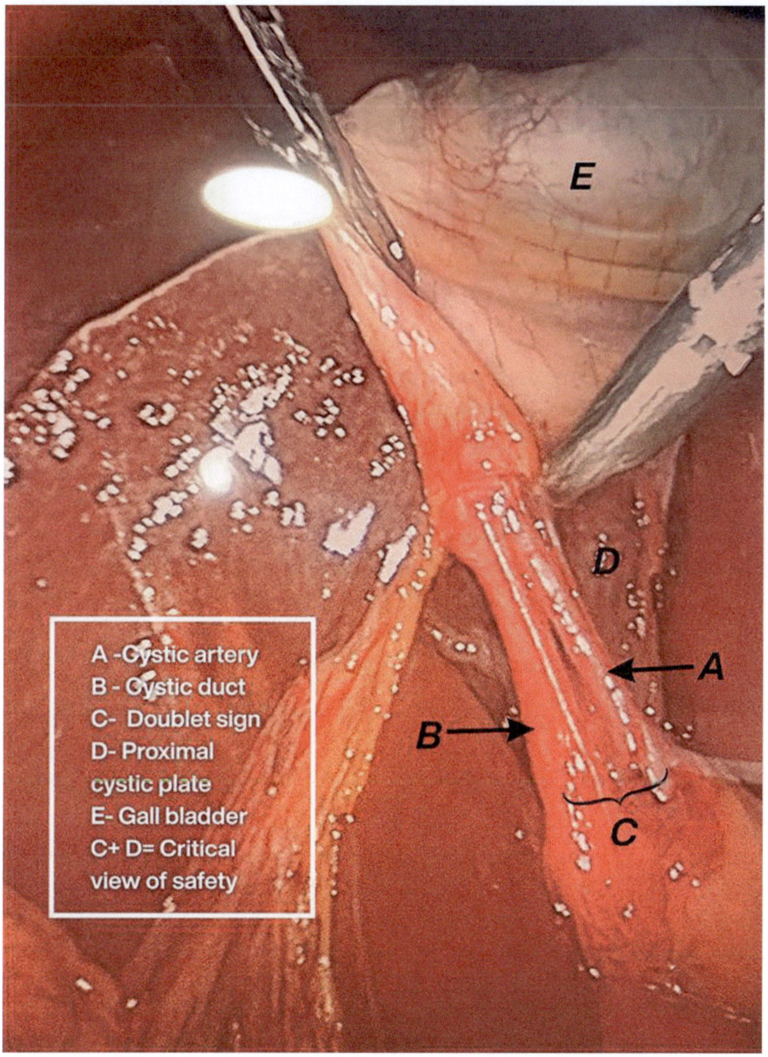

Fig. 15.2 Illustrates the critical view of safety during a laparoscopic cholecystectomy

either cut through it or not occlude completely. Consequently, the surgeon should be familiar with techniques for ligating the duct with either intracorporeal or extracorporeal ties. It is extremely helpful to know how to tie extracorporeal knots so that the cystic duct can be ligated in continuity before it is divided.

7. Rarely, an *endoscopic stapler* could be used to transect an unusually large cystic duct after ensuring that the structure is not, in fact, the common bile duct.
8. If the inflammation is significant and further dissection is considered risky an *intra-operative cholangiogram (IOC)* should be done to define biliary anatomy.
9. *Bail-out procedures:* This should be embarked upon if the gallbladder surface and/or the anatomy of the Calot's triangle is unclear. This could either be laparoscopic or open cholecystectomy and surgeons should make appropriate judgments based on intraoperative findings.

The critical view of safety has been achieved with only two structures (the cystic duct and artery) entering directly into the gall bladder and the proximal cystic plate dissected.

Severe Chronic Cholecystitis

Repeated episodes of biliary colic may lead to chronic inflammation and dense scarring in the hepatocystic triangle with biliary inflammatory fusion (BIF). The inflammation may extend to the porta hepatis. There may be a fusion of CBD and the neck of the gall bladder. The gall bladder may be shrunken, contracted, and intrahepatic. The risk factors for chronic cholecystitis are multiple previous attacks of biliary colic (> 10 attacks), male sex, previous upper abdominal surgery, obesity, and thickened gallbladder wall on abdominal ultrasound. In these patients, adherence to the principles of safe LC should be employed however, if there are problems with exposure of the hepatocystic triangle, either a subtotal cholecystectomy or conversion to open cholecystectomy should be performed. Topdown cholecystectomy should be used with caution in the setting of biliary inflammatory fusion (BIF).

Cirrhosis and Portal Hypertension

Cholelithiasis in cirrhotic patients is commoner than in the general population due to several reasons; increased intravascular hemolysis from hypersplenism, reduced gallbladder motility and emptying due to high oestrogen levels, and metabolic liver failure. In cirrhosis, there is a fibrotic and stiff liver with profuse collaterals from portal hypertension and a woody and friable intrahepatic gallbladder. The stiff liver is difficult to retract cranially, diminishing the retraction of the gallbladder fundus that is needed to expose the triangle of Calot [28].

Patients with cirrhosis and symptomatic gallstones are at increased risk during cholecystectomy for several reasons:

1. Increased collaterals and portal hypertension increase the risk of bleeding.
2. Risk of deterioration in liver function with surgery and anesthesia.
3. Increased difficulty of exposure due to the fibrosis in the liver

Historically, LC has been contraindicated in cirrhotic patients due to post-operative deaths from post-operative liver failure, sepsis, and hemorrhage [29]. However, with the advent of better and advanced laparoscopic devices such as ultrasonic shears, LC can be undertaken in selected patients (Child-Pugh A and B), with the caveat the patients must be managed by surgeons adept at providing peri-operative care of cirrhotic patients [30].

Pre-evaluation of the cirrhotic patient requires the following:

1. Determine the Child-Pugh classification and Model for End Stage Liver Disease (MELD) score
2. Computerized tomography with portal phase to identify potential varices: umbilicus (recanalized umbilical vein), porta hepatitis, gall bladder bed
3. Optimize liver function
4. Coagulation parameters and crossmatching for blood.

The major difficulties encountered during LC in cirrhotic patients can be predominately classified into 5 areas [31, 32]:

1. Adhesions with increased neovascularity around the gallbladder
2. Difficulty with retraction of the liver.
3. Inadequate exposure of the cholecystohepatic triangle
4. A high-risk gallbladder bed: Tortuous, dilated vessels may occur in the gallbladder bed that are easily injured and bleed profusely.
5. A high-risk hilum: A cavernous transformation of the portal vein or neovascularity around the hilum renders hilar dissection dangerous.

LC in Cirrhotic Patients

1. Insertion of the primary trocar may be done subumbilically as opposed to through the umbilicus to avoid collaterals using a Veress Needle. If possible, there should be an initial transillumination of the abdominal wall to look out for collaterals. Alternatively, an open access of peritoneal entry may be done. In the event sectioning of the recanalized umbilical vein during trocar insertion occurs a transmural ligation of the injured parietal vessels should be done.
2. CO_2 pneumoperitoneum should be done with lower pressures to preclude damage to the liver and kidney because of reperfusion injury. The pressure should be maintained at about 1.33KPa and gradually relieved after LC. In addition, reduced pressure will reduce venous bleeding.

3. Standard 4-trocar technique can be used but an extra 5mm trocar to the right of the epigastric port may be needed to allow passage of a blunt retractor to elevate or lift the right lobe cranially. Furthermore, in the event the quadrate lobe is large and obscures the operative area an additional blunt retractor should be passed through a left lumbar port at the level of the umbilicus. All these maneuvers will ensure effective exposure to the hepatocystic triangle. If all these fail the retraction of the gallbladder should be done on the body just above the infundibulum rather than the fundus or a fundus first technique is done.
4. Careful dissection of vascular adhesions and dilated tortuous collaterals around the gallbladder and vascularised omental adhesions should be done using advanced energy devices like Harmonic scalpel or Ligasure.
5. High-risk gallbladder bed: laparoscopic subtotal cholecystectomy with the posterior wall intact with the liver. The remnant mucosa is removed either by mucosectomy in patients with acute cholecystitis or by electrofulguration in those with chronic cholecystitis [31, 32].
6. High-risk hilum: laparoscopic subtotal cholecystectomy.
7. Haemostasis at the gallbladder bed may be secured with an Argon device, oxidized cellulose, or surgicel.

Mirizzi Syndrome

Mirizzi syndrome (MS) is defined as a common hepatic duct obstruction caused by extrinsic compression from an impacted stone in the cystic duct or infundibulum of the gallbladder [33, 34]. It is estimated to occur in 0.05–4% of patients undergoing surgery for cholelithiasis [35, 36].

Patients with Mirizzi syndrome may present with right upper quadrant pain, jaundice, and fever. However, all three symptoms are present in 44% to 71% of patients [37]. Abdominal pain is the most common presenting symptom followed by jaundice, and less commonly with the classical triad of cholangitis [38]. Crucially, symptoms are similar to that of acute and chronic cholecystitis, with or without jaundice [39, 40]. Notably, however, preoperative diagnosis on clinical presentation and investigations is not possible in a majority of patients [41].

The principal abnormality in Mirizzi syndrome starts with an inflammatory response to an impacted gallstone in Hartmann's pouch or the cystic duct. Repeated bouts of cholecystitis cause inflammation and fibrosis, Mirizzi syndrome type I. The recurrent inflammation results in pressure necrosis of the common bile duct and resultant cholecystocholedochal fistula, Mirizzi syndrome type II [42]. The dense adhesions and edematous inflammatory tissue in the hepatocystic triangle or cystic pedicle in MS can distort the normal anatomy and increase the risk of biliary injury, particularly with laparoscopic surgery. Given the foregoing, Mirizzi Syndrome (MS) represents one of the most complex pathologies that can be encountered during laparoscopic cholecystectomy [43]. Not unexpectedly, it is associated with surgical difficulty, a high conversion rate, and a high risk of operative complications, particularly bile duct injury [43].

Management of MS Diagnosed Intra-Operatively

1. Recognition of a suspected Mirizzi syndrome is an important tactical first step in its management. A wide and thickened cystic duct with or without stones can be the first sign of a Type I abnormality. Dissection around the body of the gallbladder can safely identify the neck of the gallbladder
2. Blunt dissection of the cystic pedicle is the mainstay in suspected MS to isolate the cystic duct and cystic artery. This is usually not possible in the context of Mirizzi syndrome. Swab dissection is the safest method of blunt dissection.
3. Once it is concluded that a critical view of safety is not possible, alternative approaches are used including infundibular identification and dissection, transvesical access, and removal of stones or subtotal cholecystectomy as a last resort.
4. Removal of palpable pedicle stone/stones by opening the neck of the gallbladder can facilitate safe cystic duct dissection and help to prepare it for cholangiography.
5. Following an intraoperative cholangiography, a subtotal cholecystectomy should be undertaken.
6. An Intraoperative cholangiogram is mandatory to define the anatomy of the ducts and to rule out common bile duct stones. Mirizzi type I anomalies are suspected or confirmed when there is difficulty in passing the cholangiography catheter or when cannulation is impossible. The cystic duct may be dilated and surrounded by inflammatory tissue. In MS type II it is usually performed through the fistula after stones have been dislodged during swab dissection of the cystic pedicle and may show the presence of further stones in the bile duct.
7. In MS type I if it is possible to dissect the cystic pedicle the cystic duct stump is closed with an endoloop or intracorporeal suturing. While in MS type II a T-tube is placed through the fistula after removing CBD stones with no attempts to suture or patch the fistula.

Previous Operations

With previous upper abdominal operations, there could be adhesions that would compromise access to the operative field, hence, consider alternate initial access sites other than the umbilicus. Options include any of the following:

1. Veress needle access in the left upper quadrant (Palmer's point).
2. Open epigastric region: The liver will preclude bowel adhesions to the abdominal wall. An important principle is to perform initial access in a quadrant of the abdomen expected to be free from prior procedures. For example, avoid the right upper quadrant in a patient who has had a right colectomy. Furthermore, adhesiolysis should be done without energy to minimize the risk of thermal injury to the bowel. Finally, the surgeon should have a low threshold for conversion. In addition, optical trocars could be used for primary access to minimize the likeli-

hood of bowel injury. Optical trocars enable controlled access under vision and ensure the safety of entry. They can easily be retracted from adhesions before gas insufflation.

Subtotal Cholecystectomy

Subtotal cholecystectomy is a bail-out procedure that is undertaken in difficult cases to minimize the likelihood of complications. In these difficult situations, safe identification of the cystic duct and artery is not possible on account of acute local inflammation or chronic cholecystitis with biliary inflammatory fusion (BIF). Tokyo Guidelines 2018 (TG18) advocate subtotal cholecystectomy for difficult situations as a bail-out procedure to avoid serious damage to the bile duct. Strasberg *et al* clarified the subtypes of subtotal cholecystectomy: fenestrated versus reconstituting [44]. In the reconstituted subtype, the lower end of the gallbladder is closed off, thus reducing the incidence of postoperative fistula, but creates a remnant neo gallbladder, which may result in recurrence of symptomatic cholecystolithiasis and occasionally the need for a second and more difficult completion cholecystectomy. Fenestrating subtotal cholecystectomy does not occlude the gallbladder but may suture the cyst duct internally. It has a high incidence of postoperative biliary fistula but does not appear to be associated with recurrent cholecystolithiasis. However, recent systematic reviews demonstrated the safety of these procedures [45, 46].

Once the decision is made to proceed with subtotal cholecystectomy, the surgeon should consider his/ her expertise and whether to convert to an open procedure or continue laparoscopically. Laparoscopic subtotal cholecystectomy is a safe and alternative procedure to total cholecystectomy, but it may require advanced laparoscopic skills. A systematic review and a meta-analysis revealed that although postoperative bile leakage was more common following laparoscopic subtotal cholecystectomy compared with open conversion, rates of BDI, postoperative complications, reoperation, and mortality were all lower [47, 48].

Steps of Laparoscopic Fenestrating Subtotal Cholecystectomy

(a) Incision of the anterior (perationalized) wall of the gall bladder in the fundus.
(b) Contents of the gall bladder should be evacuated into an Endobag.
(c) Incision is further continued down toward the infundibulum removing most of the anterior wall of the gall bladder. A portion of the anterior wall of the infundibulum must be left to avoid inadvertent entry into the hepatoduodenal ligament (Shield of McElmoyle) [49].

(d) Most of the anterior wall of the gallbladder should be removed and all stones evacuated, then the inner aspect of the gall bladder examined. It is important to check for biliary drainage from the gallbladder. Furthermore, if the internal orifice of the cystic duct is patent and bile is draining from it, it should be closed from the inside with an absorbable suture.
(e) A drain should be left in the hepatorenal recess and monitored for biliary drainage.

Error Traps

When the Infundibular technique is used for cystic duct identification based on the appearance of the infundibulum-cystic junction as a funnel, it can become an error trap in the following circumstances because the hepatocystic triangle has not been completely dissected:

1. Cystic duct is fused with common hepatic duct (CHD) due to acute or chronic inflammation.
2. The cystic duct is effaced by a large stone impacted in the infundibulum.
3. Difficulty exposing the hepatocystic triangle due to inadequate retraction (e.g., due to fibrosis) the CBD may be identified as the cystic duct.

In the above situations, circumferential dissection goes around the CHD/CBD rather than the cystic duct and leads to the classical BDI where the bile duct is divided twice before the gallbladder can be separated from the liver. It thus becomes an error trap.

Fundus First Technique or Dome-Down Technique

Used commonly in open cholecystectomy but rarely used in LC as it poses technical challenges as the gallbladder tends to twist once separated completely from the liver. Moreover, there is difficulty in retracting the liver. It becomes an error trap for the unwary surgeon in the following circumstances:

1. Chronic cholecystitis (shrunken gallbladder and shortened cystic plate)- the distance between the fundus and right portal pedicle is shortened hence the risk of vasculobiliary injury.
2. Chronic cholecystitis (fused planes and distorted anatomy)- the operator may dissect close to the liver rather than the gallbladder in the HC triangle which puts hilar structures at risk.

References

1. Elshaer M, Gravante G, Thomas K, Sorge R, Al-Hamali S, Ebdewi H. Subtotal cholecystectomy for "difficult gallbladders": systematic review and meta-analysis. JAMA Surg. 2015;150(2):159–68.
2. Panni RZ, Strasberg SM. Preoperative predictors of conversion as indicators of local inflammation in acute cholecystitis: strategies for future studies to develop quantitative predictors. J Hepatobiliary Pancreat Sci. 2018;25:101–8.
3. Philip Rothman J, Burcharth J, Pommergaard HC, Viereck S, Rosenberg J. Preoperative risk factors for conversion of laparoscopic cholecystectomy to open surgery—a systematic review and meta-analysis of observational studies. Dig Surg. 2016;33:414–23.
4. Santos BF, Brunt LM, Pucci MJ. The difficult gallbladder: a safe approach to a dangerous problem. J Laparoendosc Adv Surg Tech A. 2017;27:571–8.
5. Sakuramoto S, Sato S, Okuri T, Sato K, Hiki Y, Kakita A. Pre-operative evaluation to predict technical difficulties of laparoscopic cholecystectomy based on histological inflammation findings on the resected gallbladder. Am J Surg. 2000;179:114–21.
6. Hiromatsu T, Hasegawa H, Salamoto E, Komatsu S, Kawai K, Tabata T, et al. Preoperative evaluation of difficulty of laparoscopic cholecystectomy (in Japanese). J Gastroenterol Surg. 2007;40:1449–55.
7. Wakabayashi G, Iwashita Y, Hibi T, Takada T, Strasberg SM, Asbun HJ, Endo I, et al. Tokyo guidelines 2018: surgical management of acute cholecystitis: safe steps in laparoscopic cholecystectomy for acute cholecystitis (with videos). J Hepatobiliary Pancreat Sci. 2018;25(1):73–86. https://doi.org/10.1002/jhbp.517. Epub 2018 Jan 10
8. Strasberg SM. A teaching program for the "culture of safety in cholecystectomy" and avoidance of bile duct injury. J Am Coll Surg. 2013;217:751.
9. Stender S, Nordestgaard BG, Tybjaerg-Hansen A. Elevated body mass index as a causal risk factor for symptomatic gallstone disease: a Mendelian randomization study. Hepatology. 2013;58(6):2133–41. https://doi.org/10.1002/hep.26563. Epub 2013 Oct 11
10. Liu CL, Fan ST, Lai EC, Lo CM, Chu KM. Factors affecting conversion of laparoscopic cholecystectomy to open surgery. Arch Surg. 1996;131:98–101.
11. Unger SW, Unger HM, Edelman DS, Scott JS, Rosenbaum G. Obesity: an indication rather than contraindication to laparoscopic cholecystectomy. Obes Surg. 1992;2(1):29–31.
12. Simopoulos C, Polychronidis A, Botaitis S, Perente S, Pitiakoudis M. Laparoscopic cholecystectomy in obese patients. Obes Surg. 2005;15:243–6.
13. Ammori BJ, Vezakis A, Davides D, Martin IG, Larvin M, McMahon MJ. Laparoscopic cholecystectomy in morbidly obese patients. Surg Endosc. 2001;15:1336–9.
14. Paajanen H, Kakela P, Suuronen S, Paajanen J, Juvonen P, Pihlajamaki J. Impact of obesity and associated diseases on outcome after laparoscopic cholecystectomy. Surg Laparosc Endosc Percutan Tech. 2012;22:509–13.
15. Strasberg SM. Clinical practice. Acute calculous cholecystitis. N Engl J Med. 2008;358(26):2804–11.
16. Ansaloni L, Pisano M, Coccolini F, Peitzmann AB, Fingerhut A, Catena F, et al. 2016 WSES guidelines on acute calculous cholecystitis. World J Emerg Surg. 2016;11:25.
17. Okamoto K, Suzuki K, Takada T, Strasberg SM, Asbun HJ, Endo I, et al. Tokyo Guidelines 2018: flowchart for the management of acute cholecystitis. J Hepatobiliary Pancreat Sci. 2018;25(1):55–72. https://doi.org/10.1002/jhbp.516. Epub 2017 Dec 20. Erratum in: J Hepatobiliary Pancreat Sci. 2019 Nov;26(11):534
18. Gutt CN, Encke J, Köninger J, et al. Acute cholecystitis: early versus delayed cholecystectomy, a multicenter randomized trial (ACDC study, NCT00447304). Ann Surg. 2013;258:385.
19. de Mestral C, Rotstein OD, Laupacis A, et al. Comparative operative outcomes of early and delayed cholecystectomy for acute cholecystitis: a population-based propensity score analysis. Ann Surg. 2014;259:10–5.

20. Zafar SN, Obirieze A, Adesibikan B, et al. Optimal time for early laparoscopic cholecystectomy for acute cholecystitis. JAMA Surg. 2015;150:129.
21. Roulin D, Saadi A, Di Mare L, et al. Early versus delayed cholecystectomy for acute Cholecystitis, are the 72 hours still the rule?: a randomized trial. Ann Surg. 2016;264:717.
22. Cao AM, Eslick GD, Cox MR. Early cholecystectomy is superior to delayed cholecystectomy for acute Cholecystitis: a meta-analysis. J Gastrointest Surg. 2015;19:848.
23. Tornqvist B, Waage A, Zheng Z, Ye W, Nilsson M. Severity of acute cholecystitis and risk of iatrogenic bile duct injury during cholecystectomy, a population-based case-control study. World J Surg. 2016;40:1060–7.
24. Hirota M, Takada T, Kawarada Y, Nimura Y, Miura F, Hirata K, Mayumi T. Y diagnostic criteria and severity assessment of acute cholecystitis: Tokyo guidelines. J Hepato-Biliary-Pancreat Surg. 2007;14(1):78–82. https://doi.org/10.1007/s00534-006-1159-4. Epub 2007 Jan 30
25. Madni TD, Leshikar DE, Minshall CT, Nakonezny PA, Cornelius CC, Imran JB, Clark AT, Williams BH, Eastman AL, Minei JP, Phelan HA, Cripps MW. The parkland grading scale for cholecystitis. Am J Surg. 2018;215(4):625–30.
26. Madni TD, Nakonezny PA, Barrios E, Imran JB, Clark AT, Taveras L, Cunningham HB, Christie A, Eastman AL, Minshall CT, Luk S, Minei JP, Phelan HA, Cripps MW. Prospective validation of the parkland grading scale for Cholecystitis. Am J Surg. 2019;217(1):90–7.
27. Madni TD, Nakonezny PA, Imran JB, Taveras L, Cunningham HB, Vela R, Clark AT, Minshall CT, Eastman AL, Luk S, Phelan HA, Cripps MW. A comparison of cholecystitis grading scales. J Trauma Acute Care Surg. 2019;86(3):471–8.
28. de Goede B, Klitsie PJ, Hagen SM, et al. Meta-analysis of laparoscopic versus open cholecystectomy for patients with liver cirrhosis and symptomatic cholecystolithiasis. Br J Surg. 2013;100(2):209–16.
29. Delis S, Bakoyiannis A, Madariaga J, Bramis J, Tassopoulos N, Dervenis C. Laparoscopic cholecystectomy in cirrhotic patients: the value of MELD score and child-Pugh classification in predicting outcome. Surg Endosc. 2010;24(2):407–12.
30. Quillin RC 3rd, Burns JM, Pineda JA, Hanseman D, Rudich SM, Edwards MJ, Tevar AD. Laparoscopic cholecystectomy in the cirrhotic patient: predictors of outcome. Surgery. 2013;153(5):634–40.
31. Palanivelu C, Rajan PS, Jani K, et al. Laparoscopic cholecystectomy in cirrhotic patients: the role of subtotal cholecystectomy and its variants. J Am Coll Surg. 2006;203(2):145–51.
32. Bessa SS, Abdel-Razek AH, Sharaan MA, Bassiouni AE, El-Khishen MA, El-Kayal el SA. Laparoscopic cholecystectomy in cirrhosis: a prospective randomized study comparing the conventional diathermy and the harmonic scalpel for gall bladder dissection. J Laproendosc Adv Surg Tech A. 2011;21(1):1–5.
33. Witte CL. Choledochal obstruction by cystic duct stone. Mirizzi's syndrome Am Surg. 1984;50(5):241–3. PMID: 6721287
34. Alberti-Flor JJ, Iskandarani M, Jeffers L, Schiff ER. Mirizzi syndrome. Am J Gastroenterol. 1985;80(10):822–3.
35. Mishra MC, Vashishtha S, Tandon R. Biliobiliary fistula: preoperative diagnosis and management implications. Surgery. 1990;108(5):835–9. PMID: 2237763
36. Beltran MA, Csendes A, Cruces KS. The relationship of Mirizzi syndrome and cholecystoenteric fistula: validation of a modified classification. World J Surg. 2008;32(10):2237–43.
37. Ibrarullah M, Mishra T, Das AP. Mirizzi syndrome. Indian J Surg. 2008;70(6):281–7.
38. Uppara M, Rasheed A. Systematic review of Mirizzi's syndrome's management. JOP J Pancreas (Online). 2017;18:1–8.
39. Hsu YB, Yu SC, Lee PH, Wei TC. An uncommon cause of biliary obstruction (Mirizzi syndrome): report of five cases. J Formos Med Assoc. 1994;93(4):314–9.
40. Kuerer HM, Forman D, Divino CM, Wasserman EJ, Brower ST, Cunningham JD. Cholecystocholedochal fistula associated with the Mirizzi syndrome: presentation, diagnosis, and surgical management. Contemp Surg. 1996;49:131–4.

41. Kumar A, Senthil G, Prakash A, Behari A, Singh RK, Kapoor VK, Saxena R. Mirizzi's syndrome: lessons learnt from 169 patients at a single center. Korean J Hepatob Pancreat Surg. 2016;20(1):17–22.
42. Yvergneaux JP, Kint M, Kuppens E. Pitfalls in laparoscopic cholecystectomy. Acta Chir Belg. 1994;94(3):123–8.
43. Nassar AHM, Nassar MK, Gil IC, et al. One-session laparoscopic management of Mirizzi syndrome: feasible and safe in specialist units. Surg Endosc. 2021;35:3286–95. https://doi.org/10.1007/s00464-020-07765-4.
44. Strasberg SM, et al. Subtotal cholecystectomy-“fenestrating” vs “reconstituting” subtypes and the prevention of bile duct injury: definition of the optimal procedure in difficult operative conditions. J Am Coll Surg. 2016;222:89–96.
45. Elshaer M, et al. Subtotal cholecystectomy for “difficult gallbladders”: systematic review and meta-analysis. JAMA Surg. 2015;150:159–68.
46. Henneman D, et al. Laparoscopic partial cholecystectomy for the difficult gallbladder: a systematic review. Surg Endosc. 2013;27:351–35.
47. Elshaer M, Gravante G, Thomas K, Sorge R, Al-Hamali S, Ebdewi H. Subtotal cholecystectomy for “difficult gallbladders”: systematic review and meta-analysis. JAMA Surg. 2015;150:159–68.
48. Henneman D, da Costa DW, Vrouenraets BC, van Wagensveld BA, Lagarde SM. Laparoscopic partial cholecystectomy for the difficult gallbladder: a systematic review. Surg Endosc. 2013;27:351–8.
49. McElmoyle W. Cholecystectomy: a method for the difficult gallbladder. Lancet. 1954;266:1320–3.

Chapter 16
Laparoscopy in Pediatric Surgery

Lukman O. Abdur-Rahman, Kristine Griffin, and Benedict Nwomeh

Introduction

The early 1970s witnessed the growth of Minimal Access Surgery in the care of pediatric patients. Initially, interest in this innovative approach for children was limited to a few enthusiasts, while the broader pediatric surgical community adopted a “wait and see” attitude. For more than two decades, pediatric laparoscopy was restricted mainly to diagnostic use [1].

Resistance to its adoption in pediatric populations stemmed from several factors. These included the traditional belief that children do not experience pain, concerns about the high costs of laparoscopy, and the lack of appropriately sized equipment for infants and children. Early attempts to produce smaller telescopes often resulted in substandard optics and poor visualization. Furthermore, there was a widespread perception that the technique was too difficult to learn, with lengthy setup and procedure times. Compounding these issues was the belief that laparoscopy offered minimal benefit to children and pediatric surgeons, who already prided themselves on achieving excellent outcomes with small incisions [1].

L. O. Abdur-Rahman
Division of Paediatric Surgery, Department of Surgery, University of Ilorin Teaching Hospital (UITH), Ilorin, Kwara State, Nigeria

Clinical Skills and Simulation Laboratory, College of Health Sciences, University of Ilorin, Ilorin, Kwara State, Nigeria

K. Griffin
Nationwide Children’s Hospital, Columbus, OH, USA

B. Nwomeh (✉)
Department of Surgery, The Ohio State University, Columbus, OH, USA

Department of Pediatric Surgery, Nationwide Children’s Hospital, Columbus, OH, USA
e-mail: benedict.nwomeh@nationwidechildrens.org

E. Ray-Offor, R. J. Rosenthal (eds.), *Principles and Practice of Laparoscopic Surgery*, https://doi.org/10.1007/978-3-031-96321-6_16

Despite these challenges, the benefits of laparoscopy—such as reduced postoperative pain, quicker recovery, shorter hospital stays, and improved quality of life—eventually attracted both practitioners and patients. Advances in technology, including miniaturized instruments and improved optics, allowed surgeons to perform increasingly complex procedures, making laparoscopy integral to pediatric surgical practice. Today, nearly every pediatric surgeon incorporates laparoscopic techniques, and their adoption continues to grow, even in low- and middle-income countries (LMICs) [1, 2].

This chapter highlights the principles and techniques of pediatric minimally invasive surgery, emphasizing its transformative impact on surgical care. It explores perioperative considerations, common and advanced procedures, and emerging innovations such as robotic surgery and fetoscopy. Additionally, the chapter addresses postoperative strategies and provides insights to equip practitioners with the tools to navigate the challenges and maximize the benefits of minimally invasive surgery for children.

Core Considerations

Anatomic Considerations

In pediatric patients, the anatomy evolves significantly compared to adults, as growth alters the relative sizes, positions, and relations of structures. Awareness of these differences is crucial for guiding the selection and application of equipment tailored to the needs of children. For instance, port placement can be influenced by the shifting position of the umbilicus, which moves relatively farther from the xiphisternum and closer to the pubis during growth and development (Fig. 16.1). Also, as the child grows, the abdomen becomes relatively narrower, the abdominal wall thinner, and the volume of the abdominal cavity smaller. These anatomical differences necessitate careful consideration to minimize the risk of organ injury. For this reason, some surgeons routinely adopt the Hasson (open) technique for port placement for safe peritoneal access [2, 3].

Physiological Considerations

Pediatric patients present unique physiological challenges during laparoscopy, including differences in respiratory and cardiovascular systems [2, 3]:

Respiratory Changes:

- Infants' ribs are horizontal, and their diaphragms are less domed, limiting respiratory excursion. Consequently, minute ventilation depends on changes in respiratory rate, as tidal volume remains fixed.

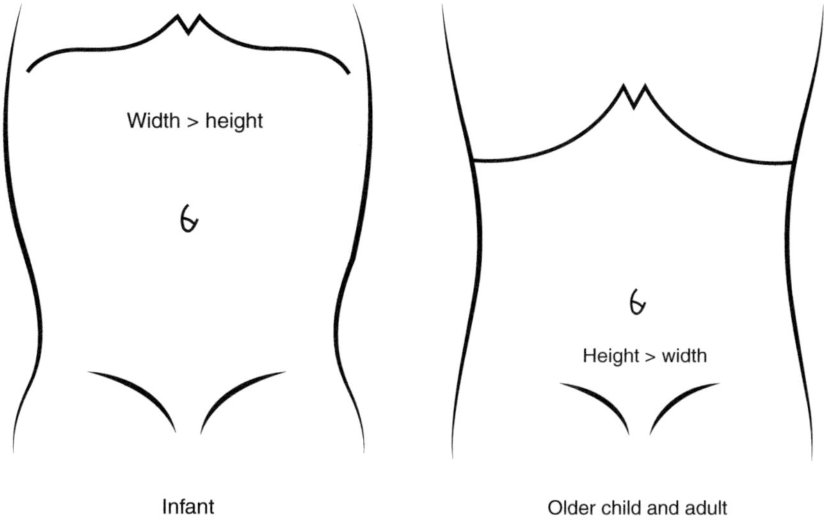

Fig. 16.1 Relative growth of longitudinal length (xiphisternum to pubis)

- Functional residual capacity (FRC) serves as a vital oxygen reservoir but is reduced by general anesthesia and insufflation pressures. This reduction may lead to airway collapse, shunting, and hypoxia.
  Cardiovascular Changes:
- Insufflation pressures can compress major intra-abdominal veins, reducing venous return and cardiac output.
- Increased systemic vascular resistance may result from mechanical compression of the aorta and splanchnic vessels and the release of humoral factors.
  Thermal and Metabolic Considerations:
- Hypothermia can result from exposure and the Joule-Thomson cooling effect of insufflated gas.
- Elevated basal oxygen consumption in children increases their susceptibility to hypoxemia, particularly during CO_2 absorption.

Physiological Changes During Laparoscopy

Key factors affecting physiological stability include [1, 3]:

1. *Surgical Manipulation:*
   - Tissue handling and organ compression may result in transient cardiopulmonary and intestinal dysfunction.

2. *Postural Adjustments:*
   - Trendelenburg or reverse Trendelenburg positioning can alter venous return, cardiac output, and pulmonary compliance, requiring careful monitoring.
3. *Gas Insufflation:*
   - Low-flow insufflation rates and pressures tailored to the patient's size (6–8 mmHg for infants, 8–12 mmHg for older children) mitigate risks such as hypercarbia and reduced lung volumes.

Preoperative Preparation and Safety

Effective preoperative preparation minimizes risks and ensures procedural success. Key steps include patient screening for contraindications, securing proper positioning, and verifying equipment functionality. General anesthesia with endotracheal intubation is standard, and careful management of insufflation pressures is critical to maintaining physiological stability [3, 4]

1. *Patient Screening:*
   - Assess for contraindications such as hemodynamic instability, severe cardiopulmonary disease, or increased intracranial pressure.
   - Obtaining informed consent for both laparoscopic and open approaches in case conversion is recommended.
2. *Equipment and Instrumentation:*
   - Verify the availability and functionality of all laparoscopic and open surgery instruments.
   - Ensure compatibility of adjunct devices like electrocautery, ultrasound, and radiologic tools.
3. *Anesthetic Management:*
   - General anesthesia with endotracheal intubation is standard, with neuromuscular blockade to facilitate intra-abdominal insufflation.
   - Avoid halothane due to its arrhythmogenic potential in the presence of CO_2.
4. *Positioning*
   - Position patients based on procedural needs (e.g., Trendelenburg for pelvic access, reverse Trendelenburg for upper abdominal surgeries).
   - Secure patients to the operating table to prevent falls during positional changes, using padding to avoid pressure injuries.

5. *Key Safety Measures:*

   - **Preoxygenation**: Prevent gastric distension by keeping the neck in a neutral position.
   - **Monitoring**: Use multiparameter monitoring, including capnography, to detect hypercarbia or hypoxia early.
   - **Thermal Management**: Utilize warmed insufflation gas to mitigate hypothermia.

6. *Intraoperative Adjustments:*

   - Minimize insufflation volumes to reduce risks to hollow organs and maintain low pressures for adequate visualization.
   - For brief procedures, a laryngeal mask airway (LMA) may suffice, but prolonged surgeries require endotracheal intubation to prevent aspiration.

Risk Mitigation Strategies

1. ***Gas Embolism***

   - A rare but serious complication, gas embolism occurs when gas inadvertently enters the vascular system. Preventive measures include careful cannula placement and vigilant monitoring during insufflation.
   - Early detection through signs like arrhythmias or cardiovascular collapse is critical.

2. ***Post-procedure Considerations***:

   - Fully deflate the pneumoperitoneum to reduce postoperative shoulder pain
   - Assess for complications such as nerve injury or hollow organ stress.

By understanding and addressing these physiological and preoperative considerations, pediatric laparoscopic procedures can be conducted safely and effectively, ensuring optimal outcomes for young patients [3, 4].

Technical Considerations

Positioning of Patients

Careful positioning of the patient, equipment, and staff is essential for optimal access and ergonomic use of the surgical field. Patient's positioning depends on the specific procedure [2, 3]:

- **Neonates**: Due to their small size, neonates can be placed transversally or at the end of the operating table. This arrangement allows a perfect inline position for the surgeon, operative field, and monitor, promoting ergonomic efficiency, for example during pyloromyotomy
- **Fundoplication**: Place the patient at the far end of the operating table.
- **Pelvic Laparoscopy**: Use a Trendelenburg position for pelvic laparoscopy.
- **Upper Abdominal Laparoscopy**: Use a reverse Trendelenburg position.
- **Splenic, Renal, or Retroperitoneal Procedures**: A lateral tilt position may be required.

To prevent pressure injuries, use gel-filled flexible or rigid molds, and adhesive materials to secure the patient in the desired position. Ensure that the airway circuit and IV tubing are of adequate lengths to avoid tension or accidental dislodgement of endotracheal tubes and IV lines.

Creating the greatest possible degrees of freedom for the surgeon is critical to performing a three-dimensional procedure with two-dimensional visualization.

Peritoneal Access and Port Placement

Peritoneal access and the placement of ports are critical steps in pediatric laparoscopy and must be tailored to minimize risks of injury to vessels and viscera. In infants, the liver and spleen are relatively large and may extend below the right costal margins, occupying much of the epigastrium. However, their soft consistency often makes their edges indistinct, rendering them less palpable in the upper abdomen. Also, due to the shallow pelvis in newborns and young children, the urinary bladder functions as an abdominal organ and is at increased risk of iatrogenic injury during suprapubic port placement. Recognizing these anatomical peculiarities is essential for safe peritoneal access. Placing trocars under laparoscopic (optical) view is the most reliable method to minimize the risk of injury to these vulnerable organs [2].

A pneumoperitoneum may be established using one of three techniques [2]:

1. ***Closed Method***: Involves the insertion of a Veress needle; however, this blind approach carries a rare but significant risk of visceral and vascular injury.
2. ***Open Hasson Method:*** The preferred technique involves a cut-down approach to insert the primary cannula (telescope) under direct vision. This method is particularly advantageous in pediatric patients for reducing injury risks.
3. ***Optical Entry Technique:*** Uses an optical trocar for direct visualization during entry, an increasingly popular option in pediatric practice.

For an unscarred abdomen, the primary cannula is typically inserted through a small incision at the umbilicus, sized to fit the cannula. Insufflation pressures and flow rates must be carefully adjusted according to the age and size of the child [1, 2]:

- ***Neonates and Infants:*** 6–8 mmHg at a CO_2 flow rate of 0.1–0.5 L/min.
- ***Small Children:*** 8–10 mmHg at a CO_2 flow rate of 0.5–1 L/min.
- ***Older Children and Adolescents:*** 12–15 mmHg at a CO_2 flow rate of 1–2 L/min.

To minimize complications such as postoperative shoulder pain and cardiac arrhythmias, the insufflation rate should initially be low (0.5 L/min) and then gradually increase. Working cannulas are placed under direct telescopic vision to ensure precise placement and to reduce the risk of intra-abdominal, vascular, or visceral injury. The positioning of ports should be adapted to the procedure, the patient's anatomy, and size. Optimal working angles (45°–90°) should be achieved using the principles of triangulation and sector action, with 60° being the most ergonomically preferred manipulation angle (Fig. 16.2) [2].

The instruments should be kept in front of the scope and the target organ or tissue, maintaining a reasonable distance that considers the patient's size and anatomy of the organ being operated on. This arrangement enhances visibility, precision, and control. Recommended positions for ports for abdominal, pelvic, and thoracic procedures are shown in Fig. 16.3a–f below:

During laparoscopy, hand-held instruments hold greater importance than open surgery due to the reliance on indirect visualization and the absence of direct tactile feedback. Many instruments originally designed for open surgery have been adapted for laparoscopy, incorporating advancements in sophistication, miniaturization, and articulation. These innovations have significantly enhanced the precision, efficiency, and overall experience of laparoscopic surgery [2].

In infants, 3 mm instruments are frequently used to accommodate their smaller anatomy. In some instances, these instruments can be employed without a trocar because of their small caliber. However, a trocar is still essential at the umbilicus to enable insufflation and provide access to the camera port, ensuring adequate visualization of the operative field [3, 4]. These adaptations highlight the critical role of appropriately designed instruments in overcoming the unique challenges of pediatric laparoscopy while maintaining safety and effectiveness.

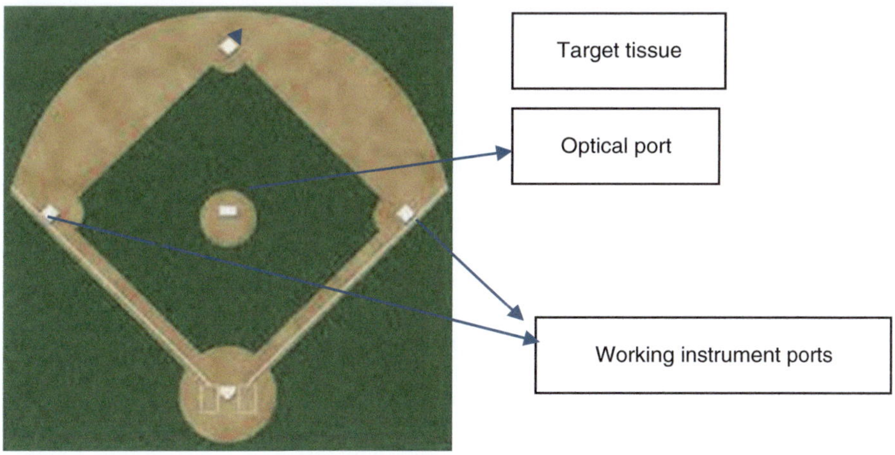

Fig. 16.2 Baseball diamond shape approach to port placement

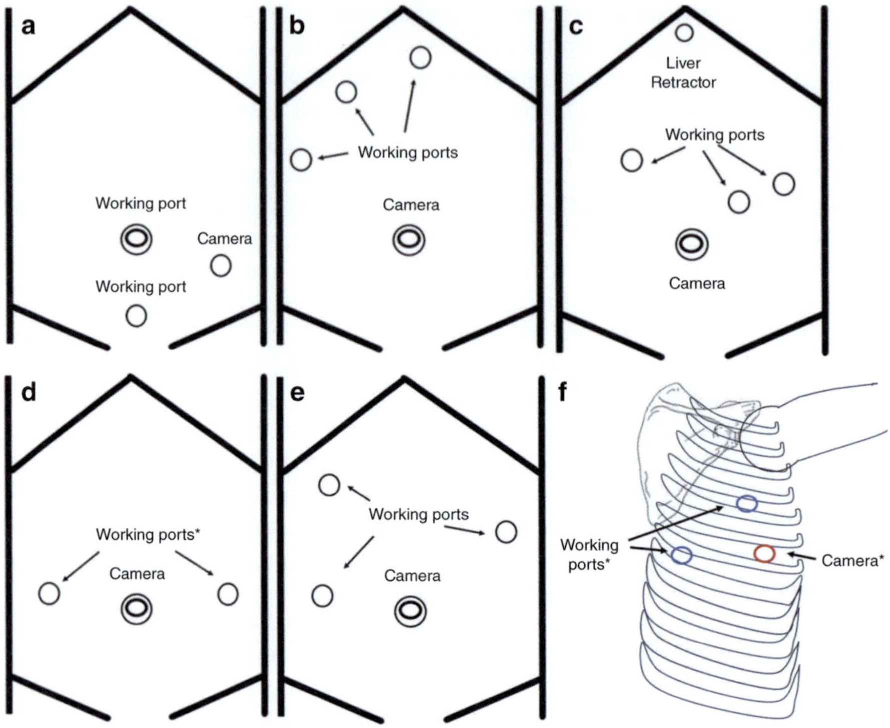

Fig. 16.3 (**a**) Port sites for laparoscopic appendectomy (**b**) Port sites for laparoscopic cholecystectomy (**c**) Port sites for Nissen fundoplication or foregut operations. *second working port is optional (**d**) Port sites for laparoscopic ovarian surgery or inguinal hernia repair *second working port is optional (**e**) Port sites for pull-through for Hirschsprung disease (**f**) Port sites for thoracoscopy *camera and working port sites interchangable depending on target anatomy

Monitoring and Preventing Adverse Effects

Increased intra-abdominal pressure, postural changes, and CO_2 absorption can lead to significant physiological changes in pediatric patients, including [2, 3]:

1. *Pulmonary Effects:* Reduced pulmonary compliance, basal alveolar collapse, and reduced total lung volume.
2. *Hypercarbia:* Stimulates the sympathetic nervous system, leading to tachycardia, hypertension, and arrhythmia [2, 3]
3. *Cardiovascular Effects:* Reduced venous return from inferior venal cava compression decreases cardiac output and organ perfusion.

Additional concerns include the leftward shift of the oxy-hemoglobin saturation curve due to carboxyhemoglobin formation (with 20–240 times higher oxygen affinity) and methemoglobin production, which is incapable of oxygen transport. Excessive carbon monoxide can exacerbate cardiac arrhythmias [3].

Using a multiparameter monitor with ECG and capnography is critical for early detection of homeostatic changes and prompt intervention.

Common Procedures

Pediatric laparoscopy encompasses a range of abdominal, pelvic, and thoracic procedures [4–12]. Abdominal surgeries, such as appendectomy and fundoplication, benefit from enhanced visualization and precision [6, 7, 9]. Pelvic interventions, including inguinal hernia repair and ovarian surgery, minimize recovery time and morbidity [1, 4]. Thoracic procedures, such as lobectomy and pectus excavatum repair, provide superior outcomes compared to open approaches [1, 4].

Abdominal Procedures

We have reached a point where virtually every intra-abdominal procedure can be performed with laparoscopy. However, certain scenarios still require open surgery such as significant intra-peritoneal adhesions, the need for wide exposure—particularly for complex oncologic resections—or technical challenges that prevent the operating surgeon from completing the procedure with minimally invasive techniques [1]. Despite these limitations, laparoscopic techniques continue to expand, including **single-incision laparoscopic surgery (SILS)**, which allows for minimally invasive procedures through a single access point. Procedures, such as ileocecectomy, cholecystectomy, Meckel's diverticulectomy, and small bowel resections, can often be successfully performed using the SILS technique [12]. Common pediatric laparoscopic procedures include [2–12]:

(a) Appendectomy (Figs. 16.3a and 16.4)
(b) Cholecystectomy (Fig. 16.3b)

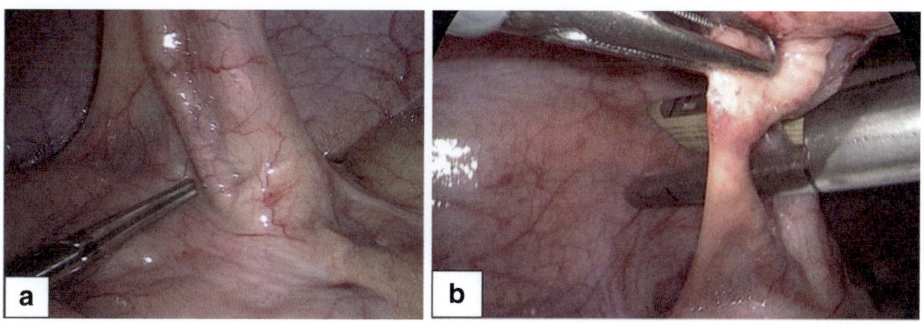

Fig. 16.4 Laparoscopic appendectomy: (**a**) Identification of appendiceal base; (**b**) Division of appendix with laparoscopic stapler

(c) Diagnostic laparoscopy
(d) Meckel's diverticulectomy
(e) Anti-reflux surgery (Nissen, Dor, and Thal Fundoplication) (Fig. 16.3c)
(f) Pyloromyotomy
(g) Laparoscopically assisted percutaneous endoscopic gastrostomy (PEG)
(h) Gastrostomy (Fig. 16.5)
(i) Jejunostomy
(j) Surgery for intestinal rotation anomalies
(k) Small bowel resection
(l) Colectomy
(m) Splenectomy
(n) Ventriculo-peritoneal shunt placement
(o) Aspiration or removal of cysts (liver, ovary, etc.)
(p) Adrenalectomy
(q) Nephrectomy
(r) Heminephrectomy
(s) Pyelo-ureteral anastomosis (pyeloplasty)

These procedures demonstrate the versatility and effectiveness of laparoscopic techniques (Fig. 16.6).

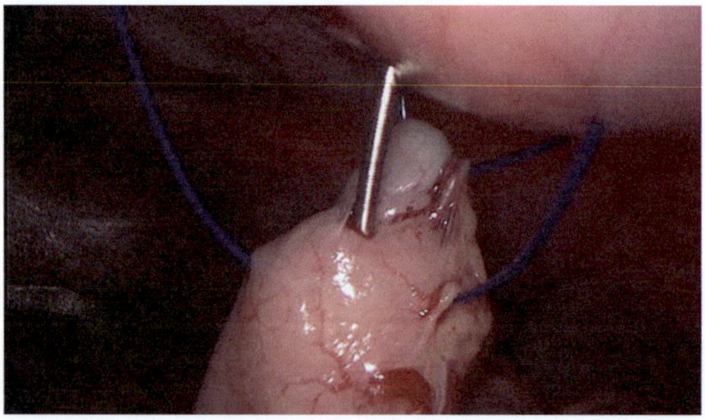

Fig. 16.5 Laparoscopic gastrostomy tube insertion using Seldinger technique

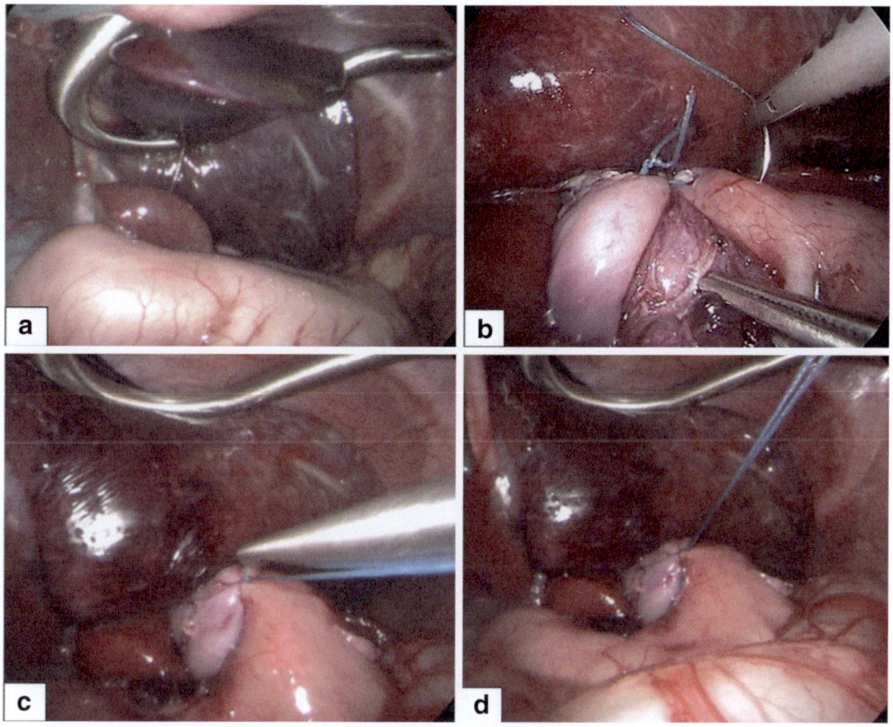

Fig. 16.6 Nissen fundoplication: (**a**) Positioning of liver retractor; (**b**) Placement of fundoplication sutures; (**c**) Extracorporeal knot-tying; (**d**) Completed fundoplication

Pelvic Procedures

The pelvis is readily accessible via laparoscopy, offering visualization of deep pelvic structures, such as the ureters and gynecologic organs, which may be less easily visualized in an open approach. This minimally invasive technique provides precise access and reduces the need for extensive dissection in many procedures.

Common laparoscopic pelvic procedures include:

- ***Ovarian Surgery:*** Ovarian masses can be mobilized laparoscopically and extracted through an extended port incision (Fig. 16.3d). Depending on the pathology and clinical indication, either laparoscopic oophorectomy or ovarian-sparing resections are performed (Fig. 16.7) [1, 4, 13]
- ***Pull-through Procedures for Hirschsprung Disease:*** Laparoscopy enables full thickness colon biopsy, colon mobilization, and deep pelvic dissection (Fig. 16.3e and 16.8). This technique reduces the transanal dissection required compared to traditional transanal or open pull-throughs, improving recovery and reducing morbidity [4, 14]

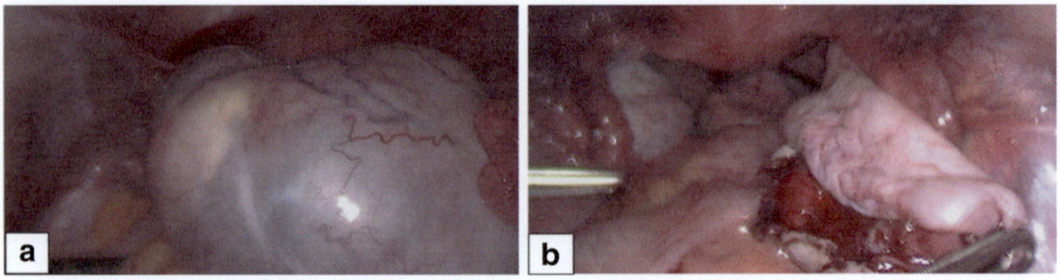

Fig. 16.7 Ovarian dermoid tumor resection: (**a**) Dermoid pre-resection; (**b**) Ovary post ovarian-sparing resection

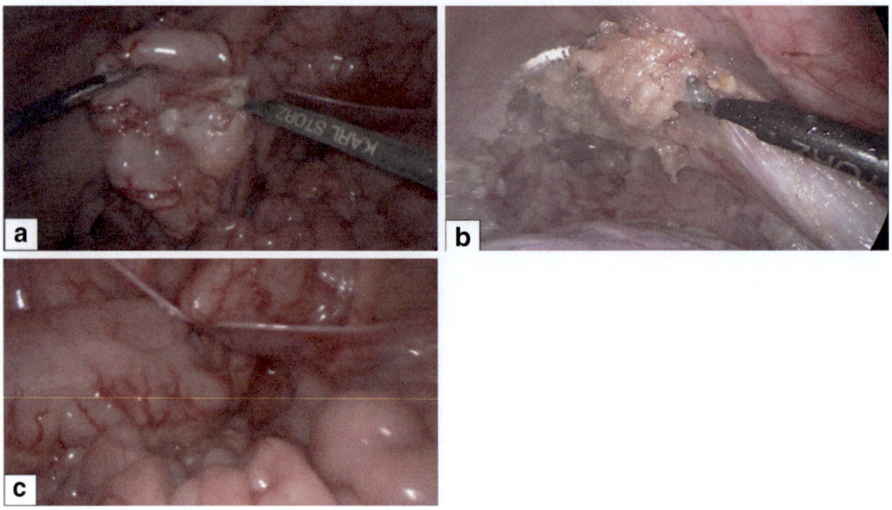

Fig. 16.8 Laparoscopic-assisted pull through for Hirschsprung: (**a**) Colon mobilization; (**b**) Pelvic dissection of rectum; (**c**) Completed pull-through

- ***Anorectal Malformations:*** In cases where the fistula lies above the levator muscles, laparoscopy facilitates precise dissection, identification, and ligation of the fistula. When necessary, laparoscopy can also be utilized for more extensive colonic mobilization [4, 15].
- ***Inguinal Hernia Repair:*** Laparoscopy provides excellent visualization of the vas deferens in males, and evaluation of the contralateral side, allowing for simultaneous repair (Figs. 16.3d and 16.9). Outcomes of laparoscopic inguinal hernia repairs in pediatric patients are comparable to those achieved with the open approach [16]
- ***Other Pelvic Procedures***: Varicocelectomy, orchidopexy, and gonadectomy for dysgenic gonads are also effectively performed laparoscopically, benefiting from the enhanced visualization and reduced invasiveness of this technique [1]

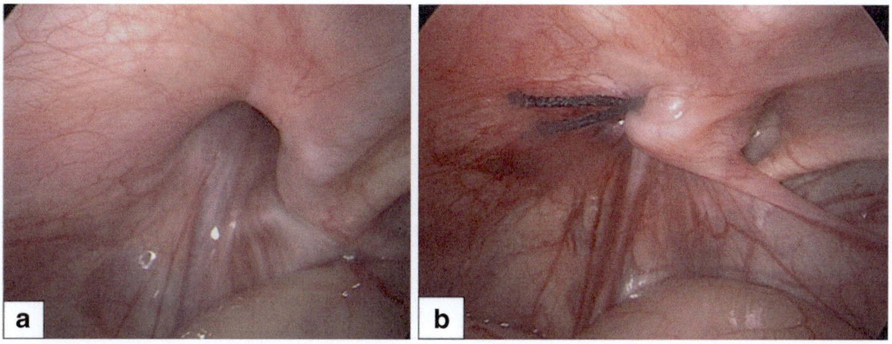

Fig. 16.9 Laparoscopic inguinal hernia repair (male patient): (**a**) Left inguinal hernia (**b**) Left inguinal hernia post-repair

Thoracic Procedures

Minimally invasive techniques using thoracoscopy have revolutionized thoracic surgery in children. Thoracoscopy provides superior visualization of thoracic structures compared to open approaches, making it particularly valuable in pediatric cases (Fig. 16.3f). Thoracoscopic procedures also result in less postoperative pain, shorter hospital stays, and reduced risks of long-term complications, such as scoliosis, when compared to thoracotomy [1, 4, 17].

Thoracoscopic procedures require close collaboration with an experienced anesthesia team familiar with single-lung ventilation to ensure adequate visualization and working space to complete the procedure. Conversion thoracotomy may be necessary if thoracic insufflation cannot be tolerated or in the event of major vascular bleeding. Surgeons must prepare for immediate conversion to open surgery when necessary to ensure patient safety [1, 4, 17].

Common pediatric thoracoscopic procedures include:

- ***Pulmonary Procedures:*** Thoracoscopic lung biopsy is increasingly used over thoracotomy, offering a minimally invasive option. Once the area of interest is localized, endoscopic staplers are used to divide the lung parenchyma. Also, wedge resection, segmentectomy, and lobectomy for congenital lung lesions or neoplasms can be performed thoracoscopically using small-diameter vesselsealing devices to divide pulmonary vasculature safely and efficiently [17]
- ***Tracheo-esophageal Fistula (TEF) and Esophageal Atresia Repair:*** Thoracoscopic repairs are gaining popularity in specialized centers, requiring proficiency in intracorporeal knot-tying. Outcomes are comparable to thoracotomy when performed by experienced teams [17]
- ***Congenital Diaphragmatic Hernia (CDH) Repair:*** Thoracoscopy offers a minimally invasive alternative to the open abdominal approach. Positive pressure insufflation aids in the reduction of herniated bowel, and the thoracoscope excellent visualization of the diaphragm defect (Fig. 16.10) [17]

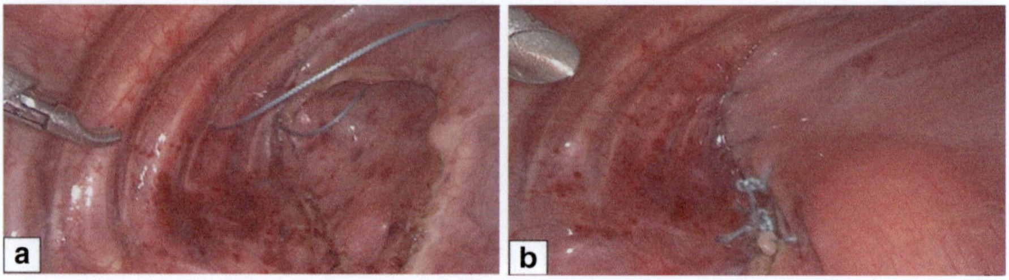

Fig. 16.10 Thoracoscopic congenital diaphragmatic hernia repair: (**a**) Diaphragm defect pre-repair; (**b**) Defect post-repair

- ***Pectus Excavatum Repair:*** The minimally invasive Nuss procedure is the gold standard for this condition. Intrathoracic bars are placed through small, lateral incisions while the patient is supine. Compared to the open Ravitch procedure, the Nuss technique results in less pain with similar long-term outcomes [17]
- ***Other Thoracic Procedures:*** Thoracoscopy is utilized for a variety of conditions, including [17]:
  (a) Bronchogenic cyst resection
  (b) Decortication for empyema
  (c) Pleurectomy and/or bleb resection for pneumothorax
  (d) Tracheo-esophageal fistula or esophageal atresia repair
  (e) Mediastinal mass resection
  (f) Pericardial window
  (g) Aortopexy
  (h) Diaphragmatic eventration plication

Advanced Techniques and Innovations

The field of pediatric minimally invasive surgery (MIS) has been transformed by advancements in technology and technique, enabling increasingly complex and precise interventions. This section highlights three key areas of innovation—assisted laparoscopic surgery, operative fetoscopy, and robotic surgery—and addresses the unique post-operative considerations necessary to optimize outcomes in pediatric patients.

Assisted Laparoscopic Surgery

The MIS approach can be challenging and often requires significant expertise from the surgeon. In situations where the procedure becomes too complex or unsafe to continue laparoscopically, it can be augmented with a laparoscopic-assisted approach, minilaparotomy, or even formal laparotomy. This is particularly useful in managing conditions such as adhesive bowel obstruction, intestinal duplication, intestinal atresia, and intussusception [11]. By combining the benefits of minimally invasive and open surgery, these techniques allow for safer and more controlled management of challenging cases.

Operative Fetoscopy

Open fetoscopy represents a groundbreaking advancement in the management of life-threatening fetal anomalies, offering a less invasive approach to managing life threatening congenital anomalies. By utilizing a specialized endoscope (fetoscope) to access the amniotic cavity, this technique minimizes uterine trauma, reduces the risk of preterm labor, and preserves the intrinsic physiologic environment. Despite its promise, fetoscopy poses unique challenges and requires a high level of technical expertise [4, 11].

Common Applications

Fetoscopy is particularly effective for addressing specific congenital anomalies, including [4, 11]:

1. **Twin-to-Twin Transfusion Syndrome (TTTS)**:
   - Fetoscopic laser photocoagulation is used to ablate shared placental vessels, thereby restoring balanced blood flow between twins. o This procedure has significantly improved survival rates and reduced neurological complications in affected fetuses.
2. **Congenital Diaphragmatic Hernia (CDH)**:
   - Fetoscopic tracheal occlusion involves the placement of a balloon in the fetal trachea to stimulate lung growth by trapping fluid within the lungs.
   - This approach enhances pulmonary development, improving postnatal outcomes for infants with severe CDH.
3. **Amniotic Band Syndrome**:
   - Fetoscopy allows for the release of constrictive amniotic bands that can cause limb deformities or amputations. The procedure helps preserve limb unctionality and improve cosmetic outcomes.

Technical Details

The success of fetoscopy relies on careful planning and execution [4, 11]:

- **Equipment**: Procedures are performed using a rigid or flexible fetoscope, often equipped with laser devices, graspers, or balloons for specific interventions.

- **Procedure**:
    1. Under ultrasound guidance, the fetoscope is inserted through a small maternal incision into the amniotic sac.
    2. The target area is visualized directly, and the necessary intervention (e.g., laser ablation or tracheal occlusion) is performed.
    3. Post-procedure, the instruments are removed, and the maternal incision is closed.

Challenges and Limitations

While promising, operative fetoscopy faces several challenges [4, 11]:

- **Placental Location**: Variable placental positioning can complicate entry and visualization.
- **Fetal Safety**: Operating within a fluid medium presents difficulties in maintaining precise control of instruments and protecting the fetus.
- **Monitoring**: Limited fetal monitoring capabilities, including the lack of intravenous access, require careful perioperative management.
- **Learning Curve**: The complexity of the procedure demands specialized training and experience.

While fetoscopy represents a promising advancement, ongoing research, and technological improvements are needed to overcome these limitations and expand its applications.

Robotic Surgery

Robotic surgery has become a significant innovation in pediatric minimally invasive surgery, heralding a new era of precision and versatility. The first robotic Nissen fundoplication in a child was reported in 2001, and since then, the technology has seen rapid growth and adoption. Technical advantages of robotic surgery over laparoscopy include articulating instruments which mimic human wrist movements and motion scaling technology which limits large hand movements, ensuring precision in small operative spaces. In addition, 3-dimensional console displays provide enhanced depth perception and improved visualization [18].

Current limitations include high equipment costs, the need for specialized staff training, and larger equipment ports (typically 8 mm, though 5 mm ports are available on some systems). In addition, most current robotic systems lack haptic feedback, although this technology is in development for future generations of robotic platforms [18].

Nearly every procedure that can be performed with traditional laparoscopy or thoracoscopy can also be done with robot assistance. Future advancements, such as smaller instruments and improved endoscopes, will likely make robotic surgery more accessible and applicable to pediatric patients.

Post-operative Considerations

Post-operative care is critical in promoting recovery and minimizing complications. For children, effective pain management is achieved with local anesthetic infiltration at trocar sites, avoiding narcotics and epidural techniques to reduce systemic effects like respiratory depression. Adequate analgesia can also prevent stress-related complications, such as increased intra-abdominal pressure, which may exacerbate residual gas embolism risks [4, 11, 12].

The unique anatomical and physiological characteristics of younger children make access and manipulation during laparoscopic procedures more demanding compared to older children and adults. Tailored approaches and heightened vigilance are necessary to navigate these challenges safely and effectively.

Conclusion

Advances in the miniaturization of laparoscopic instruments and the decreasing costs of equipment have made minimally invasive techniques increasingly accessible and applicable to a wider range of procedures in pediatric patients. These procedures reduce postoperative pain in children, shorten hospital stays, and facilitate an earlier return to school and recreational activities. Maintaining and improving laparoscopic skills requires ongoing training and regular practice. With continued innovation and skill development, minimally invasive surgery will remain at the forefront of pediatric surgical care, offering better outcomes and faster recovery for young patients.

References

1. Tam PKH. Laparoscopic surgery in children. Arch Dis Child. 2000;82:240–3.
2. Saxena AK, Höllwarth ME, editors. Essentials of pediatric endoscopic surgery. Berlin/Heidelberg: Springer; 2009.
3. Zachariou Z, editor. Pediatric surgery digest. Berlin/Heidelberg: Springer; 2009.
4. Langer JC. In: Albaness CT, editor. Pediatric minimal access surgery. New York: Taylor & Francis Group, LLC; 2005.
5. Burge DM, Griffiths DM, Steinbrecher HA, Wheeler RA, editors. Pediatric surgery. Hodder Arnold; 2005.
6. Holcomb GW III, Murphy JP, Ostlie DJ, St. Peter SD. Aschraft's pediatric surgery. 6th ed. New York: Elservier Saunders; 2014.

7. Abdur-Rahman LO, Bamigbola KT, Nasir AA, Oyinloye AO, Abdulraheem NT, Oyedepo OO, Adeniran JO. Pediatric laparoscopic surgery in North-Central Nigeria: achievements and challenges. J Clin Sci. 2016;13(4):158–62.
8. Adisa AO, Lawal OO, Arowolo OA, Akinola DO. Laparoscopic cholecystectomy in Ile-Ife, Nigeria. Afr J Med Med Sci. 2011:40.
9. Abdur-Rahman LO, Nasir AA, Bamigbola KT, Adeniran JO. Comparison of open and Laparoscopic Appendectomy at UITH Ilorin. In: Edited Conference proceedings of Pan Africa Paediatric Surgical Associations 2016 held at Biennial Congress. Festac Town, Lagos. 19–24 September 2016: Golden Tulip Hotel; 2016.
10. Abdur-Rahman LO. Laparoscopy Trocar and Ports placement and Pnuemoperitoneum. Hugh Greenwood and British Association of Paediatric Surgeon Workshop on Minimally Invasive/ Laparoscopy Surgery at LUTH Idia-Araba. Preconference workshop of Pan Africa Paediatric Surgical Associations on 19th September 2016; 2016.
11. Esposito C, Becmeur F, Steyaert H, Szavay P, editors. ESPES manual of pediatric minimally invasive surgery. Cham: Springer; 2019. ISBN 978-3-030-00963-2, ISBN 978-3-030-00964-9 (eBook). https://doi.org/10.1007/978-3-030-00964-9.
12. Noitumyae J, Mahatharadol V, Niramis R. Single-incision pediatric laparoscopic surgery: surgical outcomes, feasibility indication, and the systematic review. J Laparoendosc Adv Surg Tech A. 2022;32(11):1190–202. https://doi.org/10.1089/lap.2021.0869. Epub 2022 Jul 27
13. Knaus ME, Onwuka AJ, Afrazi A, Breech L, Corkum KS, Dillon PA, Ehrlich PF, Fallat ME, Fraser JD, Gadepalli SK, Grabowski JE, Hertweck SP, Kabre R, Lal DR, Landman MP, Lawrence AE, Leys CM, Mak GZ, Markel TA, Merchant N, Elliott Overman R, Rademacher BL, Raiji MT, Rymeski B, Sato TT, Scannell M, Schikler AG, Sujka JA, Wright T, Aldrink JH, Hewitt GD, Minneci PC, Deans KJ, Midwest Pediatric Surgery Consortium. Laparoscopy versus laparotomy for pediatric ovarian dermoids. J Pediatr Surg. 2022;57(6):1008–12. https://doi.org/10.1016/j.jpedsurg.2022.01.053. Epub 2022 Feb 12
14. Langer JC. Laparoscopic and transanal pull-through for Hirschsprung disease. Semin Pediatr Surg. 2012;21(4):283–90. https://doi.org/10.1053/j.sempedsurg.2012.07.002.
15. Rentea RM, Halleran DR, Wood RJ, Levitt MA. The role of laparoscopy in anorectal malformations. Eur J Pediatr Surg. 2020;30(2):156–63. https://doi.org/10.1055/s-0040-1701700. Epub 2020 Mar 4
16. Feehan BP, Fromm DS. Laparoscopic pediatric inguinal hernia repair: overview of "true Herniotomy" technique and review of current evidence. S D Med. 2017;70(5):217–23.
17. Karpelowsky J. Paediatric thoracoscopic surgery. Paediatr Respir Rev. 2012;13(4):244–50. https://doi.org/10.1016/j.prrv.2012.03.004; quiz 250–1. Epub 2012 Apr 12
18. Denning NL, Kallis MP, Prince JM. Pediatric robotic surgery. Surg Clin North Am. 2020;100(2):431–43. https://doi.org/10.1016/j.suc.2019.12.004. Epub 2020 Feb 7

Chapter 17
Laparoscopy in Urology

John E. Raphael and Charles P. Okpani

Introduction

The concept of inspecting and operating within the abdominal cavity using a telescope dates back to the early twentieth century and has progressively entered various surgical subspecialties, including urology. Initially, diagnostic laparoscopy was performed for gynecological and gastroenterological indications [1]. Building on Nitze's invention of the cystoscope in 1879, Kelling utilized this instrument in 1901 to conduct diagnostic laparoscopy in animals, foreshadowing future human applications [2]. In 1910, Jacobaeus performed the first diagnostic laparoscopy in humans, marking the dawn of minimally invasive approaches [3].

Key technological developments—such as the Veress needle, trocars, carbon dioxide (CO_2) insufflation, improved optics, and powerful light sources—further propelled laparoscopic surgery [4, 5]. A significant milestone occurred in 1987 with the advent of laparoscopic cholecystectomy, rapidly becoming the gold standard for gallbladder removal [6, 7].

Urology also embraced laparoscopic techniques (Table 17.1). Schuessler et al. introduced laparoscopic pelvic lymphadenectomy for prostate cancer staging [8]. Clayman and colleagues performed the first laparoscopic nephrectomy in 1991 [9].

J. E. Raphael (✉)
Faculty of Clinical Sciences, University of Port Harcourt, Choba, Rivers State, Nigeria

Division of Urology, Department of Surgery, University of Port Harcourt Teaching Hospital (UPTH), Port Harcourt, Rivers State, Nigeria
e-mail: John.raphael@uniport.edu.ng

C. P. Okpani
Faculty of Clinical Sciences, University of Port Harcourt, Choba, Nigeria

Urology Division, Department of Surgery, University of Port Harcourt Teaching Hospital, Port Harcourt, Rivers State, Nigeria

E. Ray-Offor, R. J. Rosenthal (eds.), *Principles and Practice of Laparoscopic Surgery*, https://doi.org/10.1007/978-3-031-96321-6_17

Table 17.1 Timeline of the history of laparoscopic urologic surgery

Year	Author	First procedure
1976	Cortesi	Laparoscopy for cryptorchidism
1979	Wickham	Laparoscopic ureterolithotomy
1990	Sanchez-de-Badajoz	Laparoscopic varicocelectomy
1991	Schuessler	Staging lymphadenectomy for prostate cancer
1991	Clayman	Laparoscopic nephrectomy
1992	Schuessler	Laparoscopic prostatectomy
1992	Parra	Laparoscopic cystectomy
1992	Gagner	Laparoscopic adrenalectomy
1992	Clayman	Retroperitoneoscopy
2000	Binder and Kramer	Robotic radical prostatectomy

From there, laparoscopic urology evolved to include procedures such as adrenalectomy, donor nephrectomy, pyeloplasty, and radical prostatectomy. Laparoscopic varicocelectomy was also introduced, although its benefit over the microsurgical approach remains debatable, partly due to the risk of missed accessory veins [10]. By contrast, laparoscopic nephrectomy (via transperitoneal, retroperitoneal, or hand-assisted routes) has shown notable advantages over open surgery in selected patients [11]. With time, robotic assistance has further refined these minimally invasive techniques [12, 13].

Indications for Laparoscopy in Urology

Diagnostic Laparoscopy

Although modern imaging (e.g., CT, MRI) often suffices for diagnosis, there remain instances where diagnostic laparoscopy provides definitive insight:

- *Undescended Testis:* Laparoscopy is used to locate an intra-abdominal testis and determine feasibility for orchiopexy [12, 16]
- *Intersex Disorders / Disorders of Sex Development:* Visualizing and biopsying gonadal structures laparoscopically to guide further management [12]
- *Staging in Malignancies*: Assessment of pelvic or retroperitoneal lymph nodes if imaging is inconclusive.

Operative Laparoscopy

Operative laparoscopy in urology covers a broad spectrum of surgeries:

- *Pelvic/Retroperitoneal Lymph Node Dissection* for prostate, bladder, or testicular cancer staging and treatment [8]

- *Nephrectomy (Radical, Partial, Donor)* is widely performed with laparoscopic or robotic assistance [9, 11]
- *Adrenalectomy* for benign adrenal tumors (e.g., Conn's syndrome, pheochromocytoma) or small malignant lesions [12]
- *Prostatectomy:* Laparoscopic (pure or robot-assisted) radical prostatectomy is an established option for localized prostate cancer [13]
- *Pyeloplasty* for ureteropelvic junction obstruction [12].
- Cystectomy with intracorporeal or extracorporeal urinary diversion for muscle-invasive bladder cancer [12, 17]

These procedures often rely on advanced laparoscopic skills and specialized tools, such as robotic platforms, depending on the surgical complexity and surgeon expertise [18].

Laparoscopic Anatomy and Surgical Approaches

Minimally invasive urologic procedures generally use transperitoneal or retroperitoneal access, and selection is influenced by the pathology, patient history, and surgeon familiarity [19, 20].

Transperitoneal Anatomy and Approach

- The transperitoneal approach affords a larger working space and familiar intraperitoneal landmarks:
- *Patient*: Placed in the lateral decubitus position (operative side up).
- *Surgeon position*: The surgeon usually stands on the patient's abdominal side (or "ventral" side), facing the operative flank.
- *Assistant/Camera Operator*: Depending on port placement and personal/team preference, this person is often on the opposite side of the patient or near the patient's back.
- *Monitors:* Positioned across from the surgeon on the side where the surgeon has a direct line of sight) so the surgeon can view the screen straight on (or at a slight angle) without turning significantly.
- *Colon Mobilization:* Incise the white line of Toldt and ligaments (Kocher maneuver, hepatic flexure, and IVC on the right; phrenicocolic, splenocolic, splenorenal ligaments on the left) to reflect the colon medially.
- *Ureter and Gonadal Vessels:* The gonadal vessels typically cross anterior to the ureter. They serve as guides to the renal hilum [12, 14]
- *Bladder Dome and Umbilical Ligaments:* Key pelvic landmarks include the median umbilical ligament (urachus), medial umbilical ligament (obliterated hypogastric artery), and lateral umbilical ligament (covers inferior epigastric vessels) (Fig. 17.1).

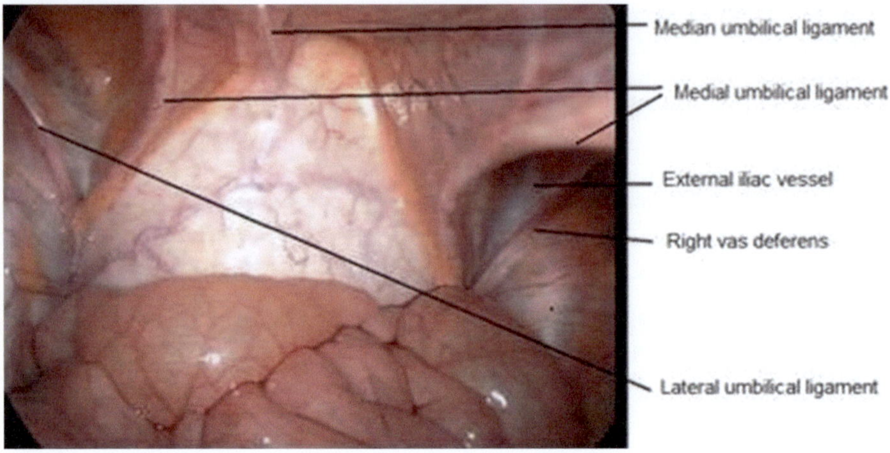

Fig. 17.1 Transperitoneal view of the abdomen at laparoscopy

- *Pouch of Douglas:* A cul-de-sac between the bladder and rectum, crucial for pelvic laparoscopic procedures [21]

Hand-Assisted Laparoscopy

This is a variant of transperitoneal surgery that enables tactile feedback through a hand port and easier specimen retrieval. It is commonly used for donor nephrectomy [12, 22].

Retroperitoneal Anatomy and Approach

The retroperitoneal laparoscopic nephrectomy avoids entering the peritoneal cavity, reducing bowel mobilization and the risk of intra-abdominal adhesions. It provides more direct access to the kidney and renal hilum, facilitating quicker control of the renal vessels and benefiting patients with prior abdominal surgeries. Working outside the peritoneum often lowers the risk of injuring intra-abdominal organs. Some studies also indicate less postoperative pain and a faster return to normal activities. However, the approach can be technically challenging due to a limited working space and potentially restricted visibility, especially in obese patients or large tumors [23].

- *Creating a Working Space:* A small open incision below the 12th rib tip, using balloon dilatation to expand the retroperitoneum.
- *Key Landmarks:* Psoas muscle (posteriorly), Gerota's fascia (enclosing the kidney), and the peritoneal reflection (anteriorly).
- *Limitations:* Less working space, more challenging orientation, and potential difficulty controlling bleeding.

Laparoscopic Technique

Regardless of the chosen approach, several common steps exist:

1. ***Equipment Checks:*** High-definition cameras, reliable CO_2 insufflators, stable light sources, and laparoscopic instruments (clip appliers, energy devices, etc.) [14].
2. ***Monitors:*** Positioned across from the surgeon on the side where the surgeon has a direct line of sight) so the surgeon can view the screen straight on (or at a slight angle) without turning significantly.
3. ***Patient Positioning*** *Transperitoneal Renal Surgery:* Modified lateral decubitus. *Retroperitoneal Surgery:* Standard flank position (90°). *Pelvic Surgery:* Supine Trendelenburg position with legs in stirrups.
4. ***Surgeon position***: The surgeon usually stands on the patient's abdominal side (or "ventral" side), facing the operative flank.
5. ***Assistant/Camera Operator*:** Depending on port placement and personal/team preference, this person is often on the opposite side of the patient or near the patient's back.
6. ***Access to cavity***

   Closed (Veress Needle) or Open (Hasson) technique for transperitoneal.
   Small open incision and balloon expansion for retroperitoneal access [4, 23].

7. ***Trocar Placement***

   The primary (camera) port is placed first, followed by additional working ports, under direct visualization to optimize instrument triangulation.

8. ***Dissection***

   Combination of blunt and sharp dissection, aided by energy devices (e.g., bipolar, ultrasonic shears).

9. ***Specimen Retrieval***

   Enclose specimens in a retrieval bag; enlarge port incisions if needed.

10. ***Closure***

    Meticulous closure of ports ≥10 mm to prevent incisional hernias.

Recent Developments

- ***3D Laparoscopy****:* Improved depth perception.
- ***Single-Port Surgery*** *(SILS):* Cosmetic benefits, though technically demanding [15]
- ***Enhanced Recovery After Surgery (ERAS)****:* Protocols to reduce hospital stay and complications [24]

Common Laparoscopic Surgeries in Urology

Laparoscopic Renal Surgery

This category includes radical nephrectomy, partial nephrectomy, and donor nephrectomy. The decision between retroperitoneal and transperitoneal routes depends on tumor location, surgeon preference, and patient factors [9, 11, 23].

Tips and Tricks in Laparoscopic Retroperitoneal Nephrectomy

1. Patient Positioning

   Place the patient in a standard 90-degree flank position with the operative side elevated. Flex the table to maximize space between the 12th rib and iliac crest.

2. Initial Access and Retroperitoneal Space Creation

   Use an open Hasson technique or a small transverse incision. Employ a balloon dilator or gentle finger dissection to expand the retroperitoneal compartment.

3. Port Placement

   Place ports widely to avoid "sword fighting."
   Displace the peritoneum anteromedially for additional working space.

4. Key Anatomical Landmarks

   The psoas muscle (posterior boundary).
   Gerota's fascia covers the kidney.
   The ureter and gonadal vessels lead to the renal hilum.

5. Renal Hilar Dissection and Control

   Identify the renal artery and renal vein carefully.
   Use a laparoscopic stapler or bulldog clamp if needed.

6. Specimen Retrieval

   Place the kidney in an Endobag.
   If the mass is large, slightly enlarge the incision.

7. Ergonomics and Visibility

   Maintain frequent suction/irrigation to clear blood and preserve the small working space.

Repair any inadvertent peritoneal tears early to maintain insufflation

Tips and Tricks in Laparoscopic Transperitoneal Nephrectomy

1. Patient Positioning

   Modified lateral decubitus (45° off supine) or pure lateral decubitus.
   Ensure adequate padding to avoid pressure injuries.

2. Trocar Placement

   Place the camera port near the lateral edge of the rectus muscle at or above the umbilicus.
   Additional working ports along the mid-clavicular and anterior axillary lines.

3. Mobilization of the Colon

   Incise the white line of Toldt; on the right, divide the right triangular ligament for upper pole access; on the left, incise the phrenicocolic, splenocolic, and splenorenal ligaments.

4. Identification of Renal Hilum

   Track the ureter and gonadal vessels cephalad.
   Dissect carefully around Gerota's fascia to avoid bleeding.

5. Hilar Control

   The renal vein is anterior, and the artery is posterior.
   Employ careful use of clips, staplers, or bulldog clamps.

6. Specimen Removal

   Use an Endobag; may enlarge a port site or use a hand-assisted incision.

7. Hemostasis and Closure

   Thoroughly inspect for bleeding.

Close all ports ≥10 mm to prevent hernias.

Laparoscopic Adrenalectomy

Laparoscopic adrenalectomy is the gold standard for most benign adrenal lesions and selected malignant pathologies [12, 25]. Depending on the tumor size, location, and surgeon preference, the procedure can be performed transperitoneally or retroperitoneally.

Key Points

- Control the adrenal vein early (especially for pheochromocytoma).
- Use gentle manipulation to prevent catecholamine surge.
- Typically, a transperitoneal approach is favored for larger or right-sided tumors because of better visualization.

Laparoscopic Pyeloplasty

A widely accepted minimally invasive solution for ureteropelvic junction (UPJ) obstruction. Success rates exceed 90% [12]. Options include:

- The transperitoneal or retroperitoneal approach is chosen based on surgeon preference and patient anatomy.
- Robotic Pyeloplasty, which can reduce suturing difficulty and operative time.

Key Points
- Precise dissection of the UPJ segment.
- Spatulated ureteral anastomosis for a watertight repair.
- A double-J stent is usually placed to ensure drainage.

Laparoscopic Varicocelectomy

Laparoscopic varicocelectomy is an alternative to the microsurgical subinguinal approach, especially when treating bilateral varicoceles or performing concurrent abdominal procedures [10]. However, the microsurgical technique often has lower recurrence rates.

Tips and Tricks in Laparoscopic Varicocelectomy

1. Patient Selection

   Useful in bilateral disease or if other intra-abdominal surgeries are planned.
   Counsel patients on possible higher recurrence compared to microsurgery.

2. Patient Positioning

   Supine with slight Trendelenburg.
   Alternatively, lithotomy positioning if combining other pelvic procedures.

3. Trocar Placement

   A typical 3-port technique: 10 mm camera port infra-umbilically and two 5 mm working ports in the lower quadrants.

4. Identification of Testicular Vessels

   Mobilize the colon medially.
   Carefully separate the testicular artery if performing an artery-sparing technique.

5. Ligation of Veins

   Use clips or a reliable energy device on the gonadal veins.
   Meticulously search for collateral or accessory veins to minimize recurrence.

6. Preservation of Lymphatics

   Consider indocyanine green (ICG) or methylene blue injection to identify lymphatic channels if feasible.
   Minimizing lymphatic disruption reduces hydrocele formation.

7. Postoperative Considerations

   Secure hemostasis.
   Close ≥10 mm port sites.

Laparoscopic Radical Prostatectomy

Laparoscopic radical prostatectomy is a minimally invasive option for localized prostate cancer. Although robotic assistance is now standard, pure laparoscopic radical prostatectomy remains viable with experienced laparoscopic surgeons [13, 18].

Tips and Tricks in Laparoscopic Radical Prostatectomy

1. Patient Positioning and Port Placement

   Supine with steep Trendelenburg (25°–30°).
   A midline camera port (12 mm) about 2–3 cm above the umbilicus.
   Two or more additional working ports (a 12 mm stapler and one or two 5 mm) on each side at the level of the umbilicus.

2. The surgeon stands on one flank (depending on handedness, while the assistant stands on the opposite side to manage ports or instruments.
3. Bladder Mobilization and Space of Retzius

   Incise the endopelvic fascia to visualize the puboprostatic ligaments.
   Develop Retzius' space with care, controlling small perforating vessels.

4. Dorsal Venous Complex Control

   Preplace sutures or clips on the dorsal venous complex (DVC) to reduce bleeding.

5. Dissection of the Seminal Vesicles and vas Deferens

   Identify and ligate the vas; skeletonize the seminal vesicles using minimal energy.

6. Neurovascular Bundle Preservation

   For nerve-sparing, avoid excessive cautery.
   Remain in the correct fascial planes (e.g., "veil of Aphrodite").

7. Prostatic Apex and Urethral Division

   Carefully incise near the apex to preserve maximal urethral length.

8. Vesicourethral Anastomosis

   Use a running or interrupted suture technique.
   Barbed sutures can facilitate a watertight, tension-free anastomosis.

9. Final Check

   Inspect the prostatic fossa for hemostasis.

Place a drain as necessary.**Future Directions**

- *Robotics & Advanced Imaging:* Refining laparoscopic surgery with enhanced dexterity, near-infrared fluorescence, and augmented reality [26]
- *Single-Incision Laparoscopic Surgery (SILS):* Potential for improved cosmesis though technically challenging [15]
- *Artificial Intelligence and Machine Learning:* Real-time surgical guidance and analytics [26]
- *Global Training and Simulation:* Virtual reality, wet labs, and tele-mentoring to expedite skill acquisition.

References

1. Vecchio R, MacFayden BV, Palazzo F. History of laparoscopic surgery. Panminerva Med. 2000;42(1):87–90.
2. Moran ME, Moll FH. History of cystoscopy. In: The history of technologic advancements in urology. Cham: Springer; 2018. p. 3–20.
3. Hatzinger M, Fesenko A, Sohn M. The first human laparoscopy and NOTES operation: Dimitrij Oscarovic Ott (1855–1929). Urol Int. 2014;92(4):387–91.
4. Semm K, Semm I. Safe insertion of trocars and the Veress needle using standard equipment and the 11 security steps. Gynaecol Endosc. 1999;8(6):339–47.
5. Holthausen UH, Nagelschmidt M, Troidl H. CO2 pneumoperitoneum: what we know and what we need to know. World J Surg. 1999;23:794–800.
6. Blum CA, Adams DB. Who did the first laparoscopic cholecystectomy? J Minim Access Surg. 2011;7(3):165–8.
7. Evans L, et al. Latrogenic gallbladder perforation during laparoscopic cholecystectomy and outcomes: a systematic review and meta-analysis. Langenbeck's Arch Surg. 2022;407(3):937–46.
8. Vargas-Rocha VE, Segales-Rojas P, Vargas Rocha BE. Is laparoscopic oncological surgery after an open surgery possible? Urol Res. 2023;1(1):1–7.
9. Clayman RV, Kavoussi LR, Soper NJ, et al. Laparoscopic nephrectomy. N Engl J Med. 1991;324(19):1370–1.
10. Al-Said S, Al-Naimi A, Al-Ansari A, et al. Varicocelectomy for male infertility: a comparative study of open, laparoscopic and microsurgical approaches. J Urol. 2008;180(1):266–70.

11. Liu Z, Qi L, Yang W, et al. Completely laparoscopic versus open radical nephrectomy and intrahepatic tumor thrombectomy: comparison of surgical complexity and prognosis. Asian J Surg. 2021;44(4):641–8.
12. Soputro NA, Al-Badr W, Moinuddin R, Aboumarzouk OM. A historical perspective of the evolution of laparoscopic surgeries in urology. J Endourol. 2022;36(10):1277–84.
13. Bansal D, Yadav SS, Tandon S, et al. Role of laparoscopy in the era of robotic surgery in urology in developing countries. Indian J Urol. 2021;37(1):32–41.
14. Gill IS, Clayman RV, McDougall EM. Advances in urological laparoscopy. J Urol. 1995;154(4):1275–94.
15. Autorino R, Kaouk JH, Stolzenburg JU, et al. Current status and future perspectives in single-port urological laparoendoscopic surgery. World J Urol. 2013;31(3):605–12.
16. Denes FT, Saito FJ, Silva FA, et al. Laparoscopic diagnosis and treatment of nonpalpable testis. Int Braz J Urol. 2008;34(3):329–35.
17. Bochner BH, Dalbagni G, Sjoberg DD, et al. Comparing open radical cystectomy and robot-assisted laparoscopic radical cystectomy: a randomized clinical trial. Eur Urol. 2018;74(4):465–71.
18. Rassweiler J, Frede T, Seemann O, Stock C, Sentker L. Telesurgical laparoscopic radical prostatectomy. Initial experience. Eur Urol. 2001;40(1):75–83.
19. Abbou CC, Hoznek A, Salomon L, et al. Laparoscopic radical cystectomy: a novel approach to bladder cancer management. Urology. 2001;57(2):204–7.
20. Breda G, Millan F, Liao J. Surgical approach to renal masses: laparoscopic versus open. Curr Opin Urol. 2018;28(4):345–50.
21. Menon M, Tewari A, Peabody JO, et al. Vattikuti institute prostatectomy: technical modifications in the first 100 cases. J Urol. 2002;167(4):1989–94.
22. Ratner LE, Kavoussi LR, Sroka M, et al. Laparoscopic live donor nephrectomy. Transplantation. 1997;60(9):1047–9.
23. Rassweiler J, Frede T, Seemann O, Stock C, Sentker L. Retroperitoneoscopy: experience with 200 cases. J Urol. 1998;160(4):1265–9.
24. Baheti AD, Varghese A, Gaitonde K. Enhanced recovery after surgery (ERAS) in laparoscopic urological procedures. J Minim Access Surg. 2019;15(3):201–6.
25. Fu B, Zhang X, Yang Y, et al. Laparoscopic adrenalectomy for pheochromocytoma: a decade of surgical experience in China. J Endourol. 2014;28(3):278–83.
26. Hung AJ, Chen J, Che Z, Gill IS. AI, machine learning, and robotics in surgery: the future is here. Am J Surg. 2023;225(2):305–13.

Chapter 18
Laparoscopic Surgery in Gynecology and Pregnancy

Emeka Ray-Offor, Tamunomie K. Nyengidiki, and Jude E. Okohue

Introduction

The past two decades have witnessed a revolution in gynecological surgeries with the advent of minimally invasive techniques. Notable gynecologists who pioneered the advancement of gynecological endo-laparoscopy include Raoul Palmer, a strong advocate of intrabdominal pressure monitoring and introducing Palmer's point [1]. Kurt Semm invented the automated insufflator to create pneumoperitoneum, thermocoagulation loops, endoscopic knot techniques, and various laparoscopic techniques [2]. Hitherto, laparoscopic procedures were largely diagnostic and for sterilization- tubal ligation. Innovative modifications in equipment and technique have facilitated more complex laparoscopic gynecological procedures such as

E. Ray-Offor
College of Health Sciences, University of Port Harcourt, Choba, Rivers State, Nigeria

Minimal Access Surgery Program, University of Port Harcourt Teaching Hospital (UPTH), Port Harcourt, Rivers State, Nigeria

Department of Surgery, UPTH, Port Harcourt, Rivers State, Nigeria

Oak Endoscopy Centre and Radiodiagnostics, Port Harcourt, Rivers State, Nigeria

T. K. Nyengidiki (✉)
Department of Obstetrics and Gynaecology, Faculty of Clinical Sciences, University of Port Harcourt, Choba, Rivers State, Nigeria

Gynaecological Oncology Unit, University of Port Harcourt Teaching Hospital (UPTH), Port Harcourt, Rivers State, Nigeria
e-mail: tamunomie.nyengidiki@uniport.edu.ng; emeka.ray-offor@uniport.edu.ng

J. E. Okohue
Madonna University, Elele, Rivers State, Nigeria

Gynescope Specialist Hospital, Port Harcourt, Rivers State, Nigeria

E. Ray-Offor, R. J. Rosenthal (eds.), *Principles and Practice of Laparoscopic Surgery*, https://doi.org/10.1007/978-3-031-96321-6_18

ovarian cystectomies, myomectomies, hysterectomies, excision, and ablation of endometriotic lesions.

The conventional multiport laparoscopic approach has evolved into innovative methods such as natural orifice transluminal endoscopic surgeries (NOTES), single incision laparoscopic surgeries (SILS), and robot-assisted laparoscopy. The benefits of these novel techniques of closed cavity surgery include better cosmesis, the potential for decreased blood loss, reduced postoperative pain, perioperative complications, shorter hospitalization, and faster recovery compared with laparotomy [3, 4]. The surgeon's skill, preference, and availability of the relevant equipment are often the most influential factors in determining which modality is utilized in the surgical management of any gynecologic case, either benign or malignant.

An obstetrics and gynecology specialist with modern practice should have in his/her armamentarium the skills of laparoscopic surgery for carefully selected cases. Moreover, pelvic pathologies are incidental or primary diagnoses in laparoscopic surgery performed by General surgeons hence the need for their familiarity with the treatment of common gynecologic disease in the setting of an emergency or elective surgery. This chapter describes the various applications of laparoscopic surgery to gynecology and important considerations related to non-obstetrics laparoscopic surgery in pregnancy.

Relevant Anatomy

A laparoscope in the abdomen facilitates illumination and magnification of the pelvis with a panoramic view of the pelvis. This enables an easier assessment of the nature and extent of the disease (Fig. 18.1). Anatomical considerations are made from the point of abdominal entry and identification of special structures

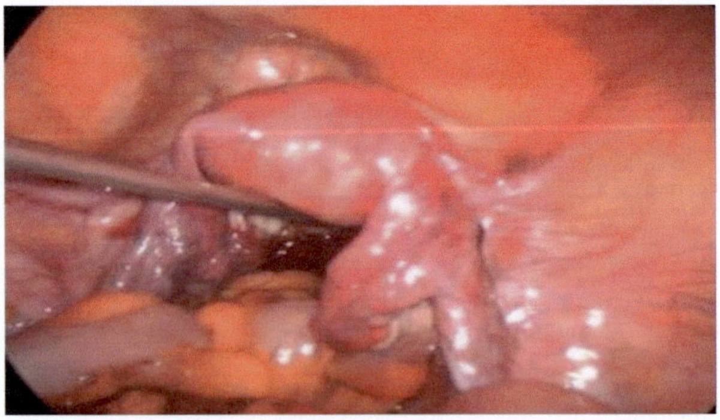

Fig. 18.1 Pelvic view with uterine manipulation

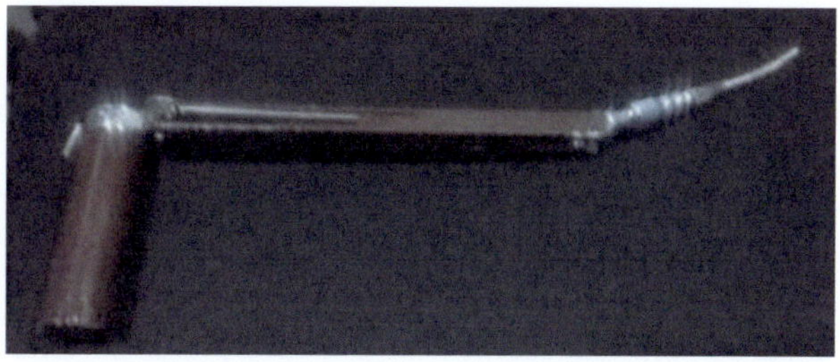

Fig. 18.2 Uterine manipulator

related to the pelvic organs such as the ureters and major pelvic vessels to avoid morbidity to the patient. From the point of insertion of the Veress needle or using the open technique through the umbilicus, it must be remembered that the peritoneal cavity is separated by a layer of skin and peritoneum less than 10 mm thick in some cases. This information is crucial to avoid injury to the intestines during the pneumoperitoneum and trocar insertion. In the absence of an abdominal pannus, endoscopic identification of the lateral umbilical folds/ligaments, harboring the inferior epigastric vessels, via transillumination of the abdominal wall will reduce the risk of vascular injury at the point of abdominal entry. The inferior epigastric vessels are branches of the external iliac vessels and are about 5.5 cm away from the midline bilaterally and superior to the suprapubic bone. Understanding the vascular anatomy is important for carrying out complex surgical procedures such as radical hysterectomy and lymphadenectomy associated with gynecological oncology cases.

Identifying the ureters in the ovarian fossa as it crosses the bifurcation of the common iliac vessels is important to avoid injury during procedures such as hysterectomy. Identifying visible peristatic motions of the ureter will assist in differentiating it from the external iliac vessels. A uterine manipulator inserted through the vagina plays an indispensable role in gynecological laparoscopy (Fig. 18.2). It brings the uterus and adnexa into clear view with a critical range of anterior, posterior, and lateral flexion of the uterus. Specific difficulties may be encountered especially in the presence of severe endometriosis where the uterus is retroverted and fixed because of adhesions from endometriotic lesions.

Indications for Gynecological Laparoscopy

The indications for laparoscopic surgery in gynecology can be broadly divided into benign and malignant conditions. This closed cavity surgical technique is for diagnostic or therapeutic purposes.

Applications of Laparoscopic Surgery in Benign Gynecologic Conditions

Ovary

Ovarian Cysts

Laparoscopic management of ovarian cysts is a veritable alternative to traditional laparotomy because of the reduced surgical morbidity, reduction in pelvic adhesions, shorter recovery period, and reduced cost [5, 6]. Benign ovarian cysts include physiological cysts such as follicular cysts; active or persistent corpus luteum cysts; hemorrhagic ovarian cysts; benign neoplasms of epithelial origin; and endometriotic cysts. The differential diagnosis is adnexal masses including the para-ovarian cyst, ectopic pregnancy, hydrosalpinx, and tubo-ovarian abscess whose differentiation can be made during diagnostic laparoscopy. The ultrasonographic features of thin, smooth ovarian cyst walls, and an absence of septations or solid components associated with a size less than 5 cm, suggest benign lesions. These benign lesions can be removed at laparoscopy by stripping and hemostatic suturing or bipolar electrocoagulation; in the latter hemostatic method, more adverse effects on ovarian volume and reserves are incurred [7]. Even for bigger cysts, aspiration for its contents is feasible while limiting content spillage (in-bag aspiration). In the event of spillage, copious irrigation with Ringer's lactate is advised. The spillage of mucinous content of a malignant cyst is associated with the dissemination of malignancy. Also, the spillage of dermoid cyst contents may result in the peritoneal deposition of a sebaceous substance. This should be avoided. The collection of sections of the cyst for a frozen section can be achieved during the surgery. Persistent ovarian cysts with acute or indolent presentation require surgical intervention ranging from ovarian cystectomy to oophorectomy. Pathologic tissues are extracted through a 12 or 15-mm port using retrieval bags or a colpotomy.

Prophylactic antibiotics should be administered if tissues are extracted via colpotomy.

Polycystic Ovary Syndrome (PCOS)

According to the Rotterdam consensus, PCOS is defined by the presence of two of the three criteria: oligo-anovulation, clinical and/or biochemical signs of hyperandrogenism; and polycystic ovaries ($\geq$ 12 follicles measuring 2–9 mm in diameter; and/or ovarian volume $^{>}$ 10mls in at least one ovary [8]. Traditionally, surgical treatment for this condition was ovarian wedge resection with a risk of converting an endocrine problem to a mechanical one from peri-adnexal adhesion formation. The laparoscopic option is commonly reserved for patients who have medically resistant PCOS [9]. The procedure can be done on an outpatient basis with less trauma and fewer postoperative adhesions than with traditional surgical approaches.

Laparoscopic ovarian drilling (LOD) destroys ovarian follicles and disrupts stroma. Reduction in the production of inhibin and androgen is associated with the destruction of follicles and a resultant increase in follicle-stimulating hormone and subsequent ovulation. Several surgeons have used various energy sources for drilling such as multi-needle intervention, harmonic scalpel, monopolar hook electrode, and office micro laparoscopic ovarian drills [10]. The classical instruction utilizes a unipolar needle with a non-insulated 1–2 cm end. The process commonly involves drilling holes into the ovarian capsule. This can be done using electrocautery, laser unipolar energy at 40 watts at four points for 4 s (rule of 4) [11]. Occasionally, bipolar energy probes are used for LOD. In such situations, continuous saline irrigation of the ovaries at the time of LOD is important to improve effectiveness. This method could also potentially reduce ovarian adhesion formation [12, 13]. The advantages of this often successful "one-off" procedure (ovarian drilling) include the prevalence of mono-follicular ovulation without the need for intensive monitoring to minimize the risks of multiple pregnancies and other adverse effects of gonadotrophin therapy. In cases of failed ovulation within 2–3 months following LOD, ovulation induction can often be more successful than when employed before the operation [10]. This procedure is however associated with a risk of iatrogenic ovarian adhesions and reduction of ovarian reserves hence the need for its use in selected cases especially for clomiphene-resistant patients. Evidence from metanalysis of RCTs after carefully weighing up the well-known benefits of bilateral vs unilateral LOD against a potential risk to ovarian reserve, advises clinicians to offer the latter to their infertile patients with clomiphene-resistant PCOS [14].

Borderline Ovarian Tumors

Histological features of borderline ovarian tumors are like malignant tumors but without identifiable destructive stromal invasion. These low malignant-potential tumors predominantly occur among women of reproductive age thus fertility sparing is important. Following intraoperative histology, laparoscopic salpingo-oophorectomy is the recommended treatment depending on the stage of the disease. The fertility-sparing options include laparoscopic cystectomy and adnexectomy. However, these options are associated with a significant risk of relapse [15].

Adnexa

Chronic Pelvic Inflammatory Disease/Infertility

The assessment of the adnexa is usually in situations of infertility and patients with acute/chronic pelvic pain. About 50 to 70% of gynecological consultations are due to infertility of which a large proportion are due to tubal factors [16]. As sequelae of pelvic inflammatory disease affect the fallopian tube, varying degrees of pathologies can be identified which could be classified as mild, moderate, or severe. A superficial vascular pattern that is suggestive of congestion, inflammation, minimal kinking, or minimal fibrosis is seen in the mild variety. For moderate-type salpingitis isthmica nodosum, distal phimosis, high degrees of vascular change, fibrosis, and ampullary dilation are noted. The findings of obstruction of the tube proximally or distally are severe. These features can be identified during diagnostic laparoscopy and further assessment via chromopertubation can be done which is the gold standard for tubal patency assessment. Interventional procedures such as excision of tubo-ovarian masses, hydrosalpinxes, and adhesiolysis have been practiced to improve pregnancy success rates either during assisted or natural conception with varying degrees of success [17].

Ectopic Pregnancy

The fallopian tube is the most common location for extrauterine pregnancy. Surgical options for management include laparoscopic salpingectomy or organ-preserving surgery such as salpingostomy. The choice of organ-preserving surgery is considered based on the skill of the surgeon, size of the tubal pregnancy, degree of damage to the affected and contralateral fallopian tubes, intensity of bleeding, any prior history of infertility or tubal pregnancy, not the least of all is the patient's wishes about future fertility [18]. A laparoscopic salpingostomy is a consideration involving a linear incision using a monopolar needle into the tube on the anti-mesenteric border directly over the pregnancy for evacuation with minimal tissue destruction. Rarely, distal tubal pregnancy can be non-forcibly expressed through the ampulla ("milked out") with the aid of atraumatic grasping forceps. Laparoscopic management of ectopic pregnancy is not limited to unruptured gestational sacs; the major determining factor is the hemodynamic stability of the patient. Prompt resuscitation and rapid evacuation of hemoperitoneum are critical to improving vision and performing the requisite procedure. A laparoscopic salpingectomy is indicated when a large tubal pregnancy has partly destroyed the involved tube with a normal contralateral tube. Different energy sources can be used for these procedures, preferably either a Harmonic scalpel or newer bipolar energy electrosurgical devices like the Enseal of LigaSure for minimal damage to adjacent tissues or organs. A re-anastomosis of segmental resection is needed if the patient desires a future pregnancy with an absent or diseased contralateral tube. However, it should be borne in mind that there is a subsequent risk of ectopic pregnancy in the affected tube with varying degrees of success following reanastomosis.

Tubal Sterilization and Tubal Surgery

The tubal sterilization procedure involves either the application of an occlusive material or the excision of a fallopian tube segment from the cornua of the uterus. Tubal sterilization outcomes are influenced by the patient's age, time from sterilization, technique, and tubal length. The outcomes are better when the residual tubal length exceeds 4 cm. The methods include electrocoagulation, mechanical occlusion with silicone rubber bands, spring or titanium clips, and partial or total salpingectomy. The serious complications of unipolar cautery, which was associated with thermal bowel injury, led to the development of alternative techniques. The Falope rings, Filshie, and Hulka-Clemens clips are safely applied laparoscopically; however, with a 1–3% pregnancy rate over 10 years [19]. Tubal surgery initially had poor results with laparotomy and macrosurgical repair techniques. Later, microsurgical repairs with small sutures and less tissue handling yielded better results. Sterilization reversal is the most successful surgical reconstructive procedure for improving fertility [20]. However, surgical repair of the fallopian tube has been largely replaced by assisted reproductive therapy (ART). Pregnancy rates after laparoscopic tubal anastomosis and conventional microsurgical anastomosis are equivalent but the results are dismal with tubo-cornual re-anastomosis. The presence of hydrosalpinx fluid is known to reduce the IVF pregnancy rates significantly [21]. Undergoing laparoscopic treatment of the hydrosalpinx, either by salpingectomy or tubal ligation before an IVF improves pregnancy rates [20].

Uterus

Uterovaginal Prolapse

Laparoscopic sacro-colpopexy is a treatment for vaginal vault prolapse with similar long-term outcomes to the open abdominal approach in quality of life, anatomical results, complications, or reintervention [22]. Hence, the laparoscopic approach is preferable, considering the short-term advantages. Major steps of the procedure are opening the peritoneum at the level of the sacral promontory, identification of the fibers of the superior hypogastric plexus, deep anterior and posterior dissection with attachment of the mesh to the vagina, displacement of the nerve fibers to the left side during suturing of the mesh to the longitudinal ligament, and reperitonealization.

Uterine Fibroids

Uterine fibroids are the most common pelvic tumors (Fig. 18.3). The indications for treatment of uterine fibroids include metrorrhagia with anemia, pelvic pain or pelvic pressure that interferes with daily life, ureteral compression, rapid tumor growth, tumor growth following menopause, and infertility. Hysterectomy is the definitive surgical treatment for uterine fibroids. However, for patients who wish to preserve fertility, a myomectomy is offered. The choice between the open or laparoscopic approach is based on the location, size, and number of fibroids. Relative contraindications for laparoscopic myomectomy include diffuse leiomyomata; women who have completed childbearing and who desire hysterectomy; any medical condition that is not suitable for anesthesia or prolonged laparoscopic surgery. Laparoscopic myomectomy is primarily used to remove intramural and subserosa fibroids. A large

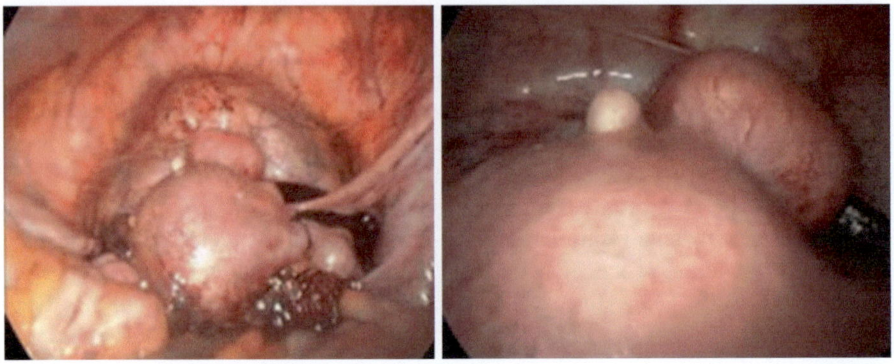

Fig. 18.3 Uterine fibroids

prospective multicenter study of 2050 women found that fibroid characteristics associated with major complications such as blood transfusion or conversion to open surgery were in cases when a single fibroid measured more than 5 cm or when more than 3 fibroid seedlings were removed [23]. The skill of the laparoscopic surgeon is a major determinant of the size of the myoma to be handled. With more experience, larger fibroids and greater numbers can be removed.

Preoperative preparations to reduce the size of myoma involve the use of GnRH analogs; however, cleavage lines are difficult to delineate following its administration with increased risk of bleeding and prolonged operating time. Vasopressin injection is a pharmacological agent that mitigates blood loss in myoma surgery. While the optimal dose of vasopressin is controversial, an upper limit of 4–6 units was proposed in a study [24]. Approximately 0.05–0.3iu/ml is injected between the fibroid and the myometrium;10 units of vasopressin is commonly diluted in 100mls of normal saline. Care must however be taken in its administration since episodes of bradycardia, cardiovascular collapse, and death have been observed with its usage. The anesthetist should always be informed before the administration of vasopressin. Suturing of enucleated dead spaces is required using conventional polyglactin sutures with good suturing techniques. Alternatively, barbed sutures such as Stratafix or V-lock can ensure good suture integrity and reduced operation time. However, this is more expensive. Enucleated myomas can be retrieved via a colpotomy or mechanical morcellation using a morcellator. The Regulatory Agency in the USA (FDA) 2020 update recommends performing laparoscopic power morcellation for myomectomy or hysterectomy with a tissue containment system only in appropriately selected patients [25, 26]. There is a theoretical risk of uterine rupture following laparoscopic myomectomy. The causes include difficulty in closing the uterine wound adequately, excess dead space, tissue strangulation during suturing, and the excessive use of energy causing necrosis. To reduce postoperative adhesions, antiadhesive materials can be placed over the incision sites, meticulous hemostasis control can be maintained, and evacuation of the intra-abdominal postsurgical blood collection.

Endometriosis

Endometriosis is a disease in which cells similar to the uterine endometrium grow outside the uterus and can affect up to 15% of reproductive-age women [27, 28]. It is a menstrual cycle-dependent chronic inflammatory systemic disease with most patients presenting with chronic pelvic pain and infertility. The deposition of endometrial tissues inside the abdominal and pelvic cavities is associated with fertility challenges and chronic or acute pelvic pain which can reduce fertility and quality of life of the patient. Endometriomas can release toxic cyst contents into the adjacent ovarian parenchyma leading to severe oxidative stress, fibrosis, loss of cortical stroma, impaired vascularization, and impaired oocyte quality [29]. Also, they reduce anti-Mullerian hormone (AMH) levels and result in a greater decline in AMH over time especially in women with cyst size greater than 3 cm [29]. There are three phenotypes of endometriosis: superficial, ovarian endometrioma, and deep endometriosis. Those with superficial endometriosis can undergo surgery to improve natural conception, ovulation induction with intrauterine insemination, and in-vitro fertilization [30]. Depending on the grade of endometriosis and the reproductive wishes of the patient various laparoscopic options are available which may involve ablation, excision, prophylactic oophorectomies, and colonic resection. The European Society of Human Reproduction and Embryology (ESHRE) guidelines recommend the removal of ovarian endometriomas greater than 3 cm in diameter before IVR treatment [31]. Deep infiltrating endometriosis (DIE) distorts the pelvic anatomy due to severe adhesions. There is a marked improvement in sexual life and reduced pain after laparoscopic management of DIE.

Retrieval of Missing Intrauterine Device

Migration of intrauterine devices to the abdominal cavity has been encountered following insertion into the uterine cavity. This migration may be asymptomatic or symptomatic depending on the location and nature of the device. A resort to laparoscopic retrieval of missing IUD reduced patient hospital stay, better cosmesis, and pain control. There are some instances where retrieval is unsuccessful, however, the success rate of IUD retrieval between 44 and 100% has been recorded depending on surgeons' expertise and the presenting complications [32].

Applications of Laparoscopy Surgery in Gynecological Malignancy

The key tenets of oncological surgery are tissue diagnosis, staging, and treatment. Laparoscopy in gynecological oncology, when applied, is associated with decreased patient discomfort, improved overall quality of life, early initiation of adjuvant therapies, and good cancer control without compromising patient safety [33, 34]. For the oncologist, minimal access surgery provides good optimal exposure, and an opportunity for meticulous tissue dissection. The surgeon needs good anatomical knowledge in addition to understanding the natural history of the disease to achieve successful laparoscopy. Despite these listed benefits, there are some limitations to the extent of deployment of this advancement related to patient and non-patient factors. The non-patient-related factors include the available 2D vision technology, counterintuitive motions, difficulty and long learning curve, surgical training and experience, and longer operation time. The patient-related limitations include obesity, extent of disease, and history of previous surgeries. All gynecological oncology surgeries can be performed via a laparoscopic approach with appropriate case selection (Fig. 18.4).

Lymph Node Detection and Lymphadenectomy

In most cases, imaging techniques cannot reliably evaluate lymphatic spread. The lymph nodes mostly involved in gynecological oncology practice include the common iliac, the external iliac, the internal iliac, the obturator nodes (pelvic lymph nodes), and the para-aortic lymph nodes; they are sampled bilaterally to the level of

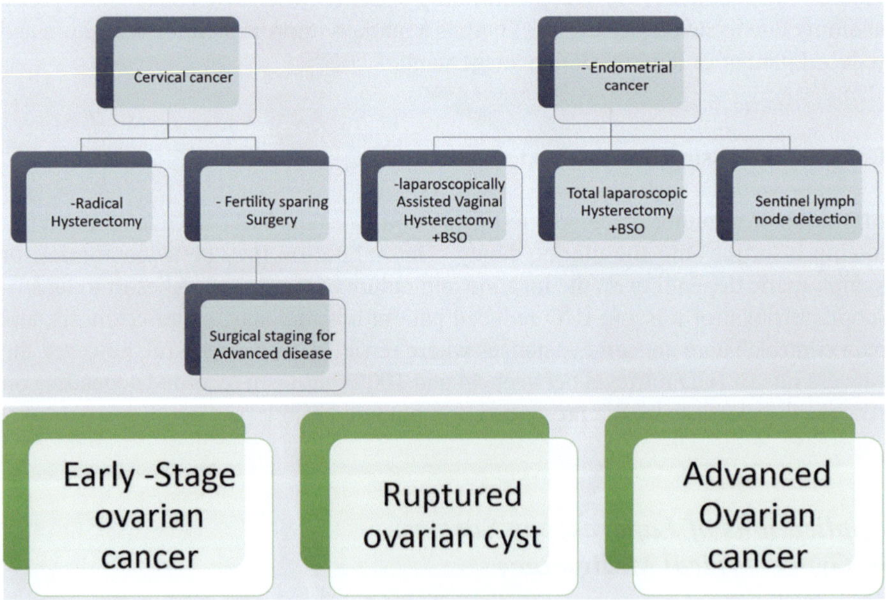

Fig. 18.4 Applications of laparoscopic surgery in gynecological oncology

the inferior mesenteric artery. The use of sentinel lymph node biopsy techniques in the staging of cervical and endometrial cancer has demonstrated promising results from available literature. The advantages are improved positive lymph node detection, reduced intraoperative complications, and postoperative morbidities including lymphedema.

To avoid comprehensive lymph node dissection complications, the sentinel lymph node mapping technique has been employed with good outcomes in endometrial cancer.

Several substances are used for sentinel mapping including isosulfan blue, methylene blue(commonly), indocyanine green, and radiolabeled technetium 99. The newer indocyanine green has a unique fluorescence characteristic in the near-infrared spectrum. A special camera system has been developed that alters the wavelength of light between the normal and reveals the location of the dye by its fluorescence. There are several sites of injection to enhance tumor detection - hysteroscopic tumor injection, subserosa, fundal, and cervical sites. The intracervical route has been associated with a higher sentinel node detection; an injection of 1 ml of any type chosen at 3 and 9 o'clock positions has a detection rate of 80–95% [35]. However, there are concerns that patients with high-grade lesions involvement of the paraaortic nodes may be missed with reliance on only sentinel node detection.

Cervical Cancer

Ever since the first total laparoscopic radical hysterectomy with pelvic and para-aortic lymph node dissection for early-stage cervical carcinoma was reported in 1992, this surgery has gained prominence in gynecologic oncological surgery [36]. The standard treatment of early-stage cervical carcinoma is radical hysterectomy. Patients with tumors less than 4 cm, negative lymph nodes, and the absence of combined angiovascular and lymphovascular space involvement can be identified by laparoscopic surgery and are ideal candidates for laparoscopic-assisted radical hysterectomy. The short-term surgical outcomes of intraoperative or post-operative adverse events for early-stage cervical cancer are the same for both open and laparoscopy routes [37]. Nevertheless, the LACC trial final analysis reported better outcomes for open surgery in terms of overall survival and disease-free period for patients undergoing open surgery [38]. There are limited roles for patients with advanced diseases. Laparoscopic vaginal radical trachelectomy (LVRT) is suited for patients with confirmed stage 1A1 with lymphovascular invasion but desirous of fertility, with cervical length greater than 2 cm or with tumor size of <2 cm with no other impediment to fertility [39]. Laparoscopy is also important in staging and in assisting the radiation oncologist in the safe placement of interstitial brachytherapy implants in patients with cervical cancer. In addition, laparoscopic resection of visibly enlarged lymph nodes has been known to improve survival instead of only radiotherapy but has marked difficulty when attached to the great vessels.

Endometrial Cancer

The surgical approach in the treatment of endometrial cancer includes washing cytology, hysterectomy, bilateral salpingo-oophorectomy, and lymphadenectomy. A Cochrane review on the overall survival and disease-free survival for women with earlystage endometrial cancer undergoing hysterectomy by laparoscopy versus laparotomy concluded that laparoscopy is associated with lower blood loss, less operative morbidities, and postoperative complications as well as faster recovery than laparotomy [40]. Disease-free and overall survival are similar in the laparoscopic and laparotomy groups [41]. One of the major risk factors for endometrial cancer is obesity which many patients may have, and this factor is associated with a higher conversion rate. This is mitigated by the introduction of robotic surgery in the management of this cohort of patients.

Ovarian Cancer

Laparoscopy is useful in diagnosing early-stage ovarian cancer with a panoramic visualization of pelvic structures, abdominal peritoneum, and bowel mesentery thus confirming organ-confined cancer with no evidence of gross metastatic disease. It is a useful decision-making tool to identify high-risk patients for suboptimal primary debulking surgery [42, 43]. The choice of neoadjuvant chemotherapy followed by an interval debulking surgery can be made in such cases. In advanced stages, primary debulking surgery often requires bowel resections and extensive upper abdominal surgery, these are better resolved by open surgery. A further role of laparoscopy is in isolated ovarian recurrences where secondary cytoreduction by this minimally invasive approach is safe and feasible in carefully selected patients [44]. Laparoscopy in early ovarian cancer enables the surgeon to evaluate patients with subclinical metastasis and enables the extraction of peritoneal washouts or ascitic fluid for cytology as an aid in the staging process. It enables proper visualization of the diaphragm, omentum, and the various groups of lymph nodes. However, limitations of assessment may be noted around the intestinal mesenteries and abdominal peritoneum with a 3–5% risk of under-staging.

Non-obstetrics Laparoscopic Surgery in Pregnancy

About 1 in 500 women require intra-abdominal general surgery during pregnancy [45]. The most common non-obstetric surgical emergencies complicating pregnancy are acute appendicitis, ovarian cysts, masses or torsion, symptomatic cholelithiasis, and other rare conditions. Favorable outcomes for the mother and fetus depend on accurate and timely diagnosis with prompt intervention. Surgery in pregnancy is associated with the risk of premature labor and miscarriage. In recent literature, there is an emerging role of laparoscopic surgery in pregnancy especially in the second trimester considered to be the safest period in terms of least risk to the fetus (Fig. 18.5) [46]. However, there are peculiar challenges that call on the expertise of an experienced laparoscopic surgeon and obstetric anesthetist for favorable outcomes.

Preoperative Preparation

Ultrasonography with high sensitivity and specificity is a safe diagnostic tool for acute painful abdominal conditions in pregnancy. However, the use of plain X-ray investigations is a decision that requires caution. Lead shielding of the fetus cannot be overemphasized as 5 mGy of radiation is known to cause teratogenicity in early pregnancy and a high risk of childhood malignancies in later pregnancy [47]. For further radiological assessment magnetic resonance imaging without intravenous contrast is safer than CT. There is a need for careful analysis of potential risks and benefits of potential diagnostic methods and therapy not only to the mother but also to the fetus. Though it is preferable to operate in the second trimester, current literature reports safe laparoscopic procedures in all trimesters of pregnancy.

Anesthesia

An experienced obstetric anesthetist is needed for a favorable outcome at surgery. Deep vein thrombosis prophylaxis with pressure stockings and pneumatic compression devices is essential. There may be impedance of venous return through the vena cava from pressure effects of a prolonged pneumoperitoneum and gravid uterus after the second trimester. To avoid the latter, the patient is positioned on the operating table in a left lateral position or supine with a lateral tilt. Carbon dioxide is the preferred insufflation gas since it is easily absorbed and non-combustible. A

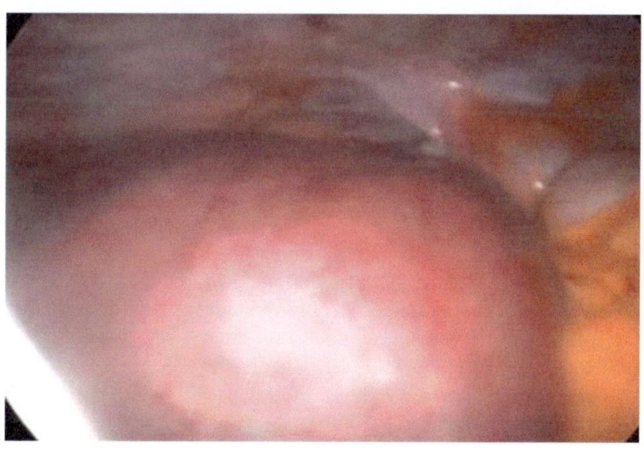

Fig. 18.5 Gravid uterus at laparoscopy (Cecum to the right of image)

pressure of 9–14 mmHg is considered safe with clear visualization of structures. However, an excessive absorption of this gas can result in hypercarbia with feto-maternal physiological changes. Monitoring of end-tidal and intraarterial carbon dioxide are recommended.

Access, Port Placement, and Technique

The risk of iatrogenic uterine injury from the Veress needle is mitigated by an open (Hasson's) access technique. In the choice of site for a primary trocar, the traditional umbilical site in a virgin abdomen is unfavorable with a very gravid uterus. A selection of the insertion point according to fundal height is needed and the abdominal wall is elevated during insertion. These measures mitigate the risk of uterine injury. Favorable sites are midline fascial incisions above the umbilicus or Palmer's point. With the laparoscope in the abdomen, after careful inspection to exclude any iatrogenic injury, secondary ports are inserted under direct vision.

There should be no cervical instrumentation and with care no uterine manipulation. A quick and precise surgery is carried out. Intraoperative fetal monitoring is not compulsory but recommended pre- and post-operatively.

The choice between laparoscopic and open routes of surgery in pregnancy should be based on the available expertise, requisite infrastructure, background history, gestation, and the woman's preference [48].

References

1. Palmer R. Safety in laparoscopy. J Repro Med. 1974;13:1–5.
2. Moll FH, Marx FJ. A pioneer in laparoscopy and pelviscopy: Kurt Semm (1927–2003). J Endourol. 2005;19(3):269–71.
3. Kumar A, et al. Single incision laparoscopic surgery: a review of literature. Ind J Surg. 2014;769(4):296–304.
4. Schmitt A, Crochet P, Pivano A, Tourette C, Faust C, Baumstarck K, et al. The effects of a laparoscopy by single-port endoscopic access in benign adnexal surgery: a randomized controlled trial. J Minim Invasive Gynecol. 2024;31(5):397–405.
5. Yuen PM, Yu KM, Yip SK, Lau WC, Rogers MS, Chang A. A randomized prospective study of laparoscopy and laparotomy in the management of benign ovarian masses. Am J Obstet Gynecol. 1997;177(1):109–14.
6. Henes M, Engler T, Taran FA, Brucker S, Rall K, Janz B, et al. Ovarian cyst removal influences ovarian reserve depending on histology, size, and type of operation. Womens Health (Lond). 2018;14:1745506518778992.
7. Sahin C, Akdemir A, Ergenoglu AM, Ozgurel B, Yeniel AO, Taskiran D, et al. Which should be the preferred technique during laparoscopic ovarian cystectomy? Reprod Sci. 2017;24(3):393–9.
8. Rotterdam ESHRE/ASRM-Sponsored PCOS consensus workshop group. Revised 2003 consensus on diagnostic criteria and long-term health risks related to polycystic ovary syndrome (PCOS). Hum Reprod. 2004;19(1):41–7.

9. Bordewijk EM, Ng KYB, Rakic L, Mol BWJ, Brown J, Crawford TJ, et al. Laparoscopic ovarian drilling for ovulation induction in women with anovulatory polycystic ovary syndrome. Cochrane Database Syst Rev. 2020;2(2):CD001122.
10. Farquhar C, Lilford RJ, Marjoribanks J, Vandekerckhove P. Laparoscopic 'drilling' by diathermy or laser for ovulation induction in anovulatory polycystic ovary syndrome. Cochrane Database Syst Rev. 2007;3:CD001122. https://doi.org/10.1002/14651858.CD001122.pub3. Update in: Cochrane Database Syst Rev. 2012 Jun 13;(6): CD001122. doi: 10.1002/14651858.CD001122.pub4
11. Armar NA, McGarrigle HH, Honour J, Holownia P, Jacobs HS, Lachelin GC. Laparoscopic ovarian diathermy in the management of anovulatory infertility in women with polycystic ovaries: endocrine changes and clinical outcome. Fertil Steril. 1990;53:45–9.
12. Merchant RN. Treatment of polycystic ovary disease with laparoscopic low-watt bipolar electrocoagulation of the ovaries. J Am Gynecol laparosc. 1996;3:503–8.
13. Fernandez H, Faivre E, Gervaise A, et al. Laparoscopic ovarian drilling using a 5french bipolar energy probe. Fertil Steril. 2010;94(2):740–1.
14. Abu Hashim H, Foda O, El Rakhawy M. Unilateral or bilateral laparoscopic ovarian drilling in polycystic ovary syndrome: a meta-analysis of randomized trials. Arch Gynecol Obstet. 2018;297(4):859–70.
15. Della Corte L, Mercorio A, Serafino P, et al. The challenging management of borderline ovarian tumors (BOTs) in women of childbearing age. Front Surg. 2022;9 https://doi.org/10.3389/fsurg.2022.973034.
16. Okafor NI, Joe-Ikechebelu NN, Ikechebelu JI, et al. Perceptions of infertility and in vitro fertilization treatment among married couples in Anambra State. Nigeria Afr J Reprod Health. 2017;21(4):55–66.
17. Melo P, Georgiou EX, Johnson N, et al. Surgical treatment for tubal disease in women due to undergoing in vitro fertilisation. Cochrane Database Syst Rev. 2020;10(10):CD002125.
18. D'Hooghe T, Tomassetti C. Surgery for ectopic pregnancy: making the right choice. Lancet. 2014;383(9927):1444–5.
19. Varma R, Gupta JK. Failed sterilisation: evidence-based review and medicolegal ramifications. BJOG Int J Obstet Gynaecol. 2004;111:1322–32.
20. Bi B, Han X, Dai W, et al. Comparisons of different treatment outcomes in IVF/ET patients with hydrosalpinx: a retrospective study. Gynecol Endocrinol. 2023;39(1)
21. Okohue JE, Ikimalo JI. IVF pregnancy and delivery following ultrasound scan guided aspiration of a left hydrosalpinx. A case report. Niger Postgrad Med J. 2015;22(2):123–5.
22. van Oudheusden AMJ, Eissing J, Terink IM, Vink MDH, van Kuijk SMJ, Bongers MY, et al. Laparoscopic sacrocolpopexy versus abdominal sacrocolpopexy for vaginal vault prolapse: long-term follow-up of a randomized controlled trial. Int Urogynecol J. 2023;34(1):93–104.
23. Sizzi O, Rosetti A, Malzoni M, et al. Italian multicenter study on complications of laparoscopic myomectomy. J Minim Invasive Gynecol. 2007;14(9):453–622022. https://doi.org/10.3389/fsurg.2022.973034.
24. Frishman G. Vasopressin: if some is good, is more better? Obstet Gynecol. 2009;113(2):476–7.
25. Product labeling for laparoscopic morcellators. US Food and Drug Administration: UPDATE Published online 2020.
26. Foley C, Donnellan N, Harris J. Tissue extraction in gynecologic surgery: past, present, and future. Clin Obstet Gynecol. 2020;63(2):305–19.
27. Bulletti C, Coccia ME, Battistoni S, et al. Endometriosis and infertility. J Assist Reprod Genet. 2010;27(8):441–7.
28. Olive DL, Pritts EA. Treatment of endometriosis. N Engl J Med. 2001;345(4):26675.
29. Harb HM, Gallos ID, Chu J, Harb M, Coomarasamy A. The effect of endometriosis on in vitro fertilisation outcome: a systematic review and meta-analysis. BJOG. 2013;120(11):1308–20.
30. Bafort C, Beebeejaun Y, Tomassetti C, Bosteels J, Duffy JM. Laparoscopic surgery for endometriosis. Cochrane Database Syst Rev. 2020;10(10):CD011031.

31. Kenedy S, Bergqvist A, Chapron C, et al. ESHRE special inter group for endometriosis and endometrium guideline development group. ESHRE guideline for the diagnosis and treatment of endometriosis. Hum Reprod. 2005;20(10):2698–704.
32. Robayo-Amortegui H, Rincon-Vanegas M, Ballestas-Blanquicet A, et al. Laparoscopy approach to sigmoid colon perforation secondary to intrauterine device migration. Gynecol Surg. 2021;18:9. https://doi.org/10.1186/s10397-021-01091-w.
33. Mourits MJE, Bijen CB, Arts HJ, ter Brugge HG, van der Sijde R, Paulsen L, et al. Safety of laparoscopy versus laparotomy in early-stage endometrial cancer: a randomised trial. Lancet Oncol. 2010;11:763–71.
34. Janda M, Gebski V, Brand A, Hogg R, Jobling TW, Land R, et al. Quality of life after total laparoscopic hysterectomy versus total abdominal hysterectomy for stage I endometrial cancer (LACE): a randomised trial. Lancet Oncol. 2010;11:772–80.
35. Gezer Ş, Duman Öztürk S, et al. Cervical versus endometrial injection for sentinel lymph node detection in endometrial cancer: a randomized clinical trial. Int J Gynecol Cancer. 2020;30(3):325–31.
36. Nezhat CR, Burrell MO, Nezhat FR, Benigno BB, Welander CE. Laparoscopic radical hysterectomy with paraaortic and pelvic node dissection. Am J Obstet Gynecol. 1992;166(3):864–5.
37. Obermair A, Asher R, Pareja R, Frumovitz M, Lopez A, Moretti-Marques R, et al. Incidence of adverse events in minimally invasive vs open radical hysterectomy in early cervical cancer: results of a randomized controlled trial. Am J Obstet Gynecol. 2020;222(3):249.e1–249.e10.
38. Ramirez PT, et al. LACC trial: final analysis on overall survival comparing open versus minimally invasive radical hysterectomy for early-stage cervical cancer. JCO. 2024;42:2741–6.
39. He Z, Bian C, Xie C. Fertility-sparing surgery in early-stage cervical cancer: laparoscopic versus abdominal radical trachelectomy. BMC Womens Health. 2022;22:241.
40. Galaal K, Bryant A, Fisher AD, et al. Laparoscopy versus laparotomy for the management of early stage endometrial cancer. Cochrane Database Syst Rev. 2012;9:CD006655.
41. Fagotti A, Ferrandina G, Fanfani F, Ercoli A, Lorusso D, Rossi M, et al. A laparoscopybased score to predict surgical outcome in patients with advanced ovarian carcinoma: a pilot study. Ann Surg Oncol. 2006;13(8):1156–61.
42. Fagotti A, Ferrandina G, Fanfani F, Ercoli A, Lorusso D, Rossi M, Scambia G. A laparoscopy-based score to predict surgical outcome in patients with advanced ovarian carcinoma: a pilot study. Ann Surg Oncol. 2006;13(8):1156–61.
43. Yokoi A, Machida H, Shimada M, Matsuo K, Shigeta S, Furukawa S, et al. Efficacy and safety of minimally invasive surgery versus open laparotomy for epithelial ovarian cancer: a systematic review and meta-analysis. Gynecol Oncol. 2024;190:42–52.
44. Harter P, Sehouli J, Vergote I, Ferron G, Reuss A, Meier W, et al. DESKTOP III investigators. Randomized trial of cytoreductive surgery for relapsed ovarian cancer. N Engl J Med. 2021;385(23):2123–31.
45. Augustin G, Majerovic M. Non-obstetrical acute abdomen during pregnancy. Eur J Obstet Gynecol Reprod Biol. 2007;131:4–12.
46. Liu YX, Zhang Y, Huang JF, Wang L. Meta-analysis comparing the safety of laparoscopic and open surgical approaches for suspected adnexal mass during the second trimester. Int J Gynaecol Obstet. 2017;136(3):272–9.
47. Goldberg-Stein SA, Liu B, Hahn PF, Lee SI. Radiation dose management: part 2, estimating fetal radiation risk from CT during pregnancy. AJR Am J Roentgenol. 2012;198:W352–6.
48. Ball E, Waters N, Cooper N, Talati C, Mallick R, Rabas S, et al. Evidence-based guideline on laparoscopy in pregnancy: commissioned by the British Society for Gynaecological Endoscopy (BSGE) Endorsed by the Royal College of Obstetricians & Gynaecologists (RCOG). Facts Views Vis Obgyn. 2019;11(1):5–25. Erratum in: Facts Views Vis Obgyn. 2020 Jan 24;11(3):261

Chapter 19
Video-Assisted Thoracoscopic Surgery

Emmanuel O. Ocheli, Christian E. Amadi, and Kelechi E. Okonta

Introduction

Minimal access procedures were used early in the twentieth century, mainly for diagnosis and, rarely, therapeutic purposes. Recently, renewed interest has occurred due to breakthrough developments in optics/imaging systems, proper instrumentation, and anesthesia techniques. Video-assisted thoracoscopic surgery (VATS) is a minimally invasive surgical technique performed by inserting a telescope and special instruments into the thoracic cavity via small skin incisions placed in the lateral aspect of the chest wall or the subxiphoid anteriorly.

Earlier, in vivo, celioscopy in dogs was performed by Kelling and Dresden in 1901 [1]. Hans Christian Jacobeus performed the first human thoracoscopy in 1910, using a cystoscope to visualize and lyse the pleural adhesions in the treatment of tuberculosis [2]. The discovery of antituberculosis drugs led to a temporary loss of interest in thoracoscopy for the next 25 years. In 1937, Anton Sattler used thoracoscopy without video assistance for managing spontaneous pneumothorax. In 1946, Joao Bronco reported the use of thoracoscopy to diagnose and treat chest trauma [3, 4]. VATS was heralded by the development of solid-state systems and microcameras in the 1980s. In the presence of isolated pockets of individual efforts in thoracoscopy, the first reported thymectomy by Landreneau et al. using the VATS technique occurred in 1992 [5]. This opened the floodgates of VATS for myriads of chest conditions. Today, the indications for VATS have expanded to the vast majority of thoracic, vascular, neurological, and a few cardiac cases.

E. O. Ocheli (✉) · C. E. Amadi · K. E. Okonta
Faculty of Clinical Sciences, University of Port Harcourt, Choba, Nigeria

Cardiothoracic/Vascular Unit, Surgery Department, University of Port Harcourt Teaching Hospital, Port Harcourt, Rivers State, Nigeria
e-mail: emmanuel.ocheli@uniport.edu.ng

E. Ray-Offor, R. J. Rosenthal (eds.), *Principles and Practice of Laparoscopic Surgery*, https://doi.org/10.1007/978-3-031-96321-6_19

The benefits of using VATS include reduced postoperative pain, an earlier recovery, shorter hospital stays, better aesthetics, and improved quality of life [6–8]. It is important to point out that there is a steep learning curve before the surgeon can be proficient in VATS. This is addressed by regular multiple wet lab courses for hands-on training experiences. Understanding the anatomy of the thorax, contents, boundaries and associated regions is fundamental to successful VATS practice. Ideally, VATS practitioners should first be knowledgeable and skilled in open thoracotomy to tackle the risk of conversion [9].

Relevant Anatomy

The area of deployment of VATS is the thorax. The thorax could be described as an irregular, truncated cone with a narrower inlet superiorly in continuity with the root of the neck; and an outlet as base, separated from the abdominal cavity by the diaphragm. The thorax is bound by a rigid wall comprising, from outside inwards, the skin, subcutaneous tissue, the ribs; and, their intervening muscles (external, internal, and innermost intercostal) and the thoracic membrane. A thin membrane lines the thoracic cavity, the pleura, which appears as a double sheet covering the inner aspect of the thoracic wall (parietal pleura) posteriorly, laterally, and anteriorly including the diaphragmatic and mediastinal surfaces where it is reflected unto the lung surface as the visceral pleura. Between the two layers of the pleura is a potential space that contains about 10–15 mls of serous fluid lubricating the mobile lung surfaces on the chest wall during respiration.

The rigid chest wall and the collapsible, compressible, compliant lungs make the pleural space an ideal work environment after insufflation during thoracoscopy (Fig. 19.1).

A detailed discussion of the anatomy of the thorax, mediastinum, and constituent cultures is available in standard anatomy textbooks; however, a few highlights are herein described.

Notably, most of the lungs, the surfaces and the intrathoracic trachea up to the carina are accessible by VATS including the hilum via fissure diastasis. The lobes and bronchopulmonary segments can be very well visualized due to the magnification in VATS. Small pleural, diaphragmatic, and peripheral pulmonary lesions are identified for biopsy when compared to open surgery, and this aids diagnosis. The inner lining of the fibrous pericardium enveloping the conical heart is lined by the parietal layer of the serous pericardium which is reflected at the root of the great vessels unto the surface of the heart as the visceral pericardium or epicardium. A small amount of serous fluid can also be found within the pericardial space formed by the double fold of the visceral pericardium. Blood, air, and fluid of varying consistencies can accumulate between the layers of the pleural and pericardial spaces in disease conditions or following trauma. VATS is used to evacuate these for analysis; and, a biopsy of the pleura and pericardium can be obtained for histopathological

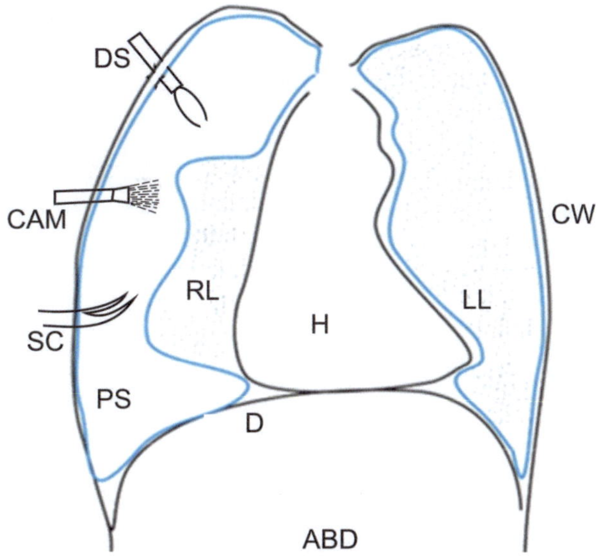

Fig. 19.1 Schematic diagram of the thorax showing the right and left lungs, the heart in-between and the diaphragmatic arch forming the base. The blue lining represents the pleural membrane and the mottled space represents lung tissues, which is collapsed on the right displaying a wide and spacious "working" pleural space (PS), penetrated by three instruments - telescopic camera (CAM), Dissecting forceps (DS) and Endoscopic scissors (SC). The dark line is the chest wall and abdomen lies below the diaphragm

tissue diagnosis. Patent ductus arteriosus (PDA), a residual patency of the embryonic/fetal ductus arteriosus connecting the aorta to any part of the pulmonary artery, can be ligated or clipped by VATS.

The fibromuscular diaphragm separates the thoracic and abdominal cavity. It comprises a peripheral muscular part that arises from the wall of the thoracic outlet with fibers running centripetally to be inserted into the dense fibrous aponeurosis referred to as the central tendon. Defects and perforations on this fibromuscular diaphragm from disease conditions or trauma can be repaired effectively by VATS. The path of the esophagus is through the diaphragmatic hiatus, bounded by the sling-like left and right crura of the diaphragm. Sliding, rolling, or combined hiatal hernias occur at this location. These can be corrected via VATS including gastroesophageal reflux disease (GERD) and achalasia.

Indications for VATS

Practically all types of open thoracic operations can now be managed by VATS depending on the surgeon's experience and the clinical condition of the patient, given the availability of all necessary and appropriate equipment and instrumentation. The magnification of visualized tissues with the use of a thoracoscope is a significant advantage in the use of VATS for these procedures. The indications for VATS just like for any other endoscopic procedure can be broadly classified into diagnostic or therapeutic indications [10]. These two classifications can be found in the management of any of the conditions listed below.

Diagnostic

Pleural Effusions or Thickening

VATS is indicated in pleural effusion where the etiology has been elusive, including recurrent episodes. A tissue biopsy of suspicious lesions of the pleura-lined thoracic cavity visualized on thoracoscopy is feasible. Such pleura-based lesions may be benign (e.g. tuberculous nodules), malignant (mesothelioma), or metastatic pleural masses (secondary deposits on the pleural membranes) (Fig. 19.2).

Lung Nodules or Masses

Indeterminate peripheral pulmonary nodules are readily accessible to VATS biopsy forceps. In addition, the cause of progressive respiratory failure in susceptible people, e.g. diffuse interstitial lung disease or fibrosis, can be confirmed using lung parenchymal tissue biopsy via thoracoscopy.

Others are mediastinal masses, cysts, or lymph node biopsy for definitive diagnosis or tumor staging.

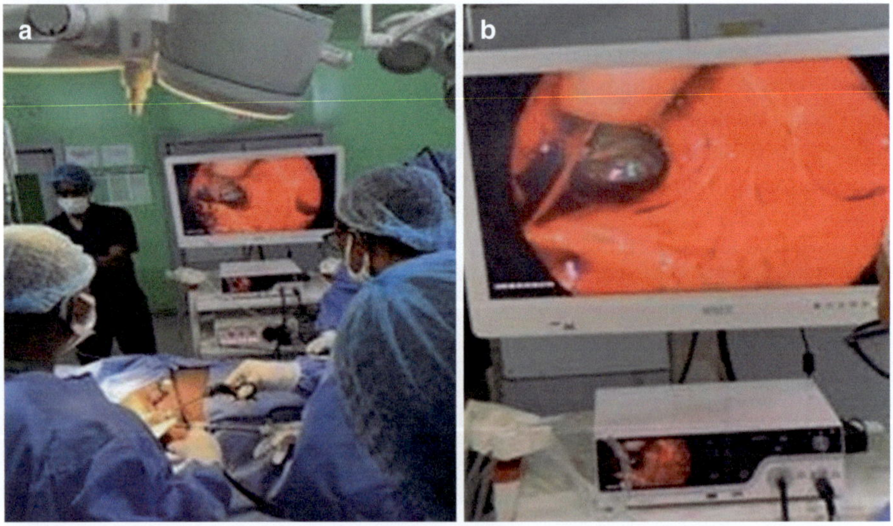

Fig. 19.2 (**a**) Panoramic view of a pleural cystic mass (**b**) Close-up view of the pleural cystic mass

Therapeutic VATS

Known therapeutic applications of VATS include:
Pleural procedures

- Evacuation of pleural effusion
- Evacuation of empyema
- Pleurodesis in selected patients (e.g. malignant effusion, recurrence, spontaneous pneumothorax, diffuse bullous lung disease).
- Pleurectomy
- Decortication

Lung procedures

- Ablation and resection of bullous lung diseases
- Lung resections for malignant, infectious, and inflammatory lung diseases (Segmentectomies, Lobectomies, and Pneumonectomies)
- Wedge resection
- Bronchopleural fistula repair
- Hydatid Cyst Resections

Esophageal

- Resection of leiomyoma
- Resection of enteric cysts
- Resection of esophageal diverticular disease
- Esophagomyotomy for motility disorders
- Antireflux procedures for GERD (Fundoplication like Belsey Mark IV)
- Video-assisted esophagectomy for early resectable esophageal cancer.

Cardiovascular

- Drainage of pericardial effusion
- Removal of pericardial cysts
- Pericardiectomy.
- Ligation of Patent ductus arteriosus (PDA).
- Harvesting internal mammary artery (IMA) for coronary artery bypass graft (CABG).

Mediastinal procedures

- Thymectomy for thymoma or in Myasthenia Gravis.
- Resection of benign mediastinal masses
- Resection of Ectopic Thyroid
- Resection of posterior mediastinal neurogenic tumors
- Removal of bronchogenic cysts
- Dorsal sympathectomy for Horner's syndrome
- Splanchnic sympathectomy for diabetic vasculitis, and hyperhidrosis.
- Drainage of Paravertebral abscess

Trauma

VATS is very useful in the management of many thoracic injuries following trauma. Most minor vascular, diaphragmatic, lung injuries and some retained foreign bodies can also be effectively managed. However, hemothorax, hemopneumothorax, penetrating chest injuries, pneumothorax, and chylothorax are managed with chest tube placement [11, 12].

Contraindications

With adequate experience and excellent anesthesia, VATS applies to virtually all types of patients. However, factors related to the patient, technicality, and equipment limit the application of this technique of thoracic surgery. Most are relative contraindications [7, 13]

A. ***Patient Factors***

- Hemodynamic instability
- Severe thoracic trauma or intrathoracic hemorrhage
- Coagulopathy
- Ventilator dependency
- Noncompliant lung
- Severe emphysema

B. ***Technical Issues***

- Dense pleural adhesions without access to the pleural space
- Moderate to large masses at the hilum extending into the superior mediastinum or the posterior paravertebral gutter
- Small (<1 cm) deeply located pulmonary nodules
- Chest wall involvement by tumor extension
- Small thoracic cavities or severe chest wall deformities (scoliosis, kyphosis, or kyphoscoliosis)
- Inability to undertake or tolerate one-lung ventilation
- Inability to achieve ipsilateral atelectasis, thus limiting exposure during operation

C. ***Equipment-Related***

- Unavailability of proper and necessary equipment and accessories.
- Inadequate visualization during the procedure.
- Some of these are no longer absolute contraindications due to progress in skills and technological advancement in VATS to improve safety and ease of executing the procedure.

Preoperative Preparation

Preoperative evaluation for patients undergoing VATS is not in any way different from patients for conventional open operations. The preoperative investigations are tailored to the diagnosis, comorbidities, type and extent of operation. These range from routine, specific/diagnostic, staging, to follow-up. All necessary investigations required in the entire management and care for the particular patients are carried out, without compromising standards.

Specific diagnostic investigations for intrathoracic diseases for which VATS is indicated include computed tomography (CT) scan with contrast enhancement, PET-CT scan, and magnetic resonance imaging for mass lesions. These may also be useful for staging malignant diseases. Contrast esophagogram, esophagoscopy, intraluminal ultrasound, high resolution and impedance monitoring, esophageal PH monitoring, and manometry are used to evaluate esophageal diseases. Bronchoscopy (rigid or flexible) and Endobronchial Ultrasound Scan (EBUS) are used for the evaluation of tracheobronchial lesions; and, can be valuable for taking biopsies and for intervention when necessary. Echocardiography, Electrocardiography (ECG), Computed Tomography Angiography (CTA), Magnetic Resonance Angiography (MRA), and conventional angiography are used when necessary to evaluate the cardiovascular status of the patient going for VATS. Occasionally, markers are placed to facilitate intraoperative localization of pulmonary nodules. This depends on the patient's clinical condition, the available support facilities and technology in the institution [14]. These include CT-guided percutaneous placement, bronchoscopy-guided placement, intraoperative ultrasonography; three-dimensional (3D) printing technology, artificial intelligence (AI) and intraoperative molecular imaging (IMI).

Routine investigations must be carried out to determine the patient's fitness for surgery and to assess comorbidities. These include hematological investigations such as full blood count, serum electrolytes, urea, creatinine levels, bleeding/clotting profile and blood lipids. Blood grouping and cross-matching are necessary in case patients need to be transfused after a significant blood loss.

Written informed consent must be obtained from patients. This involves describing what is to be done for the patient, explaining the risks and benefits of the procedure including expectations. The patient or guardian will assent to this to give the go-ahead for the surgery.

Set-up for VATS

Some of the equipment and instrumentation for VATS are similar to laparoscopy (see Chaps. 2 and 3), except for core instruments. The thoracoscopic tower comprises a high-resolution 3-chip camera, monitor, insufflator and energy device (ultrasonic Harmonic scalpel, electrocautery or LigaSure).

Other requisite instruments comprise a telescope- 0° or 30°, 10 mm or 5 mm (in some special cases), short- 5 mm and 10 mm threaded trocars (Fig. 19.3) for multi-ports VATS. Trocars are not needed for Uniportal VATS, where a single 4–5 cm utility incision is used for the procedure, and the incision is covered by an incision protector (Fig. 19.3b).

Instrumentation

The instrumentation for VATS is specifically designed to fit into the minimal incision required for the procedure and the depth of the thoracic space. They are longer, slimmer, and open closer to the tip unlike the conventional instruments for open surgeries that are shorter, bulkier, and open around the midpoint of the instruments (Fig. 19.4). Although the laparoscopic instruments are different by design, some of them can be adapted for use during some VATS procedures.

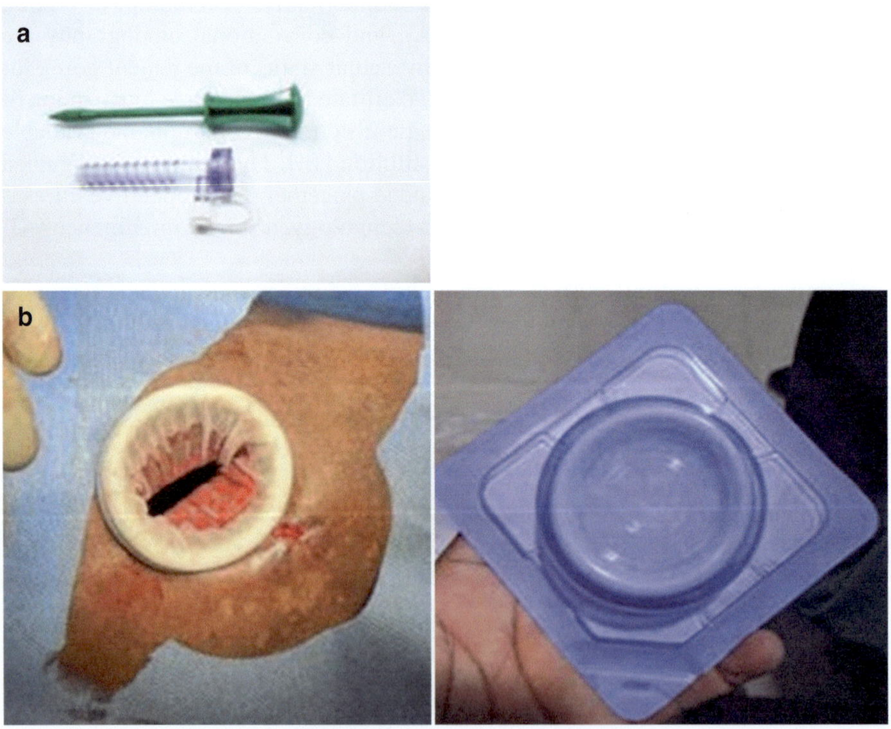

Fig. 19.3 (**a**) Trocar for thoracoscopy port (**b**) Incision/Wound Protector for Uniportal VATS

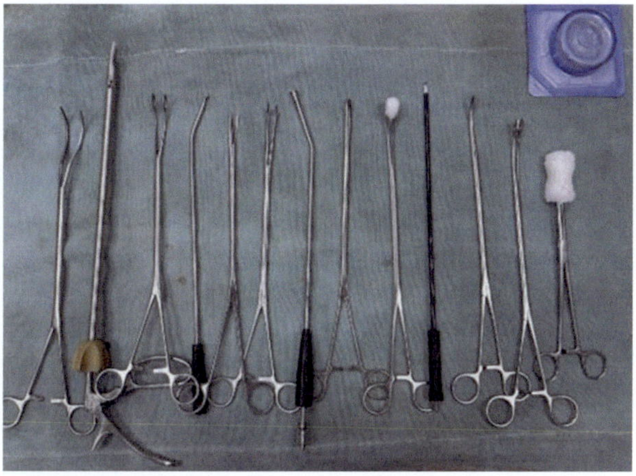

Fig. 19.4 VATS instruments

Technique

Anesthesia

VATS is mostly done under general anesthesia with one-lung ventilation (OLV) using a double lumen endobronchial tube (DLT) (Fig. 19.5). This is necessary to be able to achieve the collapse of the lung on the side of surgery to create space and ease dissections and resections. The DLT can be left-sided or right-sided and comes in different sizes. It is usually placed with the aid of an ultra-thin flexible bronchoscope to guide the placement of the tip of the DLT into the required right or left main bronchus to achieve effective lung isolation and ventilation. When the use of DLT is not feasible or Single Lumen Tube is preferred especially in some esophageal or mediastinal surgeries, an endobronchial blocker is used to achieve lung isolation and collapse or intra-pleural insufflation of carbon dioxide (CO_2). However, unlike in laparoscopy, the intra-pleural pressure should be kept lower than 10 mmHg [15]. When CO_2 is insufflated, air-tight valve trocars are used to retain the needed pressure in the pleural space. The patient is connected to monitors for continuous intraoperative monitoring of hemodynamic parameters.

Local and regional pain control can be achieved through the use of intercostal nerve blocks, thoracic paravertebral block (TPVB), erector spinae plane block (ESPB); and serratus plane block (SPB); with superior results from TPVB [16]. Prophylactic antibiotics are required before any surgical incision is made.

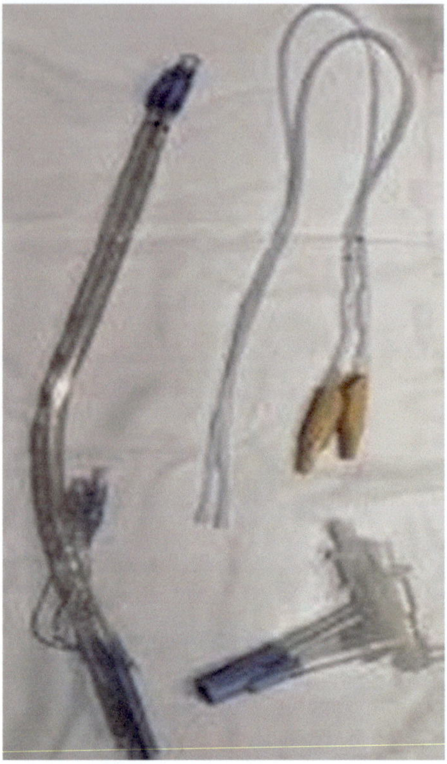

Fig. 19.5 Double Lumen Endobronchial Tube

Positioning

Patient positioning is mostly lateral decubitus position as in open surgery (Fig. 19.6). Cleaning of the chest and draping are done to allow for easy conversion to open surgery when needed. The chest is supported at the level of the tip of the scapula by a support roll or by breaking the operating table at that level. This is done to widen the rib spaces to reduce the crowding of instruments during surgery through the intercostal space. The arm on the side of access is lifted on an arm holder placed across the upper part of the patient or supported by soft paddings and is draped out of the operative field. Adequate padding is needed at major pressure points—the elbows, shoulder, hips, knees, and ankles—to prevent pain, pressure, and neurological injuries after surgery. In this lateral positioning, the surgeon and the assistant are positioned based on the preferred approach. They stay beside each other at the back for a posterior approach and stay in front of the patient for an anterior approach. Monitors are mounted facing the surgeons in direct vision.

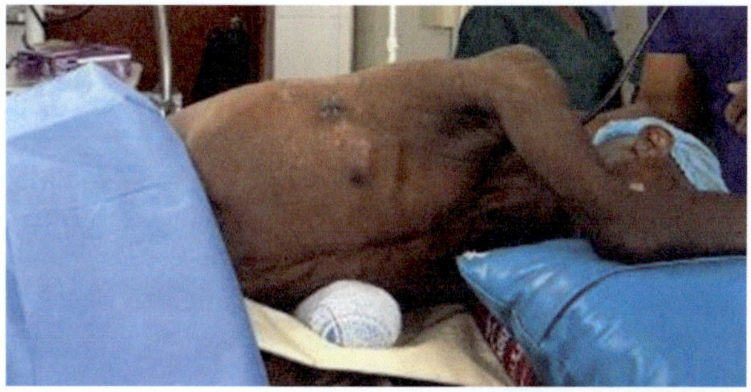

Fig. 19.6 Left lateral decubitus position for VATS with support for rib spreading

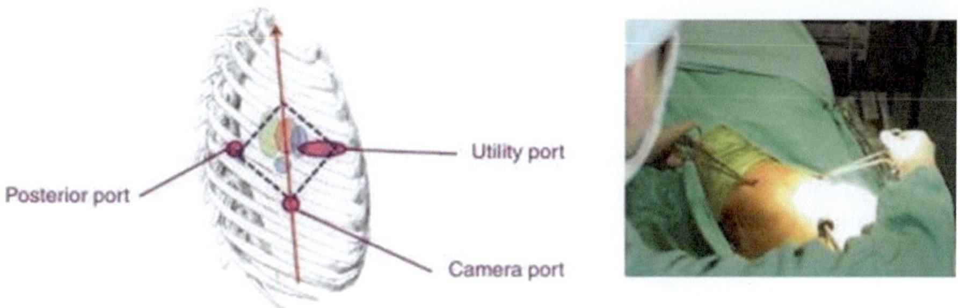

Fig. 19.7 3-ports placement for VATS access (Baseball Diamond) [15]

Access for VATS

Multiple Portal Access

Three-Port Access

Access to the chest during VATS has progressively evolved. The earlier access was through 3 ports access. This is still used by some surgeons. It has been traditionally described as a baseball diamond (Fig. 19.7). The camera port is in the 7th or 8th Intercostal space (ICS) mid-axillary line which is described as the "home base". The right port is placed in the 4th/5th ICS anterior axillary line with a 1–4 cm utility port incision and is described as the "first base". The left-hand port is placed posteriorly below the tip of the scapula with a 1 cm incision and is described as the third base while the target structure within the chest being dissected is the second base of the diamond (Fig. 19.7) [15, 17]. The ports are created after skin incision and using artery forceps or energy devices to dissect through the intercostal muscles on the upper border of the rib, avoiding injury to the neurovascular bundles. The pleura is breached, and the blunt trocar is inserted while the lung is partially collapsed to avoid injury to the underlying lung tissue. The thoracoscope/camera port is placed first, and the telescope is inserted (usually the 10 mm 30° scope). The pleural space is inspected and explored to view lesions, after which other ports are placed under vision and the underlying lung is protected. The anesthetist is then informed to collapse and isolate the lungs for the procedure to commence. Where insufflation with carbon dioxide (CO_2) is required or preferred by the surgeon, the valve-trocar is used for all ports, and intrapleural pressure is maintained between 8 and 10 mm Hg. In cases of diagnostic thoracoscopy, single port placement is sufficient after induced pneumothorax, first to conduct inspection/exploration and identification of lesion(s) on insertion of the thoracoscope.

Two-Port Access

The 3-port access evolved into the 2-port access with the elimination of the posterior port [15]. The anterior utility port becomes the main port where all instruments are placed for dissection; and, the camera port at the 7th ICS is the second port and is maintained for the thoracoscope (Fig. 19.8).

Uniportal Access

The Uniportal access is also an evolution from the 2-port access. The camera port at the 7th ICS is eliminated and a single 4–6 cm anterior utility port placed at the 4th/5th ICS anterior axillary line is used for VATS procedures (Fig. 19.9) [15]. All instruments including the thoracoscope are inserted through the Uniportal utility access. The Uniport incision is protected by a wound retractor (Fig. 19.8). This allows space for the instruments to move in and out of the small space smoothly; and, protects the wound from desiccation and injury from the multiple instruments. Almost all thoracic procedures can now be done through the Uniportal access in experienced hands.

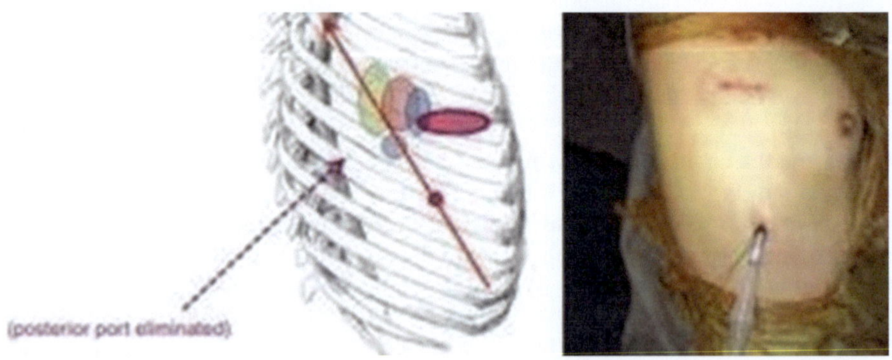

Fig. 19.8 2-port access

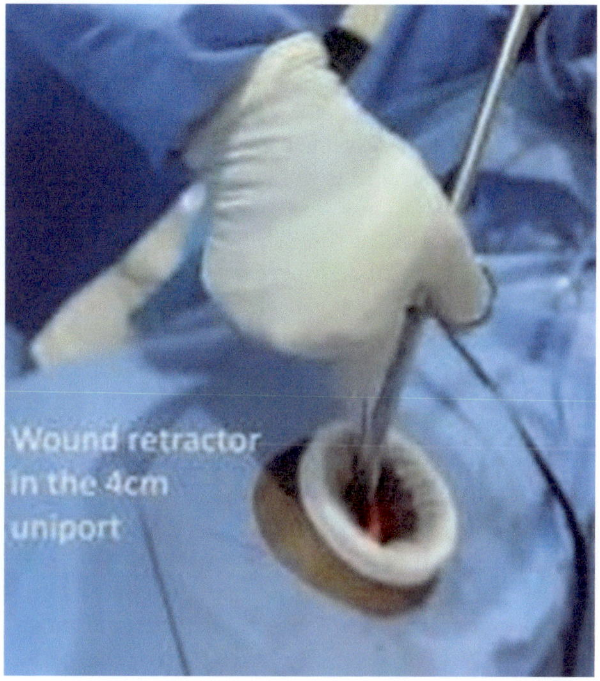

Fig. 19.9 Uniport with wound retractor/protector

Subxiphoid Approach

This involves a single incision at the subxiphoid area like a Uniportal access. It avoids the intercostal neurovascular bundles as the dissection does not go through the rib spaces. This approach is favored for thymic surgeries, anterior mediastinal tumors; and, some pulmonary vascular dissections and procedures [18]. The rectus abdominis muscle is dissected, the posterior sternal space is created by finger dissection, and a wound retractor is placed. Care must be taken not to injure the pericardium and the heart directly retrosternal. Occasionally carbon dioxide (CO_2) insufflation is used with valve trocars and a very low mediastinal pressure of 5–8 mmHg is maintained to create a retrosternal workspace without disrupting the hemodynamics. The pleural space may be breached when necessary, unilaterally or bilaterally for adequate work space to accomplish the task at hand.

Basic Principles of VATS

After careful patient selection and workup, the team ensures instrumentation and setup are put in place as mentioned above. The nurse confirms sterility and arrangement of instruments and all hardware are in good working condition. The approach and access for the VATS procedure are confirmed by the team. The surgeon and assistant ensure that the patient is well - positioned and padded, secured to the operating table, adjust the table height and angulation to their satisfaction, and affirm comfortable ergonomic positioning for instrument handling without clashing or clogging the operating field.

For Uniportal access, the camera is placed in the anterior part of the incision and the remaining instruments work from the remaining space behind. All instruments and energy devices must be tested before the commencement of surgery. The pleural space is entered after adequate lung collapse except when there are adhesions where care is taken to free such before proceeding with the surgery. The pleural space is explored first to identify and confirm the area of pathology before dissection commences. Energy devices should not be indiscriminately activated to avoid catastrophic injury to major vessels and other vital structures. Instrument clashes should be avoided as much as possible. If there is a need to convert to open surgery, the decision should not be delayed, as this is not a failure, but a necessary life-saving decision.

Most bleeding from low-pressure vessels or branches stops with applied pressure. Hence, a prepared swab-on-stick must be ready on table at all times to use for compression while the situation is being analyzed and a decision taken. Open thoracotomy should not be done in a hurry as much as possible. The use of energy devices and staplers should be mastered well before the procedure. The surgeon should be familiar with the specifications and mode of operation of the various devices to be used.

Resected tissues and specimens are carefully collected in a bag through the utility incision and sent for histology or other further analysis to confirm the final diagnosis.

End of Procedure

When surgery is concluded, adequate hemostasis is ensured, and the space is irrigated and checked for air leaks post-lung resection or tracheal surgery. A chest tube is usually placed in the space for drainage of any residual collection and the wound is closed in layers. The wound site and adjacent intercostal spaces are infiltrated with local anesthetic agents to ameliorate postoperative pain and enhance faster recovery. The patient can be extubated on the table if conditions are satisfactory and transferred to the recovery room awake or mildly sedated. Close monitoring of vital signs is done to ensure full recovery.

Postoperative Care

Post-operative pain relief ensures early recovery. Interventions of intercostal nerve block (ICNB) vs. thoracic paravertebral block (TPVB) vs. erector spinae plane block (ESPB) vs. intravenous morphine consumption at 24 h and 48 h postoperatively, showed patients who received TPVB had less demand for morphine than ICNB and ESPB [19]. A post-operative radiograph is done mostly en route to the recovery room or latest within 24 h of surgery to assess the chest for residual collections and full lung re-expansion. The patient is discharged usually on the 3rd–5th postoperative day depending on the rate of recovery.

References

1. Hatzinger M, Badawi JK, Häcker A, Langbein S, Honeck P, Alken P. Georg Kelling (1866–1945): the man who introduced modern laparoscopy into medicine. Urologe A. 2006;45(7):868–71.
2. Hatzinger M, Kwon ST, Langbein S, Kamp S, Hacker A, Alken P. Hans Christian Jacobaeus: inventor of human laparoscopy and thoracoscopy. J Endourol. 2006;20:848–50.
3. Sattler A. Zur Behandlung der Spontan-pneumothorax mit besonnnberer Berück-sichtigung der Thorakoskopie. Beitr Klin Tuberk Spezif Tuberkuloseforsch. 1937;89:394–408.
4. Martins Castello Branco J. Thoracoscopy as a method of exploration in penetrating injuries of the thorax. Dis Chest. 1946;12:330–5. https://doi.org/10.1378/chest.12.4.330.
5. Landreneau RJ, Dowling RD, Castillo WM, Ferson PF. Thoracoscopic resection of an anterior mediastinal tumor. Ann Thorac Surg. 1992;54(1):142–4. https://doi.org/10.1016/0003-4975(92)91162-3.
6. Bendixen M, Jørgensen OD, Kronborg C, Andersen C, Licht PB. Postoperative pain and quality of life after lobectomy via video-assisted thoracoscopic surgery or anterolateral thoracotomy for early-stage lung cancer: a randomised controlled trial. Lancet Oncol. 2016;17:836–44. https://doi.org/10.1016/S1470-2045(16)00173-X.
7. Manolache V, Motas N, Davidescu M, Bluoss C, Rus O, Tanase B, Jianu E, Burlacu A, Alexe V, Cioalca-Iliescu M, Nicolae G, Dobritoiu F, Saon C, Paleru C, Bosinceanu M, Horvat T, Cordos I, Gonzalez-Rivas D. Minimally invasive thoracic surgery—video assisted thoracic surgery: technique and indications. Chirurgia (Bucur). 2022;117(1):101–9. https://doi.org/10.21614/chirurgia.2608.
8. Sihoe ADL. The evolution of video assisted thoracic surgery. In: Gonzalez-Rivas D, Ng C, Rocco G, D'Amico T, editors. Atlas of Uniportal video assisted thoracic surgery. Singapore: Springer; 2019. https://doi.org/10.1007/978-981-13-2604-2_1.
9. Falase BA, Majekodunmi AA, Ismail S, Sanusi MO, Adeyeye OO. Video-assisted thoracic surgery in a Nigerian teaching hospital: experience and challenges. Niger J Clin Pract. 2016;19:233–6.
10. Okonta KE. The expected indications for video-assisted thoracoscopy surgery in SubSaharan Africa. Sub-Saharan J Endosc Proced. 2022;1:2.
11. Divisi D, Zaccagna G, De Sanctis S, et al. The role of video-assisted thoracoscopy in chest trauma: a retrospective monocentric experience. Updates Surg. 2024; https://doi.org/10.1007/s13304-024-02003-1.
12. Kakamas FH, Ali RK, Amin BJH, et al. The role of VATS in the removal of intrathoracic foreign bodies—a systematic review. Indian J Thorac Cardiovasc Surg. 2023;39(2):125–36. https://doi.org/10.1007/s12055-022-01445-9.
13. Hanna JM, Berry MF, D'Amico TA. Contraindications of video-assisted thoracoscopic surgical lobectomy and determinants of conversion to open. J Thorac Dis. 2013;5(Suppl 3):S182–9. https://doi.org/10.3978/j.issn.2072-1439.2013.07.08.
14. Tang L, Zhang Y, Wang Y. Intraoperative identification of pulmonary nodules during minimally invasive thoracic surgery: a narrative review. Quant Imaging Med Surg. 2022;12(11):5271–87.
15. Lomanto D, et al., editors. Mastering endo-laparoscopic and thoracoscopic surgery. https://doi.org/10.1007/978-981-19-3755-2_30.

16. Jo Y, Park S, Oh C, Pak Y, Jeong K, Yun S, Noh C, Chung W, Kim YH, Ko YK, Hong B. Regional analgesia techniques for video-assisted thoracic surgery: a frequentist network meta-analysis. Korean J Anesthesiol. 2022;75(3):231–44.
17. Alvarado S, Bonome C, Gonzalez-Rivas D. Anaesthesia for Uniportal VATS. In: GonzalezRivas D, Ng C, Rocco G, D'Amico T, editors. Atlas of Uniportal video assisted thoracic surgery. Singapore: Springer; 2019. https://doi.org/10.1007/978-981-13-2604-2_4.
18. Li M, Xu L, Li L, Dai Q, Xu D. The early perioperative outcomes of subxiphoid approach versus lateral intercostal approach thoracoscopic thymectomy for thymic tumors: a meta-analysis. J Laparoendosc Adv Surg Tech A. 2022;32(3):256–64. https://doi.org/10.1089/lap.2021.0036. Epub 2021 Mar 4
19. Sandeep B, Huang X, Li Y, Xiong D, Zhu B, Xiao Z. A comparison of regional anesthesia techniques in patients undergoing video-assisted thoracic surgery: a network meta-analysis. Int J Surg. 2022;105:106840. https://doi.org/10.1016/j.ijsu.2022.106840.

Part III
Newer Concepts

Chapter 20
Fluorescence-Guided Laparoscopic Surgery

Elad Boaz, Noam Kahana, Ana Pena, Samuel Szomstein, Emanuele Lo Menzo, and Raul J. Rosenthal

Introduction

Laparoscopic surgery has revolutionized the field of surgery with its minimally invasive approach, offering patients reduced postoperative pain, shorter hospital stays, and faster recovery times. Fluorescence imaging techniques have emerged as a valuable adjunct to conventional laparoscopy, providing real-time visualization of structures and processes not easily discernible under white light, improving surgical precision and patient outcomes.

E. Boaz · N. Kahana
Department of General Surgery, The Bariatric and Metabolic Institute, Ellen Leifer Shulman and Steven Shulman Digestive Disease Center, Cleveland Clinic Florida, Weston, FL, USA

Department of General Surgery, Shaare Zedek Medical Center, Faculty of Medicine, Hebrew University of Jerusalem, Jerusalem, Israel

A. Pena
Department of General Surgery, The Bariatric and Metabolic Institute, Ellen Leifer Shulman and Steven Shulman Digestive Disease Center, Cleveland Clinic Florida, Weston, FL, USA

S. Szomstein
Department of General Surgery, The Bariatric and Metabolic Institute, Ellen Leifer Shulman and Steven Shulman Digestive Disease Center, Cleveland Clinic Florida, Weston, FL, USA

Herbert Wertheim College of Medicine, Florida International University, Miami, FL, USA

E. Lo Menzo
Department of General Surgery, The Bariatric and Metabolic Institute, Ellen Leifer Shulman and Steven Shulman Digestive Disease Center, Cleveland Clinic Florida, Weston, FL, USA

Florida Atlantic University College of Medicine, Boca Raton, FL, USA

Florida International University College of Medicine, Miami, FL, USA

E. Ray-Offor, R. J. Rosenthal (eds.), *Principles and Practice of Laparoscopic Surgery*, https://doi.org/10.1007/978-3-031-96321-6_20

Indocyanine green (ICG) is a sterile, anionic, water-soluble but relatively hydrophobic, tricarbocyanine molecule with a molecular mass of 776 Daltons. ICG stands out as the cornerstone of fluorescence imaging. Initially developed for near-infrared (NIR) photography in 1955 by Kodak's research laboratories and subsequently approved for clinical use by the FDA in 1959, ICG has continually demonstrated its versatility and safety in medical applications. With its rapid hepatic clearance and minimal toxicity, ICG has been utilized since the late 1950s for various medical purposes, including cardiac output measurement, retinal vessel anatomy studies, and liver functional assessment [1–3].

Following intravenous administration, ICG is rapidly bound to plasma proteins, predominantly lipoproteins, with minimal leakage into the interstitium. ICG undergoes rapid hepatic extraction. Its exclusive excretion by the liver, primarily in unconjugated form via bile, enables multiple injections during procedures. When injected outside blood vessels, ICG migrates to the lymphatic system, reaching nearby lymph nodes within minutes and subsequently binding to macrophages [4].

Upon excitation with specific wavelengths of light, typically in the NIR spectrum (approximately 820 nm), ICG fluoresces, allowing for its detection with designated scopes and cameras. This fluorescence aids in identifying anatomical structures, such as biliary ducts, vessels, and lymph nodes, facilitating surgical navigation and precision. Commercially available systems incorporate laparoscopes and cameras capable of operating in both visible and NIR light, providing images for both conventional laparoscopy and NIR fluorescence imaging [4]. Importantly, the transition between standard light and NIR fluorescence is seamlessly controlled by the surgeon. With its low toxicity profile and exceptional tissue penetration capabilities, ICG has become a cornerstone in fluorescence imaging for minimally invasive surgery (Table 20.1). This chapter will explore the clinical uses of ICG in laparoscopic surgery, specifically examining its effectiveness in procedures related to the foregut, hepatobiliary system, small bowel, colorectal, and bariatric and metabolic surgeries.

R. J. Rosenthal (✉)
Division of General Surgery, Ronald Reagan UCLA Medical Center, David Geffen School of Medicine, Los Angeles, CA, USA
e-mail: rosentr@ccf.org

Table 20.1 Utilization of Indocyanine Green in Laparoscopic Surgery

Indications	Foregut surgery	Perfusion assessment	Gastric conduit, anastomotic margins
		Diffusion	Lymphatic drainage and sentinel lymph node visualization
	Hepatobiliary surgery	Perfusion assessment Diffusion Excretion	Visualization of liver segments Detection of primary and metastatic liver tumors Bile duct visualization
	Colorectal surgery	Perfusion assessment Diffusion Excretion	Resection/anastomotic margins Visualization of lymphatic drainage Ureter localization

Hepatobiliary Surgery

Given its predominant excretion via bile, ICG holds significant promise for visualizing the biliary tree, particularly in the context of cholecystectomy where bile duct injury remains a formidable complication. Despite meticulous dissection techniques aimed at achieving the "critical view of safety" and the potential use of intraoperative cholangiogram, the risk of inadvertent bile duct injury persists, especially in cases of anatomical complexity or inflammation. ICG-enhanced fluorescence offers a novel approach akin to "virtual" cholangiography, allowing surgeons to delineate normal anatomy or variations early in the procedure, guiding dissection and minimizing the risk of injury. Studies have shown impressive visualization rates of key structures like the cystic duct and common hepatic duct, both pre- and post-dissection, with doses typically ranging from 0.2 to 0.5 mg/kg (Table 20.2). More than 95% of ICG is captured by hepatocytes and excreted into bile within 15 minutes of injection [5, 6]. To achieve a perfect visualization of the biliary anatomy, the ideal conditions are obtained when there is very little background fluorescence in the liver parenchyma and high-intensity fluorescence in the biliary tree. Recently, Baldari et al. proposed a formula to calculate the perfect weight-based amount of ICG to be given to patients before surgery, to get the best possible visualization of the biliary tree [7].

The liver's unique metabolism of ICG is also invaluable in laparoscopic hepatectomy, a procedure increasingly favored worldwide for its benefits regarding blood loss, perioperative morbidity, and length of stay. The unique feature of liver catabolism of ICG provides a convenient tool for real-time visualization of the hepatic segments, vascular structures, and bile ducts, enabling more accurate anatomical hepatic resections. By utilizing transhepatic injection of ICG under intraoperative ultrasound (IUS) guidance, surgeons can delineate hepatic segments with precision, facilitating anatomically precise resections based on the demarcation between fluorescent and non-fluorescent areas. Moreover, ICG fluorescence

Table 20.2 Dosing and timing of indocyanine green (ICG) administration

Procedure	Purpose	Injection type	Usual dosage	Timing	ICG duration
Esophagectomy	Gastric conduit perfusion assessment	Intravenous	3 ml + 10 ml saline flush	Intraoperatively	Arterial & venous phase: min
Gastrointestinal & colorectal carcinoma	Visualization of lymphatic drainage & SLN	Peritumoral area	0.5–1 ml on each tumor quadrant	Preoperatively or intraoperatively	Remains stable during surgery
Cholecystectomy	Bile duct vvisualization	Intravenous	0.4–2.5 ml	At least 45 minutes before the procedure	Visible during surgery
Liver segmentation	Visualize liver segments	Positive staining: inject in portal branch	0.0250.25 mg/body (0.25–2.5 mg/10ml)	Prior to hepatic dissection	Remains stable during surgery
		Negative staining: Intravenous	2.5 mg/body	After portal pedicle closure	Remains stable during surgery
Liver cancer	Visualization of primary & metastatic tumors	Intravenous	0.5 mg/kg	14 days preoperatively	Remains stable during surgery
Colorectal resection	Perfusion assessment	Intravenous	3–3.5 ml + 10 ml saline	Intraoperatively	Arterial & venous phase, min
Ureter localization	Visualization of ureters	Cystoscopic guided retrograde intraureteral ICG	2.5 mg/ml 5 ml per ureter	Preoperatively/during pelvic dissection	Remains stable during surgery

SLN sentinel lymph node, *ICG* indocyanine green

imaging aids in intraoperative tumor detection and delineation, enabling the identification of tumor margins and assessment of proximity to vital structures [8–10]. This capability enhances oncological outcomes by ensuring adequate resection margins while sparing healthy liver tissue unnecessarily. Notably, ICG fluorescence imaging can visualize lesions as deep as 10 mm from the liver surface and assess their relationship with vascular and biliary structures, offering invaluable guidance during surgery.

Foregut Surgery

In laparoscopic foregut surgery, ICG fluorescence imaging is pivotal for assessing perfusion, lymph node mapping, and prophylaxis and management of surgical complications. Anastomotic leakage post-gastric or esophageal cancer surgery poses significant risks, often attributed to inadequate blood supply, which leads to higher mortality, reoperations, and increased hospital stay. Among the contributing risk factors, it has been suggested that inadequate blood supply to the stumps is the most relevant one. The use of ICG fluorescence imaging to evaluate the perfusion in real time offers a convenient way to obtain a more reliable assessment and thus may decrease the potential development of leaks associated with ischemia [11, 12]. The blood supply network of the anastomosis can be visualized immediately under the fluorescence mode after intravenous injection of 2–5 mg ICG. However, the lack of objectivity and a threshold for adequate perfusion is a major limitation.

Lymphadenectomy plays a pivotal role in oncological foregut surgery, necessitating extended dissection prone to complications. The identification of the sentinel lymph node and lymph node mapping is another major application of fluorescence imaging. This approach provides a feasible, safe, time-efficient, and reliable method with better detection rates, enabling an adequate lymphadenectomy, which could improve oncological outcomes [13]. Furthermore, it may facilitate the recollection of small fluorescent lymph nodes that otherwise wouldn't be identified with usual methods, increasing the number of lymph nodes resected. While some ICG can enter the lymphatic circulation when injected intravenously, to achieve reliable lymph nodal mapping and sentinel lymph node identification, ICG should be administered locally (endoscopically or surgically) near the tumor. Once injected, ICG is drained through the lymphatic network, reaching the first lymph node in 10–15 min and the regional lymph nodes in 1–2 h, staying in the lymphatic network for about 24–48 h. These time frames could guide the lymph node mapping and the sentinel lymph node identification, respectively. Intraoperative ICG lymphography offers real-time localization and management, especially beneficial in reoperations or post-radiation scenarios.

One of the possible complications following an esophagectomy is a thoracic duct injury with an estimated incidence of between 2% and 12%. Intraoperative identification of the thoracic duct can be challenging as the conventional methods of identifying the thoracic duct, including a diet rich in fat components the day before the procedure or the administration of milk/cream by nasogastric tube, are not reliable. The difficulty in detecting its location and the chyle leakage make intraoperative ICG lymphography a valuable technique. In practice, 2–3 mg ICG is injected subcutaneously in both inguinal regions approximately 30 min before the surgery. During the procedure, real-time fluorescence lymphography can be achieved, usually allowing one to locate and eventually spare or ligate the thoracic duct [14].

Small Bowel Surgery

The application of ICG fluorescence in small bowel surgery has been mostly aimed toward assessing intestinal perfusion during bowel ischemia. Presently, subjective clinical findings such as tissue coloration, pulsation of marginal vessels, temperature, bleeding from marginal arteries, peristalsis, or objective or Doppler measurements can be used to confirm the adequate perfusion of the bowel. Studies on patients undergoing emergency surgery for occlusive or non-occlusive mesenteric ischemia, employing ICG to evaluate bowel viability, indicate that ICG prompts a modification of the operative strategy in approximately one-third of cases [15]. The advantage of using ICG fluorescence is that it enables an objective perfusion assessment. As previously mentioned, the current fluorescence-based perfusion assessment is still qualitative. Similar to the colorimetric estimation under the white light images, it is based on the surgeon's visual evaluation of how bright the fluorescence becomes in the tissues after the dye is administered.

Additionally, anecdotal reports suggest the use of ICG in other small bowel pathologies, including incarcerated abdominal wall hernias, arteriovenous malformations, and localization of obscure bleeding from the small bowel.

Colorectal Surgery

A further interesting clinical application of fluorescence is the possibility to study in real-time perfusion of organs and bowel prior to or after anastomosis. Among the risk factors for anastomotic leakage, one of the most important contributing factors is poor local tissue oxygenation secondary to inadequate anastomotic vascular perfusion. A simple injection of a few milliliters of ICG allows real-time evidence of adequate perfusion of the bowel prior to proximal transection, after division of the mesentery, and before the completion of the anastomosis. Multiple studies investigating the application of ICG fluorescence imaging to evaluate the vascularization of anastomosis show a notable decrease in the rate of anastomotic leakage and revision following colorectal surgeries, particularly left-sided colectomies and rectal resections [16–19].

Besides its common use for angiography and lymphography, like other areas of the gastrointestinal tract, ICG has also been used intraluminally for tumor localization as well as for the detection of peritoneal metastasis. In colorectal surgery, the peri-tumoral injection of ICG can be used to study lymphatic mapping that might be interesting in the case of right-sided tumors, known to have highly variable lymphatic drainage, or for sentinel lymph node biopsy in early-stage rectal cancers [20, 21].

Bariatric and Metabolic Surgery

ICG and NIR technology are increasingly recognized as valuable adjuncts in bariatric surgery. They play a role in mapping vasculature and evaluating blood supply and aberrant arterial anatomy, which can be particularly useful during revisional bariatric surgery. Detecting aberrant anatomy can prompt surgical adjustments to mitigate complications [22].

Moreover, ICG is beneficial as an intraluminal agent for leak identification. Studies suggest its superior sensitivity compared to standard methods like methylene blue and air alone [23, 24]. Given the significant revision rates in bariatric patients, in which leaks are a major concern, ICG's role in assessing vascular patterns, perfusion, and leak testing is particularly valuable. While intravenous ICG and intraluminal methylene blue have comparable leak detection rates, adding ICG to standard methylene blue may enhance sensitivity. Although ICG can be given intravenously and is useful for vascular mapping, larger-scale research with standardized ICG administration dosing and protocol still needs to be done before any changes in the standard of care can be recommended.

Advancements and Future Directions

Recent advancements in fluorescence imaging technology have expanded its applications and capabilities in laparoscopic surgery. Multispectral imaging systems allow for the simultaneous visualization of multiple fluorophores with distinct emission spectra, enabling multiplexed imaging and improved tissue characterization. Furthermore, the development of activatable fluorescent probes, which remain nonfluorescent until activated by specific enzymes or physiological conditions within the tumor microenvironment, offers enhanced tumor specificity and reduced background signal. Future directions in fluorescence imaging include the integration of artificial intelligence and machine learning algorithms to automate image analysis and interpretation, optimizing surgical decision-making.

Conclusion

ICG-enhanced laparoscopic surgery has emerged as a powerful tool in the armamentarium of laparoscopic surgeons, offering enhanced visualization, improved intraoperative decision-making, and superior patient outcomes. By offering the surgeon additional information on anatomy, perfusion, or lymphatic drainage, fluorescence-guided laparoscopic surgery continues to evolve, paving the way for safer, more precise, and more effective surgical interventions across a wide range of specialties.

References

1. Baillif S, Wolff B, Paoli V, Gastaud P, Mauget-Faÿsse M. Retinal fluorescein and indocyanine green angiography and spectral-domain optical coherence tomography findings in acute retinal pigment epitheliitis. Retina. 2011;31(6):1156–63. https://doi.org/10.1097/IAE.0b013e3181fbcea5.
2. Desai ND, Miwa S, Kodama D, et al. A randomized comparison of intraoperative indocyanine green angiography and transit-time flow measurement to detect technical errors in coronary bypass grafts. J Thorac Cardiovasc Surg. 2006;132(3):585–94. https://doi.org/10.1016/j.jtcvs.2005.09.061.
3. Lim C, Vibert E, Azoulay D, et al. Indocyanine green fluorescence imaging in the surgical management of liver cancers: current facts and future implications. J Visc Surg. 2014;151(2):117–24. https://doi.org/10.1016/j.jviscsurg.2013.11.003.
4. Alander JT, Kaartinen I, Laakso A, et al. A review of indocyanine green fluorescent imaging in surgery. Int J Biomed Imaging. 2012;2012:940585. https://doi.org/10.1155/2012/940585.
5. Ishizawa T, Tamura S, Masuda K, et al. Intraoperative fluorescent cholangiography using indocyanine green: a biliary road map for safe surgery. J Am Coll Surg. 2009;208(1):e1–4. https://doi.org/10.1016/j.jamcollsurg.2008.09.024.
6. Dip FD, Asbun D, Rosales-Velderrain A, et al. Cost analysis and effectiveness comparing the routine use of intraoperative fluorescent cholangiography with fluoroscopic cholangiogram in patients undergoing laparoscopic cholecystectomy. Surg Endosc. 2014;28(6):1838–43. https://doi.org/10.1007/s00464-013-3394-5.
7. Baldari L, Boni L, Kurihara H, Cassinotti E. Identification of the ideal weightbased indocyanine green dose for fluorescent cholangiography. Surg Endosc. 2023;37(10):7616–24.
8. Aoki T, Yasuda D, Shimizu Y, et al. Image-guided liver mapping using fluorescence navigation system with indocyanine green for anatomical hepatic resection. World J Surg. 2008;32(8):1763–7. https://doi.org/10.1007/s00268-008-9620-y.
9. Inoue Y, Arita J, Sakamoto T, et al. Anatomical liver resections guided by 3Dimensional parenchymal staining using fusion Indocyanine green fluorescence imaging. Ann Surg. 2015;262(1):105–11. https://doi.org/10.1097/SLA.0000000000000775.
10. Wang X, Teh CSC, Ishizawa T, et al. Consensus guidelines for the use of fluorescence imaging in hepatobiliary surgery. Ann Surg. 2021;274(1):97–106. https://doi.org/10.1097/SLA.0000000000004718.
11. Luo RJ, Zhu ZY, He ZF, Xu Y, Wang YZ, Chen P. Efficacy of Indocyanine green fluorescence angiography in preventing anastomotic leakage after McKeown minimally invasive Esophagectomy. Front Oncologia. 2021;10:619822. Published 2021 Jan 8. https://doi.org/10.3389/fonc.2020.619822.

12. Mori M, Shuto K, Hirano A, et al. A novel parameter identified using Indocyanine green fluorescence angiography may contribute to predicting anastomotic leakage in gastric cancer surgery. World J Surg. 2020;44(8):2699–708. https://doi.org/10.1007/s00268-020-05488-0.
13. Chen QY, Xie JW, Zhong Q, et al. Safety and efficacy of Indocyanine green tracer-guided lymph node dissection during laparoscopic radical gastrectomy in patients with gastric cancer: a randomized clinical trial. JAMA Surg. 2020;155(4):300–11. https://doi.org/10.1001/jamasurg.2019.6033.
14. Vecchiato M, Martino A, Sponza M, et al. Thoracic duct identification with indocyanine green fluorescence during minimally invasive esophagectomy with the patient in the prone position. Dis Esophagus. 2020;33(12):doaa030. https://doi.org/10.1093/dote/doaa030.
15. Fransvea P, Fico V, Puccioni C, et al. Application of fluorescence-guided surgery in the acute care setting: a systematic literature review. Langenbecks Arch Surg. 2023;408(1):375. Published 2023 Sep 25. https://doi.org/10.1007/s00423-023-03109-7.
16. Watanabe J, Takemasa I, Kotake M, et al. Blood perfusion assessment by Indocyanine green fluorescence imaging for minimally invasive rectal cancer surgery (EssentiAL trial): a randomized clinical trial. Ann Surg. 2023;278(4):e688–94. https://doi.org/10.1097/SLA.0000000000005907.
17. Meijer RPJ, Faber RA, Bijlstra OD, et al. AVOID; phase III randomised controlled trial using indocyanine green for the prevention of anastomotic leakage in colorectal surgery. BMJ Open. 2022;12(4):e051144.
18. Jafari MD, Pigazzi A, McLemore EC, et al. Perfusion assessment in LeftSided/low anterior resection (PILLAR III): a randomized, controlled, parallel, multicenter study assessing perfusion outcomes with PINPOINT near-infrared fluorescence imaging in low anterior resection. Dis Colon Rectum. 2021;64(8):995–1002.
19. Blanco-Colino R, Espin-Basany E. Intraoperative use of ICG fluorescence imaging to reduce the risk of anastomotic leakage in colorectal surgery: a systematic review and meta-analysis. Tech Coloproctol. 2018;22(1):15–23. https://doi.org/10.1007/s10151-017-1731-8.
20. Emile SH, Elfeki H, Shalaby M, et al. Sensitivity and specificity of indocyanine green near-infrared fluorescence imaging in detection of metastatic lymph nodes in colorectal cancer: systematic review and meta-analysis. J Surg Oncol. 2017;116(6):730–40. https://doi.org/10.1002/jso.24701.
21. Yeung TM, Wang LM, Colling R, et al. Intraoperative identification and analysis of lymph nodes at laparoscopic colorectal cancer surgery using fluorescence imaging combined with rapid OSNA pathological assessment. Surg Endosc. 2018;32:1073–6.
22. Ortega CB, Guerron AD, Yoo JS. The use of fluorescence angiography during laparoscopic sleeve gastrectomy. JSLS. 2018;22(2):e2018.00005. https://doi.org/10.4293/JSLS.2018.00005.
23. Hagen ME, Diaper J, Douissard J, et al. Early experience with intraoperative leak test using a blend of methylene blue and Indocyanine green during robotic gastric bypass surgery. Obes Surg. 2019;29(3):949–52. https://doi.org/10.1007/s11695-018-03625-2.
24. Kalmar CL, Reed CM, Peery CL, Salzberg AD. Intraluminal indocyanine green for intraoperative staple line leak testing in bariatric surgery. Surg Endosc. 2020;34(9):4194–9. https://doi.org/10.1007/s00464-020-07606-4.

Chapter 21
Fundamentals of Robot-Assisted Laparoscopic Surgery

Olusegun Komolafe and Emeka Ray-Offor

Introduction

Man has always used tools, which have evolved with increasing knowledge and technology, from the simplest of farming tools like hoes or sickles to current sophisticated farming equipment like combine harvesters! Therefore, it is logical that implementations that improve surgical procedure performance will be developed parallel to advances in knowledge and technology. The use of automated machines for precise processes has gradually found its way into medical practice. Certainly, current RAS procedures, which can seem so advanced, and complex, are merely a staging post on advancing humankind's knowledge and skill. What seems so impressive to us now, will be old-fashioned and outdated to our grandchildren.

In the 1970s and 1980s as technology improved enough to allow quick long-distance transmission of instructions to control machines remotely, platforms for use in the military, and in space programs were developed [1]. The Programmable Universal Manipulation Arm (PUMA) was a robotic arm used in the motor manufacturing industry to perform various tasks [2]. One such device, the PUMA 560 was modified and used for a stereotactic brain biopsy in 1985 [3]. Over the next

O. Komolafe (✉)
NHS Lanarkshire, University Hospital Wishaw, Wishaw, Scotland, UK
e-mail: Segun.komolafe@lanarkshire.scot.nhs.uk

E. Ray-Offor
College of Health Sciences, University of Port Harcourt, Choba, Rivers State, Nigeria

Minimal Access Surgery Program, University of Port Harcourt Teaching Hospital (UPTH), Port Harcourt, Rivers State, Nigeria

Department of Surgery, UPTH, Choba, Rivers State, Nigeria

Oak Endoscopy Centre and Radiodiagnostics, Port Harcourt, Rivers State, Nigeria
e-mail: emeka.ray-offor@uniport.edu.ng

E. Ray-Offor, R. J. Rosenthal (eds.), *Principles and Practice of Laparoscopic Surgery*, https://doi.org/10.1007/978-3-031-96321-6_21

decade, further procedures were performed with robotic systems such as the PROBOT for prostatic surgery, and robotic surgery platforms became commercially available [4]. The AESOP (Automated Endoscopic System for Optimal Positioning) (Computer Motion, Inc., Goleta, CA) was a platform for laparoscopic cameras, and the ZRSS (ZEUS robotic surgery system) incorporated AESOP and two arms to mimic the surgeon's movements [5]. The main commercial competitor for the ZRSS was the da Vinci surgical system, and by 2003, both companies merged with the ZRSS being phased out. Other robotic surgery systems are commercially available now, though the Intuitive da Vinci robotic surgery system is the market leader and most widely used RAS platform [6].

The variety of RAS devices and platforms means that use is widespread across the breadth of surgery. A quick literature search will confirm that all surgical specialties have adopted RAS [7]. The evidence for minimally invasive surgery over open surgery is no longer in debate. Employing RAS, especially in inaccessible confined anatomical areas such as the mediastinum, and bony pelvis, expands the role of MIS in these specialties with improved visibility, ergonomics, and dexterity in confined spaces. There are now scientific journals dedicated to RAS, and a quick read through the contents of any recent issue demonstrates the breadth of the practice of RAS in all surgical specialties.

The drive towards RAS is also fuelled by evidence of patients having a better outcome—reduced length of stay, reduced complications, and reduced inflammatory response [8]. The reasons for these findings seem intuitive—a better view means more precise surgery, which means less trauma, and less "collateral" damage, and patients do better. There is also evidence that operating sitting down, for example, results in less surgeon fatigue, which also correlates with better patient outcomes [9]. In addition, the stable platform in RAS eliminates the physiological tremors from the assistant surgeons in long procedures [10].

Indications and Contraindications

Two domains bear on the use of RAS with regard to indications and contraindications. The first domain is directly related to clinical procedures. All MIS procedures may be amenable to RAS, in simplest terms, with similar contra-indications. Procedures in confined spaces benefit significantly from RAS with improved dexterity and optics. This has been the driver for the early adoption of RAS in "pelvic" specialties—lower tract urology, gynecology oncology, and rectal surgery.

The second, more pertinent domain, is that RAS is very expensive, so requires complex supporting architecture, to maximize the surgical output—close links with manufacturers, a dedicated theatre team trained on the platform, high caseload volume, appropriately trained surgeons, regular audit of outcomes. These all aggregate and synergize as the foundation for an excellent RAS program. Conversely, when any is missing, it is difficult to have a good RAS program, and certainly not one that is cost-effective.

Procedures that can be done easily using conventional MIS with identical outcomes to RAS are better performed with MIS purely for the added cost of RAS. However, this in itself is open to debate. Many robotic surgeons maintain that once they are beyond the learning curve, the improved dexterity and optics result in better performance of straightforward MIS procedures and justify the added expense. Employing RAS, especially in inaccessible confined anatomical space expands the role of MIS in these specialties with improved visibility, ergonomics, and dexterity in confined spaces.

Urology

RAS has been a "game-changer"—the gold standard for prostatic surgery is the robotic prostatectomy. As the depth of the pelvis makes it harder to access and also because the structures that are significant in the field are very small, RAS has advantages in urological surgeries [11]. Since the first robot-assisted prostatectomy was done in 2000, RASs have been used successfully in nephrectomies, Andersen-Hyne pyeloplasty for uteropelvic junction obstruction, and adrenalectomies [12]. Some of the procedures that are now available that in the past were not possible are vasectomy reversals, sub-inguinal removal of a varicocele, and removal of innervations of the spermatic cord [13].

General Surgery

The accuracy of the current robotic systems allows for dissection in congested abdominal cavities and cases where the lymphatics and vasculature are very close together. The list of gastrointestinal organs operated with the robot ranges from the stomach, liver, gall bladder, pancreas, small bowel, adrenal, colon, and others [14, 15]. In addition, robot-assisted anterior abdominal wall surgeries are reported with noninferior outcomes to conventional laparoscopic surgery; however robotic repair has increased operative duration and healthcare costs [16]. Structured quality assessment for robotic bariatric surgery suggests that robotic bariatric surgery may enhance surgical safety compared with laparoscopic bariatric surgery [17].

Colorectal Surgery

In colorectal surgery, the three main colorectal operations where robotic surgery has found the most use are ventral mesh rectopexy, right hemicolectomy, rectal cancer surgery with increasing utilization of robotic laparoendoscopic single-site technique [18]. The ROLAR trial demonstrated the non-inferiority of robot-assisted rectal surgery to the conventional laparoscopic approach [19]. RSSs with single port site capability are increasingly utilized in rectal surgery. It is conceivable that over the next decade, in many countries with the means, certain procedures such as rectal cancer surgery will be centralized on RAS systems.

Gynecology

Robotic surgery offers an effective and safe alternative in oncologic and non-oncologic gynecological surgeries including microsurgical fallopian tube re-anastomosis [20].

Robotic Surgical Systems

The intricate human qualities of sensitivity, empathy, adaptability, and decision-making abilities exhibited by the surgeon have a delicate impact on life and death and are difficult to precisely replicate in RAS. To date, no active robotic surgical systems (RSSs) can autonomously perform predefined tasks, but mainstream semi-active platforms rely on the non-programmed actions of the surgeon, unlike purely dependent systems**.** There are now many commercially available RAS platforms. A recent review article describes over 20 different RAS systems although only 6 were in clinical use with full regulatory approval in the US at publication [21].

Generally, the robotic platforms have three components. The surgeon console is either closed (immersive) or open console with conventional screens. This component accepts input from the surgeon controlled through finger loops, laparoscopic handles, joystick handles, or foot pedals. A processing unit provides the computing resources, and a set of arms interacts with the patient. The robotic arms used for the surgical handling of tissue vary across systems. There are either single-arm (trans-abdominal or transluminal) or multi-arm systems. The latter may be boom-mounted e.g. da Vinci® (Intuitive Surgical), Bitrack System™ (Rob Surgical System). Micro Hand S® (Wego), Avatera® (Avatera Medical) etc. Other RSSs are modular with 3–5 arms mounted on individual carts e.g. Senhance® and Luna™ (Asensus Surgical), Versius® (Cambridge Medical Robots), Hugo™ (Medtronic), Dexter® (Distal Motion) Mantra® (SS Innovation), Kangdou® (Sagebot), Carina™ (Ronovo Surgical), etc. The arms also may be bed mounted like Ottava® (Johnson & Johnson) and Anovo Hominis® (Momentis Surgical). The robotic arms are fully wristed, with 7 degrees of freedom designed for single or multi-use instruments of varying sizes depending on the brand. Some systems are compatible with commercial laparoscopic instruments (Maestro® (Moon Surgical) and Revo-I® (Meerocompany). For enhanced optics, most robotic surgical platforms offer 3D visualization, which is associated with improved surgeon proficiency with greater speed to task completion and decreased errors [21]. In addition, some systems incorporate near-infrared-emitting light sources in conjunction with near-infrared cameras for fluorescence-guided imaging. This facilitates identifying anatomic structures or evaluating tissue perfusion during surgery, The da Vinci platform with over 20 years of patent rights has dominated the US and global RAS market. There have been four main iterations, initially the S, the X, the XI, then the da Vinci 5, each progressively more advanced. The boom on the S platform was fixed so did not allow multi-quadrantic operation, unlike the more current XI and 5 models which have limbs on a mobile boom that can rotate in different directions.

There are a variety of RSSs for robotic laparoendoscopic single-site techniques.

Peri-Operative Care

No specific pre-operative preparations are required for patients undergoing RAS, different from any patient undergoing a major minimally invasive surgery procedure. Many units will develop RAS patient pathways with input from the various stakeholders. At one author's institution, in the weeks leading up to surgery, Colorectal RAS pre-op patients will typically see the Enhance Recovery Nurse Specialist, attend a PreAssessment Clinic (seeing Nurses & Anaesthetists), attend "Surgery School" (input from ERAS Nurse, Physiotherapists, Nurses, Surgeons), attend Stomatherapy Clinic (Stoma Nurse). With all these ambulatory/clinic input, patients are admitted on the morning of surgery with those requiring bowel prep having taken it at home the day before.

The theatre layout requires some consideration (Fig. 21.1). The operating surgeon has his or her head in the console on certain platforms so depends on the console speaker, to be heard. Some RAS platforms have an audio amplification system built into the console to facilitate communication, though the problem can sometimes be difficulty in hearing what is said at the table when the surgeon's head

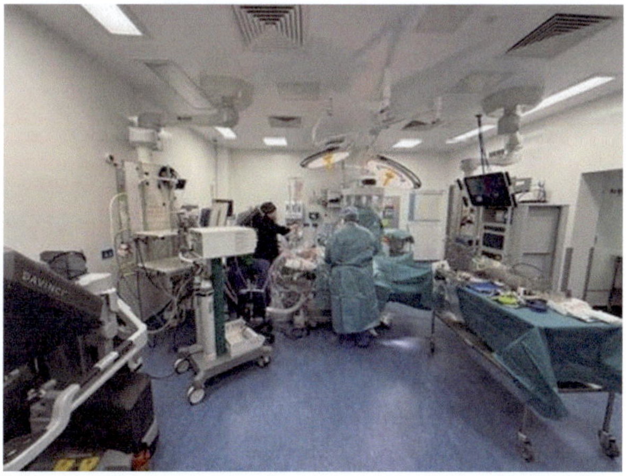

Fig. 21.1 Theatre layout, with console placed in the direction of the Anaesthetic team and surgical table, so the surgeon does not have back to table/team, in a large theatre room with enough space for two consoles, robotic platform, robotic stack as well as surgical instrument tray, etc., but still enough space for circulating team, and extra equipment eg. Endoscopy stack, to be brought in when required

is within the console. The robotic platform can represent a physical barrier to accessing the patient, Anaesthetists will want robust vascular access, with line extensions. A transparent drape is placed over the patient's upper body, with a metal frame overlying the patient's face, ensuring that the face and airway cannot be accidentally hit by robotic arms (Figs. 21.2, 21.3 and 21.4).

For safety reasons, it is advisable to have clear protocols in place for emergency undocking of the robotic platform where time-critical access to the patient is needed—for loss of airway, or catastrophic major hemorrhage, for example. One author's institution has a defined emergency undocking process: as part of the daily pre-op brief, before every robotic procedure, the theatre teams go over the defined roles in the (rare) eventuality the surgeon or anesthetist calls out "Code Red" with a view to emergency undocking in a matter of seconds (Fig. 21.5).

RAS "first" or "table" assistants are also a crucial part of RAS programs—the operating surgeon is at the console, controlling the robotic limbs, but needs a scrubbed health professional who remains sterile at the table, to change instruments, and use accessory ports for retraction, and inserting or removing items such as swabs. First assistants and dedicated robotic scrub nurses are integral, and team building is a key part of starting, and growing a good RAS program.

There are no specific post-op issues as such. Anecdotally, in an author's experience, the use of high-flow gas delivery for robotic surgery has led to some patients developing surgical emphysema. A bit more consideration may need to be given to local anesthetic agents as RAS patients have more ports than they would for MIS procedures. This however does not impact outcomes, as has been previously discussed with RAS patients having a shorter length of stay.

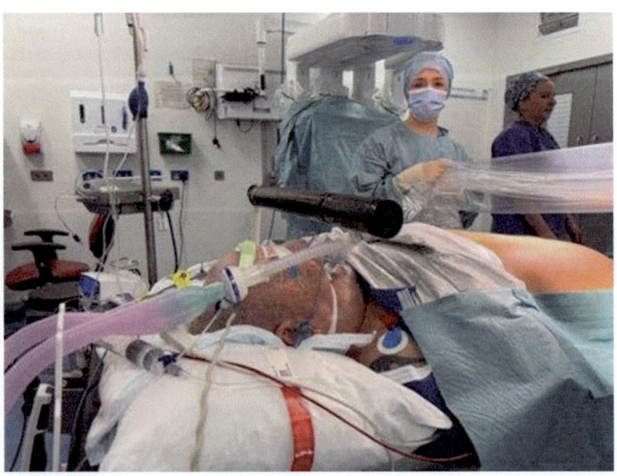

Fig. 21.2 Metallic bar across the patient's face to prevent injury from robotic limbs

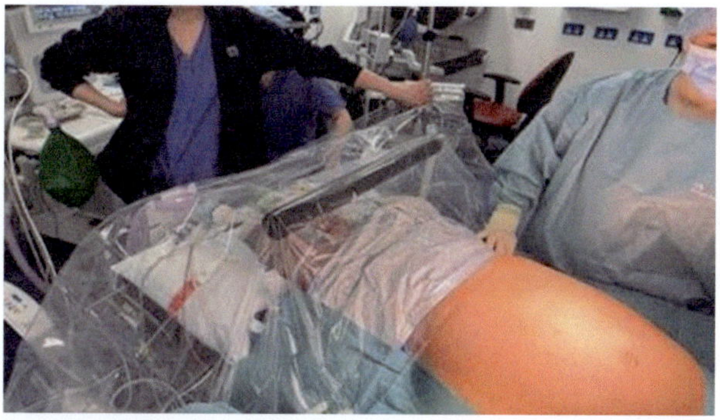

Fig. 21.3 Transparent sterile drape placed across patients face—facilitates surgical team being aware of face, airways, etc

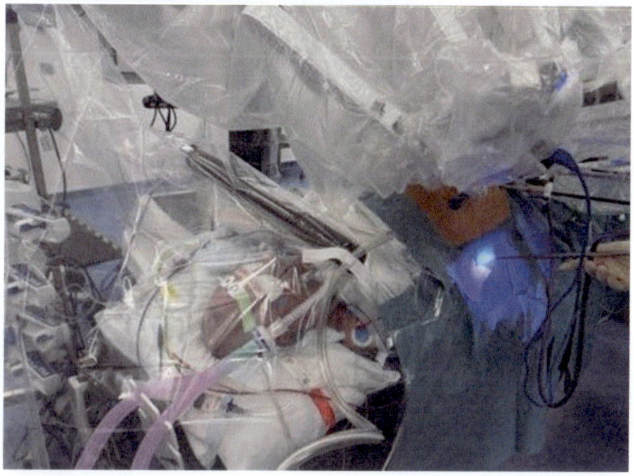

Fig. 21.4 Robot about to be docked, with ports in place

Unique Challenges/Limitations

The loss of tactile feedback is one of the major constraints of RAS. In addition, robotic systems do not allow for the feeling of temperature, pressure, tension, and vibrations. Every honest robotic surgeon will have at least one anecdote of a situation where more force than intended has been applied to tissue. There are unfortunate case reports of major injury with avulsion of vessels, perforations, etc [22, 23]. With experience, as one progresses up the learning curve, a robotic surgeon has a better appreciation of the force being applied from visual cues. However, maneuvering robotic instruments "blind" is fraught with danger in RAS. The newest robot models under creation are trying to address this haptic challenge by providing the surgeon with continuous, real-time sensory feedback [24].

Outcomes in surgery correlate directly with volume and expertise. Training in RAS must be part of a planned RAS program, with regular access to an RAS platform (Fig. 21.6), and a good volume of patients to operate on. It seems logical that robotic surgeons are effectively sub-specialists so training pathways should reflect that. This can mean that in certain contexts, experienced surgeons, and surgical

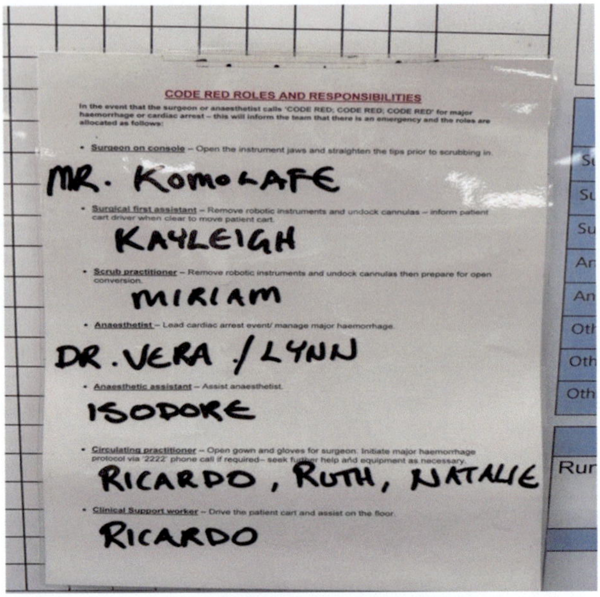

Fig. 21.5 Robotic theatre responsibilities in case of emergency undocking—defined at the start of each case, as part of the pre-operative brief

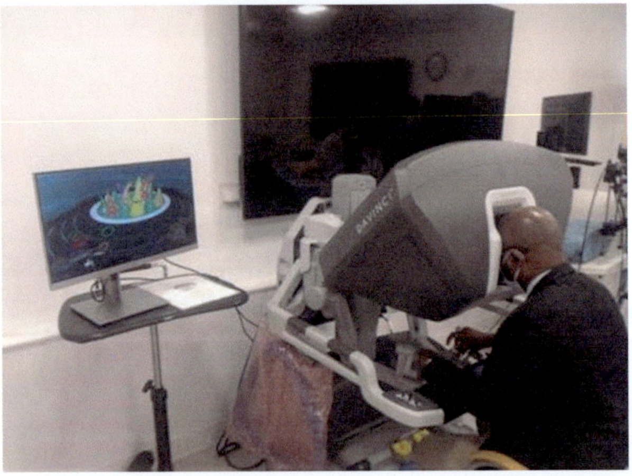

Fig. 21.6 Simulation training on robot-assisted laparoscopy

trainees, are not trained in RAS if they will not go on to have a large volume RAS practice.

RAS is "here to stay". A forecast suggests that robotic surgery may surpass laparoscopy and open surgery in colectomies, proctectomies, pancreatectomies, and esophagectomies by 2025 [25]. The main barrier of cost will come down with improved technology, and natural market forces, as more RAS systems become commercially available. Healthcare providers and the leadership of healthcare systems need to envision the future and then work with industry partners to deliver the best healthcare for their citizens, in a manner that is economically viable, and equitable for all.

References

1. Pugin F, Bucher P, Morel P. History of robotic surgery: from AESOP® and ZEUS® to da Vinci®. J Visc Surg. 2011;148(5 Suppl):e3–8.
2. PUMA. The leading edge in Robotic technology. https://digital.hagley.org/FILM_2018222_FC57. Accessed online 26 Jan 2025.
3. Kwoh YS, Hou J, Jonckheere EA, Hayati S. A robot with improved absolute positioning accuracy for CT guided stereotactic brain surgery. IEEE Trans Biomed Eng. 1988;35(2):153–60. https://doi.org/10.1109/10.1354.
4. Davies BL, Hibberd RD, Ng WS, Timoney AG, Wickham JEA. The development of a surgeon robot for prostatectomies. Proc Inst Mech Eng H. 1991;205:35–8.
5. Brassetti A, Ragusa A, Tedesco F, et al. Robotic surgery in urology: history from PROBOT® to HUGO™. Sensors (Basel). 2023;23(16):7104.
6. Marchegiani F, Siragusa L, Zadoroznyj A, Laterza V, Mangana O, Schena CA, Ammendola M, Memeo R, Bianchi PP, Spinoglio G, Gavriilidis P, de'Angelis N. New robotic platforms in general surgery: what's the current clinical scenario? Medicina (Kaunas). 2023;59(7):1264. https://doi.org/10.3390/medicina59071264. PMID: 37512075; PMCID: PMC10386395
7. Goh EZ, Ali T. Robotic surgery: an evolution in practice. J Surg Protoc Res Methodol. 2022;2022(1):snac003. https://doi.org/10.1093/jsprm/snac003.
8. Bhama AR, Obias V, Welch KB, et al. A comparison of laparoscopic and robotic colorectal surgery outcomes using the American College of Surgeons National Surgical Quality Improvement Program (ACS NSQIP) database. Surg Endosc. 2016;30(4):1576–84.
9. Zárate Rodriguez JG, Zihni AM, Ohu I, Cavallo JA, Ray S, Cho S, Awad MM. Ergonomic analysis of laparoscopic and robotic surgical task performance at various experience levels. Surg Endosc. 2019;33(6):1938–43. https://doi.org/10.1007/s00464-018-6478-4. Epub 2018 Oct 22. Erratum in: Surg Endosc. 2022; 36(1):852
10. Lanfranco AR, Castellanos AE, Desai JP, Meyers WC. Robotic surgery: a current perspective. Ann Surg. 2004;239(1):14–21. https://doi.org/10.1097/01.sla.0000103020.19595.7d.
11. Yu HY, Hevelone ND, Lipsitz SR, Kowalczyk KJ, Hu JC. Use, costs, and comparative effectiveness of robot-assisted laparoscopic and open urological surgery. J Urol. 2012;187(4):1392–8. [PubMed: 22341274]
12. Rassweiler J, Rassweiler MC, Kenngott H, Frede T, Michel MS, Alken P, Clayman R. The past, present and future of minimally invasive therapy in urology: a review and speculative outlook. Minim Invasive Ther Allied Technol. 2013;22(4):200–9. https://doi.org/10.3109/13645706.2013.816323. Epub 2013 Jun 30
13. Koukourikis P, Rha KH. Robotic surgical systems in urology: what is currently available? Investig Clin Urol. 2021;62(1):14–22. https://doi.org/10.4111/icu.20200387.
14. Marchegiani F, Siragusa L, Zadoroznyj A, et al. New robotic platforms in general surgery: what's the current clinical scenario? Medicina (Kaunas). 2023;59(7):1264. Published 2023 Jul 7. https://doi.org/10.3390/medicina59071264.
15. Sucandy I, Rayman S, Lai EC, Tang CN, Chong Y, Efanov M, Fuks D, Choi GH, Chong CC, Chiow AKH, Marino MV, Prieto M, Lee JH, Kingham TP, D'Hondt M, Troisi RI, Choi SH, Sutcliffe RP, Cheung TT, Rotellar F, Park JO, Scatton O, Han HS, Pratschke J, Wang X, Liu R, Goh BKP, International Robotic, Laparoscopic Liver Resection Study Group Investigators. Robotic versus laparoscopic left and extended left hepatectomy: an international multicenter study propensity score-matched analysis. Ann Surg Oncol. 2022;29(13):8398–406. https://doi.org/10.1245/s10434-022-12216-6. Epub 2022 Aug 23. PMID: 35997903; PMCID: PMC9649869
16. Olavarria OA, Bernardi K, Shah SK, Wilson TD, Wei S, Pedroza C, Avritscher EB, Loor MM, Ko TC, Kao LS, Liang MK. Robotic versus laparoscopic ventral hernia repair: multicenter, blinded randomized controlled trial. BMJ. 2020;370:m2457. https://doi.org/10.1136/bmj.m2457. PMID: 32665218; PMCID: PMC7359869

17. Giudicelli G, Gero D, Romulo L, Chirumamilla V, Iranmanesh P, Owen CK, Bauerle W, Garcia A, Lucas L, Mehdorn AS, Pandey D, Almuttawa A, Cabral F, Tiwari A, Lambert V, Pascotto B, De Meyere C, Yahyaoui M, Haist T, Scheffel O, Robert M, Nuytens F, Azagra S, Kow L, Prasad A, Vaz C, Vix M, Bindal V, Beckmann JH, Soussi D, Vilallonga R, El Chaar M, Wilson EB, Ahmad A, Teixeira A, Hagen ME, Toso C, Clavien PA, Puhan M, Bueter M, Jung MK. Global benchmarks in primary robotic bariatric surgery redefine quality standards for Roux-en-Y gastric bypass and sleeve gastrectomy. Br J Surg. 2024;111(1):znad374. https://doi.org/10.1093/bjs/znad374. PMID: 37981863; PMCID: PMC10771137
18. Ray-Offor E, Komolafe O. Robot-assisted laparoscopic colorectal surgery. In: Ray-Offor E, Rosenthal RJ, editors. Colorectal & hernia laparoscopic surgery. Cham: Springer; 2024. https://doi.org/10.1007/978-3-031-63490-1_4.
19. Jayne D, Pigazzi A, Marshall H, Croft J, Corrigan N, Copeland J, Quirke P, West N, Rautio T, Thomassen N, Tilney H, Gudgeon M, Bianchi PP, Edlin R, Hulme C, Brown J. Effect of robotic-assisted vs conventional laparoscopic surgery on risk of conversion to open laparotomy among patients undergoing resection for rectal cancer: the ROLARR randomized clinical trial. JAMA. 2017;318(16):1569–80. https://doi.org/10.1001/jama.2017.7219. PMID: 29067426; PMCID: PMC5818805
20. Mäenpää MM, Nieminen K, Tomás EI, Laurila M, Luukkaala TH, Mäenpää JU. Robotic-assisted vs traditional laparoscopic surgery for endometrial cancer: a randomized controlled trial. Am J Obstet Gynecol. 2016;215(5):588.e1–7. https://doi.org/10.1016/j.ajog.2016.06.005. Epub 2016 Jun 8
21. Sarin A, Samreen S, Moffett JM, et al. Upcoming multi-visceral robotic surgery systems: a SAGES review. Surg Endosc. 2024;38:6987–7010. https://doi.org/10.1007/s00464-024-11384-8.
22. Lau PJ, McGreevy JM, Thomes Pepin JA, Ramaswamy A, Faizer R. Challenges of conversion from robotic surgery for vascular complications. J Vasc Surg Cases Innov Tech. 2022;9(2):101035. https://doi.org/10.1016/j.jvscit.2022.09.010. PMID: 37013065; PMCID: PMC10066544
23. Pagès PB, Gutierrez I, Baste JM. Pulmonary artery repair during robotic lung resection: narrative review and management. J Vis Surg. 2022;8:3.
24. Intuitive da vinci 5. https://www.intuitive.com/en-us/products-and-services/davinci/5. Accessed online 8 Feb 2025.
25. Ferrari D, Violante T, Novelli M, Starlinger PP, Smoot RL, Reisenauer JS, Larson DW. The death of laparoscopy. Surg Endosc. 2024;38(5):2677–88. https://doi.org/10.1007/s00464-024-10774-2. Epub 2024 Mar 22

Chapter 22
Artificial Intelligence in Laparoscopic Surgery

Brett P. Weiss and Raul J. Rosenthal

Introduction

The integration of artificial intelligence (AI) into laparoscopic surgery marks a transformative step in surgical innovation that combines advanced computational algorithms with the surgeon's precision in minimally invasive procedures. AI enhances preoperative planning, intraoperative guidance, surgical robotics, and post-operative course modeling to improve efficiency, workflow, and patient outcomes. By enabling machine-learning algorithms for lesion detection, 3D reconstruction of complex anatomic variants, and augmented reality tools, among other uses, AI is not only refining the surgeon's capabilities but also redefining the boundaries of what is achievable in the modern operating room of the twenty-first century. This chapter introduces current applications of AI in both laparoscopic and robotic surgery as well as the critical focus on training the next generation of surgeons to leverage these new and innovative technologies into their practice.

B. P. Weiss
Miller School of Medicine, University of Miami, Miami, FL, USA

R. J. Rosenthal (✉)
Division of General Surgery, Ronald Reagan UCLA Medical Center,
David Geffen School of Medicine, Los Angeles, CA, USA
e-mail: rosentr@ccf.org

E. Ray-Offor, R. J. Rosenthal (eds.), *Principles and Practice of Laparoscopic Surgery*, https://doi.org/10.1007/978-3-031-96321-6_22

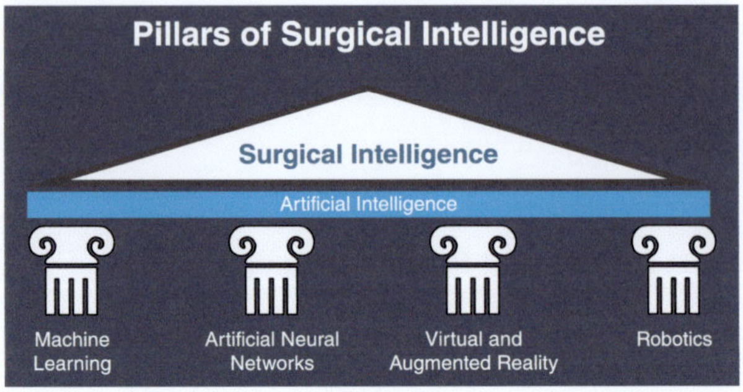

Fig. 22.1 Pillars of surgical intelligence

Surgical Intelligence

Before exploring the applications of artificial intelligence in laparoscopic surgery, it is essential to first define the concept of Surgical Intelligence.

Surgical Intelligence represents an emerging field that leverages data-driven insights to improve surgical outcomes (Fig. 22.1). AI analyzes data streams, links them to patient outcomes, and provides actionable insights to improve decision-making. Through advancements in problem-solving, object recognition, and unbiased decision-making capabilities, machine learning enables surgical systems to complement and amplify the skills of human surgeons, paving the way for smarter, more efficient procedures [1–3].

AI in the Patient's Surgical Journey

The use of AI spans the surgical care continuum for patients and can be introduced as early as the preoperative planning phase for computer-aided lesion detection, AI-generated 3D surgical navigation, and AI-generated multi-organ segmentation. When it is time to operate, AI can again be enabled for intraoperative guidance with capabilities like 3D shape instantiation, tissue feature tracking, simultaneous localization and mapping, computer vision, and augmented reality. Finally, in the postoperative period, AI can be leveraged longitudinally to support postoperative decision-making, utilized with wearable devices for real-time monitoring and analysis of patients both in the hospital and at home, and applied through machine learning models to predict sepsis, complications, and clinical outcomes, showcasing its integration across multiple facets of postoperative care.

AI-Based Preoperative Planning

AI-driven preoperative planning uses patient-specific data to tailor strategies and enhance surgical precision. Ahead of the decision to operate, the surgeon should be confident in correctly identifying abnormal lesions and the planned margins of resection to avoid omission errors, false positives, and misguided preoperative planning. AI is effective in being a 'second set of eyes' for the surgeon during preoperative screenings. One study used a dataset of 500,000 labeled endoscopic images of Barrett's Esophagus (BE) to pre-train a deep-learning computeraided detection system (CAD) in identifying both early-stage neoplasms and non-dysplastic BE. The AI tool identified lesions (if present), overlaid a heat map, and placed crosshairs at the most abnormal aspect of the lesion. With 89% accuracy, 90% sensitivity, and 88% specificity, this CAD AI system "achieved higher accuracy" than any of the individual endoscopists who reviewed the images. Evident here is the value that AI can provide surgeons in the identification of abnormal lesions, which has downstream implications as they plan for surgical intervention [4].

Anatomical variation in the structure, position, or size of organs or vessels can add significant challenges to laparoscopic surgeries by complicating the identification of landmarks and increasing the risk of iatrogenic injury to critical structures. AI offers an individualized approach to patients using detailed preoperative 3D imaging that can help surgeons effectively manage anatomical variations and aberrance. One use of AI has leveraged a registration-free deep learning algorithm that uses abdominal CT imaging to construct 3D models of abdominal organs for clear multi-organ segmentation in patients with complex anatomy for which clear anatomic differences could be visualized preoperatively. Some of these preoperative tools have significant crossover with intraoperative guidance that allows real-time navigation using the patient's 3D model as a map [5].

AI-Based Intraoperative Guidance

While AI can help surgeons gain insight into preoperative planning, it also offers significant advantages in the operating room. For example, AI-informed tissue feature tracking involves identifying, analyzing, and following specific characteristics of tissues such as their texture, elasticity, or motion over time. This tracking mechanism is important in laparoscopic surgery as it can identify abnormal motility, highlight subtle changes in tissue properties, and enhance spatial awareness intraoperatively. AI's tissue-tracking capability could enable robotics to automate tasks like suturing, cutting, and debridement, which require precise anatomical perception. As such, AI not only recognizes tissue but also the laparoscopic instruments and their dynamic pitch, roll, and yaw motions. One study that used deep learning models to track real-time tissue deformities and the spatial properties of surgical tools indicated "excellent performances", and tools like these demonstrate significant potential to enhance surgical precision, improve intraoperative decision-making, and reduce the risk of complications [6].

With approaches to laparoscopic surgery that use a monocular endoscope, there lies a challenge in generating 3D models from the 2D image sequences it produces. To overcome this challenge, a computational technique called Simultaneous Localization and Mapping (SLAM) was developed. SLAM was designed to generate a 3D map of the anatomic cavity and the monocular endoscope trajectory to create a real-time map of the surgical field. The technology behind SLAM is akin to that of robot vacuum cleaners; they must construct a map of an unknown environment while simultaneously keeping track of their location within it. SLAM generates a 3D model of the abdominal cavity intraoperatively as the surgeon simultaneously navigates through it. A study on SLAM in ventral hernia repair demonstrated its ability to map the cavity and predict endoscope trajectories. The ability to have such precision intraoperatively is important in navigating complex anatomical spaces, tracking tissue deformations as anatomy shifts from manipulation or insufflation, and providing an adaptive understanding of the surgical environment [7].

With the massive volume of available surgical image and video data, AI models have been developed to enable computers to interpret and analyze this visual information and subsequently mimic human vision by detecting, recognizing, and understanding objects and patterns. The first step is image classification, which leverages a trained deep-learning model to recognize what is in the image. For example, this may be used to identify specific steps from laparoscopic surgical videos. Next, the model detects objects or instruments and differentiates them from the tissue. This integration is quite important in avoiding injuries to contiguous and delicate anatomical structures. By integrating computer vision with machine learning, surgeons can therefore achieve finer levels of precision and support during complex operations [8].

Augmented reality (AR) has been introduced in conjunction with AI to assist with accurate and rapid localization of underlying anatomy so that surgeons can preoperatively plan reconstructive surgery or benefit from visual overlays intraoperatively. AR combines the power of AI with the advanced technology of digital overlay by generating complex 3D models and allowing surgeons to visualize them on top of the real patient's anatomy intraoperatively. It is also unique in that it does not compromise operating room sterility and has enhanced capabilities like responding to hand gestures and voice commands [9].

Surgical Robotics

With the increasing practice of robotic surgery, it is important to acknowledge how it not only challenges the current laparoscopic model but also seeks novel surgical automation. Currently, surgical robotics builds on the AI foundations of laparoscopic surgery to achieve a goal state of autonomous execution of specific surgical subtasks, reduction of surgeon tedium, and the ability to continuously learn from surgeon's demonstrations [10]. However, it is essential to understand that the robot is designed to be used as an aid and not a replacement; this highlights the significance of the human-robot interaction. A study performed using a combination of laparoscopic approach and robotic surgery introduced automatic adjustment of the laparoscope based on the surgeon's gaze in the operative field. It was demonstrated that the system had an accuracy of better than 1 degree of visual angle with one gaze gesture and that could help reduce the assistant surgeon's fatigue and cramped workspaces [11]. As surgical robotics continues to evolve, its integration with advanced technologies like artificial intelligence and machine learning promises to further enhance precision, reduce complications, and redefine the boundaries of minimally invasive surgery.

AI in the Post-Operative Period

AI's role in surgical care does not end with the operation itself but rather extends into the post-operative period and beyond, where it enhances various aspects of patient care including real-time monitoring with wearable devices and predictive modeling for complications to drive continuous support throughout the recovery process.

A study evaluating wearable devices in the postoperative setting demonstrated that they capture valuable data pertaining to vital signs, physiologic measurements, and physical activity.

Many of these devices are available commercially and their ability to aggregate these fundamental data points in real-time can allow for the identification of high-risk patients before they decompensate. Changes in vitals can often be the first signs of complications, and these devices typically offer continuous monitoring whereas traditional intermittent readings may risk missing critical changes [12]. While the data from wearable devices may be valuable for informing AI and machine-learning models, it is important to acknowledge that their effectiveness depends on patient compliance and measurement accuracy.

Although wearables enhance the ability to predict complications, they are limited by the scope of the data they collect. Additionally, non-physiologic data points can also be associated with complications but may not be captured by wearables. On the other hand, electronic health records (EHRs) provide a vast repository of longitudinal data that can be leveraged to predict complications and postoperative outcomes. For example, one study focusing on the use of digital applications in medicine analyzed over 46 billion data points from an EHR, including free-text notes, to predict clinical outcomes such as mortality, readmission, and length of stay. The large neural networks tested in this study demonstrated high accuracy in predicting these outcomes, showing how big data and advanced analytics can uncover connections and associations to predict postoperative states requiring early intervention [13].

Another study evaluated the performance of various machine-learning models in predicting postoperative sepsis following laparoscopic appendectomy. These models demonstrated accuracy in predicting 30-day mortality and highlighted the value of such predictions in aiding surgical decision-making. For example, identifying a high risk of sepsis can influence surgeons to personalize postoperative care, including interventions, prescriptions, and the level of monitoring they deem appropriate [14].

Another study demonstrated that machine-learning and deep-learning algorithms have strong predictive performance in identifying patients at risk for postoperative ileus (POI), a complication of laparoscopic surgery for colon cancer occurring in 3–30% of cases. These models highlighted key factors such as duration of anesthesia, opioid use, and body weight as significant contributors to the development of POI. Such insights provide surgeons with valuable information to design postoperative care plans, helping to mitigate complications and optimize recovery [15].

By leveraging AI, big data, and machine-learning models, we can transform postoperative care—using wearable devices, EHR data, and predictive algorithms to identify risks, guide interventions, and personalize recovery plans, ultimately improving patient outcomes and advancing surgical care.

Training the Next Generation of Surgeons

Considering the way forward, it starts with the surgeon. It is critically important to adopt AI-driven solutions that can not only enhance surgical intervention within the operating room but also inform surgical training outside the OR. Currently, AI is being used to aid in surgical trainee upskilling and one study interpreted eight types of movement during minimally invasive robotic knot tying and suturing to predict surgical skill level (e.g., novice vs expert) [16, 17]. Similarly, another AI-based tool employed the use of a convolutional neural network to evaluate video footage of laparoscopic cholecystectomy operations to determine trainee skill level; good performance was determined by narrow and focused instrument handling within the operative field [16, 18]. This type of valuable insight is challenging in current models in which attending surgeons' limited time hinders trainees' opportunities to receive a timely evaluation of their technical skill sets. Likewise, AI also has the power to provide a deeper level of individualized and personalized training to surgical trainees through Intelligent Tutoring Systems (ITS). These models provide automated feedback from surgical video interpretation and subsequently curate highly personalized instructional material based on the trainee's assessed performance level. A randomized controlled trial found that trainees who received AI-generated feedback and instruction had skill acquisition 2.6× faster and achieved 36% higher performance on simulated brain tumor removal surgery than conventional teaching models that lack AI-driven insights [19]. With real-time feedback from AI, surgical trainees can engage in continuous improvement that may otherwise be challenging in the more standardized surgical training approaches typically used. Additionally, virtual reality (VR) offers the opportunity for trainees as early as their medical student years to begin learning surgical skills that can be conducted anytime and anywhere without the need for an operating room. A randomized trial investigating the effectiveness of virtual reality in training medical students in surgical technique for tibial shaft fracture intramedullary nailing showed that students who received supplementary VR training performed significantly better in time and motion, knowledge of instruments, instrument handling, knowledge of the procedure, and flow of operation/planning than the control group that only received printed materials. Evident is the great promise that VR holds in training future surgeons from as early as the undergraduate medical level and from anywhere in the world [20].

Ethical Considerations in Surgical Intelligence

An emerging technology as new and innovative as AI in the context of surgery comes with uncharted territory involving ethical dilemmas, legal considerations, and moral responsibility. Thus, it is essential to acknowledge the major ethical implications associated with its use in this area of medicine. First, AI models may exhibit a risk of bias as the algorithms are trained only on the specific types of surgery, demographics, and surgeons to which they are exposed. In other words, the output is only as good as the input. Secondly, the AI models leverage enormous datasets comprised of confidential patient data, which exposes a potential vulnerability and begs the question of privacy and security surrounding data encryption and storage. Thirdly, oversight and agency must be considered especially in the context of surgical intervention—who is accountable for surgical decision-making and possible error (surgeon or AI)? Finally, AI's ability, or lack thereof, to demonstrate non-technical skills, creativity, and 'soft skills' typically unique to humans, must be evaluated to determine to what extent AI should be permitted to take on human agency [21, 22].

Opportunities for Improvement

While the use of cases for AI in surgery is growing and advancing, this novel technology still has its limitations. As surgeons can attest, each patient's anatomy is slightly different and while AI can aid in highlighting these differences, it may not be consistently accurate in recognizing different structures such as tiny nerves covered by fat, for instance. Similarly, training sets for AI must be updated and expanded for a variety of patient factors including rare cases, severe obesity, adhesions, and other anatomical abnormalities. Finally, there is an art to surgery for which the human element is critical, and there remains uncertainty around AI's ability to respond in a crisis, such as massive bleeding or incorrect dissection planes. Thus, while the role of AI in surgery will likely continue to grow, we must challenge its abilities, recognize its limitations, and work to integrate it into practice with appropriate balance [23].

Conclusion

Artificial intelligence (AI) is revolutionizing the field of surgery by enhancing precision, decision-making, and training. In the preoperative phase, AI facilitates early detection of abnormalities, assists in planning complex procedures, and optimizes surgeon decision-making to improve surgical outcomes. During surgery, AI-driven tools enhance intraoperative guidance by improving navigation, minimizing iatrogenic injuries, and automating repetitive tasks such as suturing and cutting. In recovery, patients benefit from AI's ability to synthesize and interpret a continuous data stream from wearable devices and also appreciate its value in predicting complications and clinical outcomes. Surgical robotics further complement these advancements, empowering human surgeons to perform safer, more decision-guided operations. Beyond the operating room, AI, along with virtual and augmented reality (VR and AR), offers innovative learning opportunities for surgical trainees. However, as these technologies become more integrated into surgical practice, ethicolegal considerations must remain a priority to ensure responsible implementation and patient-centered care. Together, these advancements herald a new era in surgery, where technology and human expertise converge to deliver safer, more efficient, and patient-focused care.

References

1. Forbes Technology Council. How surgical intelligence can help eliminate variability and disparity in surgical care. Retrieved from https://www.forbes.com/councils/forbestechcouncil/2022/12/08/how-surgical-intelligence-can-help-eliminate-variability-and-disparity-in-surgical-care/.2. 2022, December 8
2. Theator. Surgical intelligence: the new frontier. Retrieved from https://theator.io/blog/surgical-intelligence-the-new-frontier/#:~:text=Surgical%20Intelligence%20is%20a%20new,can%20 unearth%20surgical%20 best%20practices. n.d.
3. Vanderbilt University Engineering. What is AI in surgery? Retrieved from https://blog.engineering.vanderbilt.edu/what-is-ai-in-surgery. n.d.
4. de Groof AJ, et al. Deep-learning system detects neoplasia in patients with Barrett's esophagus with higher accuracy than endoscopists in a multistep training and validation study with benchmarking. Gastroenterology. 2020;

5. Gibson E, et al. Automatic multi-organ segmentation on abdominal CT with dense VNetworks. IEEE Trans Med Imaging. 2018;37(8):1822–34. https://doi.org/10.1109/TMI.2018.2806309.
6. Lu J, et al. SuPer deep: a surgical perception framework for robotic tissue manipulation using deep learning for feature extraction. 2021 IEEE International Conference on Robotics and Automation (ICRA), Xi'an, China; 2021. p. 4783–9. https://doi.org/10.1109/ICRA48506.2021.9561249. Keywords: {Deep learning; Automation; Transfer learning; Training data; Surgery; Tools; Feature extraction}
7. Grasa ÓG, et al. Visual SLAM for handheld monocular endoscope. IEEE Trans Med Imaging. 2014;33(1):135–46. https://doi.org/10.1109/TMI.2013.2282997.
8. Kitaguchi D, Takeshita N, Hasegawa H, Ito M. Artificial intelligence-based computer vision in surgery: recent advances and future perspectives. Ann Gastroenterol Surg. 2021;6(1):2936. https://doi.org/10.1002/ags3.12513. PMID: 35106412; PMCID: PMC8786689
9. Pratt P, et al. Through the hololens looking glass: augmented reality for extremity reconstruction surgery using 3D vascular models with perforating vessels. Eur Radiol Exp. 2018;2(1):2.
10. Zhou XY, Guo Y, Shen M, et al. Application of artificial intelligence in surgery. Front Med. 2020;14:417–30. https://doi.org/10.1007/s11684-020-0770-0.
11. Fujii K, Gras G, Salerno A, Yang G-Z. Gaze gesture based human robot interaction for laparoscopic surgery. Med Image Anal. 2018;44:196–214. ISSN 1361-8415
12. Wells CI, Xu W, Penfold JA, Keane C, Gharibans AA, Bissett IP, O'Grady G. Wearable devices to monitor recovery after abdominal surgery: scoping review. BJS Open. 2022;6(2):zrac031. https://doi.org/10.1093/bjsopen/zrac031.
13. Rajkomar A, et., al. Scalable and accurate deep learning with electronic health records. NPJ Digit Med. 2018;1:18. https://doi.org/10.1038/s41746-018-0029-1. PMID: 31304302; PMCID: PMC6550175
14. Bunn C, et al. Application of machine learning to the prediction of postoperative sepsis after appendectomy. Surgery. 2021;169(3):671–7. https://doi.org/10.1016/j.surg.2020.07.045. ISSN 0039-6060, https://www.sciencedirect.com/science/article/pii/S0039606020305183
15. Zhou CM, Li H, Xue Q, Yang JJ, Zhu Y. Artificial intelligence algorithms for predicting post-operative ileus after laparoscopic surgery. Heliyon. 2024;10(5):e26580. https://doi.org/10.1016/j.heliyon.2024.e26580. PMID: 38439857; PMCID: PMC10909660
16. Guerrero DT, et al. Advancing surgical education: the use of artificial intelligence in surgical training. Am Surg. 2023;89(1):49–54. https://doi.org/10.1177/00031348221101503. Epub 2022 May 15. PMID: 35570822
17. Fard MJ, Ameri S, Darin Ellis R, Chinnam RB, Pandya AK, Klein MD. Automated robot-assisted surgical skill evaluation: predictive analytics approach. Int J Med Robot. 2018;14:e1850.
18. Lavanchy JL, Zindel J, Kirtac K, et al. Automation of surgical skill assessment using a threestage machine learning algorithm. Sci Rep. 2021;11:5197.
19. Julian D, Smith R. Developing an intelligent tutoring system for robotic assisted surgery instruction. Int J Med Robot Comp Assist Surg. 2019;15(6):n.
20. Blumstein G, et al. Randomized trial of a virtual reality tool to teach surgical technique for Tibial shaft fracture intramedullary nailing. J Surg Educ. 2020;77(4):969–77. https://doi.org/10.1016/j.jsurg.2020.01.002. Epub 2020 Feb 5. PMID: 32035854
21. Satapathy P, et al. Artificial intelligence in surgical education and training: opportunities, challenges, and ethical considerations—correspondence. Int J Surg. 2023;109(5):1543–4. https://doi.org/10.1097/JS9.0000000000000387. PMID: 37037597
22. Cobianchi L, et al. Artificial intelligence and surgery: ethical dilemmas and open issues. J Am Coll Surg. 2022;235(2):268–75. https://doi.org/10.1097/XCS.0000000000000242.
23. Kitaguchi D, Takeshita N, Hasegawa H, Ito M. Artificial intelligence-based computer vision in surgery: recent advances and future perspectives. Ann Gastroenterol Surg. 2021;6(1):29–36. https://doi.org/10.1002/ags3.12513. PMID: 35106412; PMCID: PMC8786689

Appendix

Trouble Shooting (Table 1)

Table 1 Society of American Gastrointestinal Endoscopic Surgeons SAGES Laparoscopy troubleshooting guide

Problem	Cause	Solution
Poor insufflation/loss of pneumoperitoneum	CO_2 tank empty or very low	Change tank
	Accessory port stopcock(s) open	Inspect all accessory ports. Open or close stopcock(s) as needed
	Leak in sealing cap, reducer	Change cap or cannula
	Excessive suctioning pressure	Allow time to re-insufflate, lower suction intensity
	Loose, disconnected or kinked insufflation tubing	Tighten connection or reconnect at source or at port, unkink tubing
	Hasson stay sutures loose	Replace or secure sutures
	CO_2 flow rate set too low	Adjust flow rate, check to be sure insufflator is set to large cavity setting
	Valve on CO_2 tank not fully open	Use valve wrench to open fully
	Leak at skin where port enters cavity	Apply penetrating towel clip or suture around port
	Patient inadequately paralyzed	Discuss with Anaesthesia colleagues to ensure appropriate relaxation and depth of anesthesia

(continued)

E. Ray-Offor, R. J. Rosenthal (eds.), *Principles and Practice of Laparoscopic Surgery*, https://doi.org/10.1007/978-3-031-96321-6

Table 1 (continued)

Problem	Cause	Solution
Excessive pressure required for insufflation (initial or subsequent)	Veress needle or cannula tip not in peritoneal space	Reposition needle or cannula under direct visualization if possible
	Occlusion of tubing (kinking, table joints, etc.)	Inspect full length of tubing
	CO_2 port stopcock turned off	Fully open stopcock
	Patient is "light" (not fully paralyzed)	Communicate with anesthesia
	Morbidly obese patient	Consider use of longer Veress needle or cannula, or any other safe method of peritoneal cavity entry
Inadequate lighting (partial/complete loss)	Light is dim	Increase gain, Check laparoscope for adequate fiberoptics. Replace light cable and or camera. If using 5 mm laparoscope, consider upsizing to 10 mm laparoscope
	Light is on standby	Take light off standby
	Loose connection of source or scope	Adjust connection
	Light is on 'manual-minimum'	Switch to automatic or increase brightness setting
	Fiber optics are damaged	Replace light cable
	Automatic iris adjusting to bright reflection from instrument	Re-position instruments, or switch to manuals setting
	Light is absorbed by blood or bile in the operative field	Remove blood with suction or switch to manual
	Monitor brightness turned down	Readjust setting
	Room brightness floods monitors	Dim room lights
	Bulb is burned out	Replace bulb
	Residue related to heat from light source of light cord	Scrape off residue or replace light cord
	Laparoscope is dark	Check white balance
Poor quality picture	Flickering electrical interference, poor cable shielding	Replace cautery cables, switch camera head, make sure cables don't cross, don't different plug points
	Color problems	White balance camera, check chrome on monitor, check printer digital capture cables
	Glare not caused by lighting	Check for loose cables not plugged in
Lighting too bright	Light is on "manual-maximum"	'Boost' on lightsource is activated
	Monitor brightness turned up	Go to 'automatic', deactivate boot' mode, readjust monitor settings

(continued)

Table 1 (continued)

Problem	Cause	Solution
No picture on monitor(s)	Camera control or other components (video recorder, printer, light source, monitor) not "on"	Make sure all power source is activated
	Cable connector between camera control unit, and/or monitors not attached properly	Cable should run from "video out" on camera control unit to "video in" on primary monitor. Use compatible cables for camera unit and light source
	Cable between monitors not connected	Cable should run from "video out" on primary monitor to "video in" on secondary monitor
	Input select button on monitor doesn't match "video in" choice	Assure matching selections
	Input selection button on monitor or video peripherals (e,g, video recorder, digital capture, printer) not selected	Adjust input.
Poor quality picture (a) fogging/haze	Condensation on lens from cold laparoscope entering warm abdomen	Use ant-fog solution or warm water, wipe lens externally
	Condensation on laparoscope eyepiece, camera lens	Detach camera from scope (or camera from coupler), inspect and clean lens as needed
	Moisture in camera cable connecting plug	Use suction or compressed air to dry out moisture (don't use cotton tip applicators on multi-pronged plug)
(b) flickering, electrical interference	Poor cable shielding	Move electrosurgical unit to different circuit or away from video-equipment, make sure cables do not cross, switch camera head;replace cables as necessary
	Unsecure connection of video cable between monitors	Reattach video cable at each monitor
(c) blurring, distortion	Camera out of focus	Adjust camera focus ring
	Cracked lens, internal moisture	Inspect scope/camera, replace if needed
	Image too grain	Adjust enhancement and/or grain settings for units with this option

(continued)

Table 1 (continued)

Problem	Cause	Solution
Inadequate suction/ irrigation	Occlusion of tubing (kinking, blood clot, etc.)	Inspect full length of tubing. If necessary, detach from instrument and flush tubing with sterile saline
	Occlusion of valves in suction/irrigator device	Detach tubing, flush device with sterile saline
	Not attached to wall suction	Inspect and secure suction & wall source connector
	Not attached to irrigation bag	Ensure spike is fully inserted into the irrigation bag
	Irrigation fluid container not pressurized	Inspect pressure bag or compressed gas source, connector, and pressure dial setting. Ensure irrigation bag is elevated to maximize gravitational effect
	Too many devices connected to suction, creating 'steal'	Turn off suction to completing devices
	No flow of irrigant despite all the above	Ensure device is turned on, adequate battery/power, may need to change out for a new irrigator
Absent or "weak" cauterization	The dispersive electrode pad is not properly in place	Ensure adequate dispersive electrode contact
	Connection between electrosurgical unit and instrument loose	Inspect both connecting points
	Foot pedal or hand switch not connected to electrosurgical unit	Ensure appropriate connection to electrosurgical unit
	Wrong output selected	Correct output choice
	Connected to the wrong socket on the electrosurgical unit	Check that cable is attached to Laparoscopic socket
	Instrument insulation failure outside of surgeon's view	Use new instrument and inspect insulation, inspect tissue around instrument for iatrogenic injury
	Continual lack of electrosurgery effect despite all the above	Completely change out the electrosurgery cable for a new one and send cable to check for defects

https://www.sages.org/laparoscopy-preparation-and-troubleshooting-guide/

Index

E. Ray-Offor, R. J. Rosenthal (eds.), *Principles and Practice of Laparoscopic Surgery*, https://doi.org/10.1007/978-3-031-96321-6